Non-communicable Diseases, Big Data and Artificial Intelligence

Non-communicable Diseases, Big Data and Artificial Intelligence

Editors

Youxin Wang
Ming Feng

MDPI • Basel • Beijing • Wuhan • Barcelona • Belgrade • Manchester • Tokyo • Cluj • Tianjin

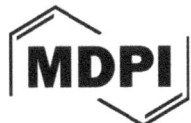

Editors
Youxin Wang
Department of Public Health,
School of Public Health
Capital Medical University
Beijing
China

Ming Feng
Peking Union Medical
College Hospital,
Peking Union Medical
College Chinese Academy of
Medical Sciences
Beijing
China

Editorial Office
MDPI
St. Alban-Anlage 66
4052 Basel, Switzerland

This is a reprint of articles from the Special Issue published online in the open access journal *Journal of Personalized Medicine* (ISSN 2075-4426) (available at: www.mdpi.com/journal/jpm/special_issues/noncommunicable_diseases_Intelligence).

For citation purposes, cite each article independently as indicated on the article page online and as indicated below:

LastName, A.A.; LastName, B.B.; LastName, C.C. Article Title. *Journal Name* **Year**, *Volume Number*, Page Range.

ISBN 978-3-0365-4848-7 (Hbk)
ISBN 978-3-0365-4847-0 (PDF)

© 2022 by the authors. Articles in this book are Open Access and distributed under the Creative Commons Attribution (CC BY) license, which allows users to download, copy and build upon published articles, as long as the author and publisher are properly credited, which ensures maximum dissemination and a wider impact of our publications.

The book as a whole is distributed by MDPI under the terms and conditions of the Creative Commons license CC BY-NC-ND.

Contents

About the Editors vii

Preface to "Non-communicable Diseases, Big Data and Artificial Intelligence" ix

Gerardo Alfonso Perez and Javier Caballero Villarraso
An Entropy Approach to Multiple Sclerosis Identification
Reprinted from: *J. Pers. Med.* **2022**, *12*, 398, doi:10.3390/jpm12030398 1

Kuo Liu, Yunyi Xie, Qian Zhao, Wenjuan Peng, Chunyue Guo and Jie Zhang et al.
Polymorphisms and Gene-Gene Interaction in AGER/IL6 Pathway Might Be Associated with Diabetic Ischemic Heart Disease
Reprinted from: *J. Pers. Med.* **2022**, *12*, 392, doi:10.3390/jpm12030392 13

Jia Zhang, Ruijuan Han, Guo Shao, Bin Lv and Kai Sun
Artificial Intelligence in Cardiovascular Atherosclerosis Imaging
Reprinted from: *J. Pers. Med.* **2022**, *12*, 420, doi:10.3390/jpm12030420 27

Qing Liu, Qing Zhou, Yifeng He, Jingui Zou, Yan Guo and Yaqiong Yan
Predicting the 2-Year Risk of Progression from Prediabetes to Diabetes Using Machine Learning among Chinese Elderly Adults
Reprinted from: *J. Pers. Med.* **2022**, *12*, 1055, doi:10.3390/jpm12071055 41

Qing Liu, Miao Zhang, Yifeng He, Lei Zhang, Jingui Zou and Yaqiong Yan et al.
Predicting the Risk of Incident Type 2 Diabetes Mellitus in Chinese Elderly Using Machine Learning Techniques
Reprinted from: *J. Pers. Med.* **2022**, *12*, 905, doi:10.3390/jpm12060905 53

Na Shi, Lan Lan, Jiawei Luo, Ping Zhu, Thomas R. W. Ward and Peter Szatmary et al.
Predicting the Need for Therapeutic Intervention and Mortality in Acute Pancreatitis: A Two-Center International Study Using Machine Learning
Reprinted from: *J. Pers. Med.* **2022**, *12*, 616, doi:10.3390/jpm12040616 69

Guanhua Dou, Dongkai Shan, Kai Wang, Xi Wang, Zinuan Liu and Wei Zhang et al.
Integrating Coronary Plaque Information from CCTA by ML Predicts MACE in Patients with Suspected CAD
Reprinted from: *J. Pers. Med.* **2022**, *12*, 596, doi:10.3390/jpm12040596 83

Xi Bai, Zhibo Zhou, Yunyun Luo, Hongbo Yang, Huijuan Zhu and Shi Chen et al.
Development and Evaluation of a Machine Learning Prediction Model for Small-for-Gestational-Age Births in Women Exposed to Radiation before Pregnancy
Reprinted from: *J. Pers. Med.* **2022**, *12*, 550, doi:10.3390/jpm12040550 97

Chan-Yang Min, Jung-Woo Lee, Bong-Cheol Kwon, Mi-Jung Kwon, Ji-Hee Kim and Joo-Hee Kim et al.
Physical Activity Is Associated with a Lower Risk of Osteoporotic Fractures in Osteoporosis: A Longitudinal Study
Reprinted from: *J. Pers. Med.* **2022**, *12*, 491, doi:10.3390/jpm12030491 111

Yuze Li, Ziming Xu, Chao An, Huijun Chen and Xiao Li
Multi-Task Deep Learning Approach for Simultaneous Objective Response Prediction and Tumor Segmentation in HCC Patients with Transarterial Chemoembolization
Reprinted from: *J. Pers. Med.* **2022**, *12*, 248, doi:10.3390/jpm12020248 125

Nidan Qiao, Yichen Ma, Xiaochen Chen, Zhao Ye, Hongying Ye and Zhaoyun Zhang et al.
Machine Learning Prediction of Visual Outcome after Surgical Decompression of Sellar Region Tumors
Reprinted from: *J. Pers. Med.* **2022**, *12*, 152, doi:10.3390/jpm12020152 . . . . **139**

Chao Lu, Jiayin Song, Hui Li, Wenxing Yu, Yangquan Hao and Ke Xu et al.
Predicting Venous Thrombosis in Osteoarthritis Using a Machine Learning Algorithm: A Population-Based Cohort Study
Reprinted from: *J. Pers. Med.* **2022**, *12*, 114, doi:10.3390/jpm12010114 . . . . **153**

Rui Guo, Renjie Zhang, Ran Liu, Yi Liu, Hao Li and Lu Ma et al.
Machine Learning-Based Approaches for Prediction of Patients' Functional Outcome and Mortality after Spontaneous Intracerebral Hemorrhage
Reprinted from: *J. Pers. Med.* **2022**, *12*, 112, doi:10.3390/jpm12010112 . . . . **163**

Jie Wang, Zhuo Wang, Ning Liu, Caiyan Liu, Chenhui Mao and Liling Dong et al.
Random Forest Model in the Diagnosis of Dementia Patients with Normal Mini-Mental State Examination Scores
Reprinted from: *J. Pers. Med.* **2022**, *12*, 37, doi:10.3390/jpm12010037 . . . . **175**

Danning Wu, Shi Chen, Yuelun Zhang, Huabing Zhang, Qing Wang and Jianqiang Li et al.
Facial Recognition Intensity in Disease Diagnosis Using Automatic Facial Recognition
Reprinted from: *J. Pers. Med.* **2021**, *11*, 1172, doi:10.3390/jpm11111172 . . . . **187**

About the Editors

Youxin Wang

WANG Youxin, male (born 1979), Professor of Capital Medical University and vice director of BeKey Laboratory of Clinical Epidemiology, award of BeNova Project Science and BeTalent Project. He is the associate editor of BMC Public Health in chronic diseases field, executive member of the China Association of Young Statisticians, and member of the Geriatrics Society of the Chinese Medical Association. He has presided over four grants from the National Natural Science Foundation of China and one grant from the National Key R&D Program of China. His research focus is on the epidemiology of non-communicable disease, including diabetes, stroke and dementia.

Ming Feng

Ming Feng, male (born 1976), staff of neurosurgery, associate professor of Peking union medical college hospital, Chinese academy of medical sciences. He served as the deputy leader of the medical big data group of the smart Medical Branch of the Chinese Medical Association, member of the Neurosurgery Branch of the BeMedical Association, member of the Chinese pituitary adenoma collaboration group, and senior member of the Chinese Stroke Society. He presided over one grant from the National Natural Science Foundation of China and two grants from the BeNational Natural Science Foundation. His research focus is on the clinical research on pituitary adenoma, medical big data and artificial intelligence.

Preface to "Non-communicable Diseases, Big Data and Artificial Intelligence"

The 2030 Agenda for Sustainable Development adopted by the United Nations in 2015 recognized non-communicable diseases (NCDs) as a major public health challenge. NCDs are usually multifactorial diseases influenced by both genetic and environmental factors, which makes them difficult to prevent and treat effectively. Medical and health big data, consisting of lifestyle, clinical, and biological data, provide an almost unlimited amount of information about diseases, far exceeding the human ability to make sense of it. Artificial intelligence (AI) offers the potential to analyze large and complex datasets in order to improve predictive, preventive, and personalized medicine (3P medicine).

This reprint included 15 articles, which overview the most recent advances in the field of AI and their application potential in 3P medicine.

Youxin Wang and Ming Feng
Editors

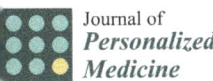

Journal of Personalized Medicine

Article

An Entropy Approach to Multiple Sclerosis Identification

Gerardo Alfonso Perez [1,*] and Javier Caballero Villarraso [1,2]

[1] Department of Biochemistry and Molecular Biology, University of Cordoba, 14071 Cordoba, Spain; bc2cavij@uco.es
[2] Biochemical Laboratory, Reina Sofia University Hospital, 14004 Cordoba, Spain
* Correspondence: ga284@cantab.net

Abstract: Multiple sclerosis (MS) is a relatively common neurodegenerative illness that frequently causes a large level of disability in patients. While its cause is not fully understood, it is likely due to a combination of genetic and environmental factors. Diagnosis of multiple sclerosis through a simple clinical examination might be challenging as the evolution of the illness varies significantly from patient to patient, with some patients experiencing long periods of remission. In this regard, having a quick and inexpensive tool to help identify the illness, such as DNA CpG (cytosine-phosphate-guanine) methylation, might be useful. In this paper, a technique is presented, based on the concept of Shannon Entropy, to select CpGs as inputs for non-linear classification algorithms. It will be shown that this approach generates accurate classifications that are a statistically significant improvement over using all the data available or randomly selecting the same number of CpGs. The analysis controlled for factors such as age, gender and smoking status of the patient. This approach managed to reduce the number of CpGs used while at the same time significantly increasing the accuracy.

Keywords: multiple sclerosis; DNA methylation; entropy

Citation: Alfonso Perez, G.; Caballero Villarraso, J. An Entropy Approach to Multiple Sclerosis Identification. *J. Pers. Med.* **2022**, *12*, 398. https://doi.org/10.3390/jpm12030398

Academic Editors: Youxin Wang and Ming Feng

Received: 21 January 2022
Accepted: 3 March 2022
Published: 4 March 2022

Publisher's Note: MDPI stays neutral with regard to jurisdictional claims in published maps and institutional affiliations.

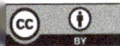

Copyright: © 2022 by the authors. Licensee MDPI, Basel, Switzerland. This article is an open access article distributed under the terms and conditions of the Creative Commons Attribution (CC BY) license (https://creativecommons.org/licenses/by/4.0/).

1. Introduction

Multiple sclerosis (MS) is a chronic autoimmune illness affecting the brain and spinal cord associated with various degrees of disability. In MS, the immune system of the patient attacks the axons, more specifically, the myelin cover; see Figure 1 for a graphical illustration [1]. Inflammation is highlighted by some researchers as one of the drivers of neurodegeneration in MS [2–4]. The evolution of the illness varies greatly from patient to patient, with some individuals experiencing long periods of remissions due to mechanisms that are not yet well understood. The usual manifestation age of the illness is from 20 to 45 years old, but it can occasionally manifest at younger ages, even in children [5]. The causes of MS remain unclear, with a complex underlying combination of genetic and environmental factors the most likely cause [6–10].

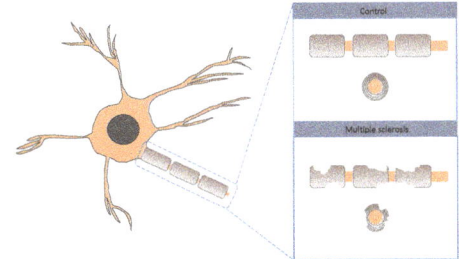

Figure 1. Graphical illustration of neurological damage in MS.

There are some gender considerations to take into account, as the illness is more common in women than men in a 3:1 ratio (and in some countries like Sweden even 5:1).

Some of the common symptoms of the illness include fatigue and numbness, typically in one side of the body [11,12]. Behavioral and cognition abnormalities are also common [13–15]. Currently there are many therapeutic approaches to control or stop the progression of the disease, but no curative treatment is available. However, a large amount of research has been generated regarding this disease. MS has a particularly high prevalence in some areas of Europe and the United States, particularly in northern regions [16].

CpG DNA methylation data has been used to analyze neurodegenerative diseases such as Alzheimer's [17–20] and Parkinson [21–23]. As can be seen in Figure 2, in the context of DNA methylation, CpG dinucleotide (or CpG) refers to cytosine followed by a guanine in the same DNA strand (typically 5' to 3'), not to be confused with cytosine and guanine pared in two complementary strands.

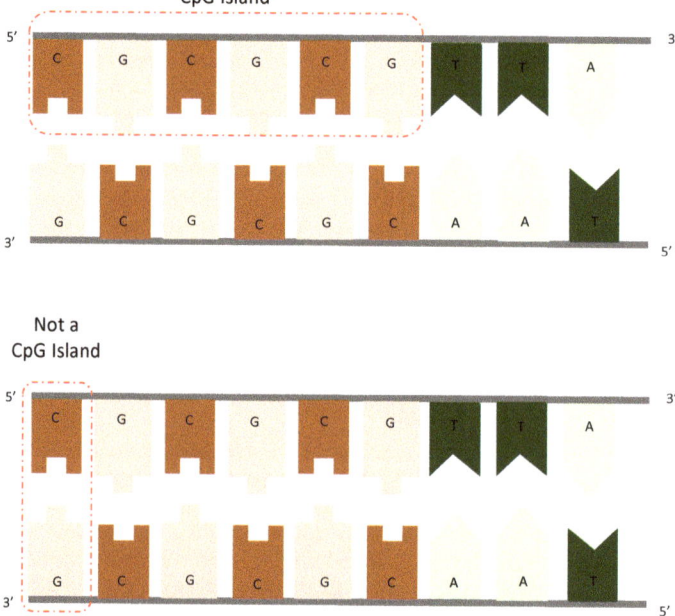

Figure 2. Illustration of CpG islands.

Methylation is simply the addition of a methyl group at the 5-carbon (see Figure 3). DNA methylation has been extensively studied in the context of aging, with several biological clocks built using such types of data. Technological advances in recent years have made possible the analysis of DNA methylation levels on thousands of CpGs in a fast and reliable way. In practice, what is obtained is the percentage level of methylation with a value ranging from 0 to 1 (100% methylated). DNA methylation for cancer diagnostics has made significant progress in the last decades, including many seminal papers [24–27]. There is also a significant body of research covering diabetes [28–32].

DNA methylation has also been used in the context of multiple sclerosis [33,34]. Most of the existing literature on the topic tends to use linear approaches. In this paper, we have followed a non-linear approach, which is in principle more generic and encompassing than a linear approach. Machine learning techniques have been successfully used in multiple applications of different types of diseases [35–38]. More specifically, neural networks have been used as an algorithm for the identification of neurodegenerative illnesses, such as Alzheimer's, using DNA methylation data as the input [39–41].

We applied the concept of Shannon Entropy in the context of DNA methylation applied to multiple sclerosis identification. As far as we are aware, this approach has not been followed before. Shannon Entropy is a concept initially developed in information theory, which attempts to quantify the amount of information contained in a certain set of data [42]. The precise mathematical definition of this concept will be introduced in the materials and methods section. It will be shown that using the concept of Shannon Entropy for CpG selection can generate accurate results.

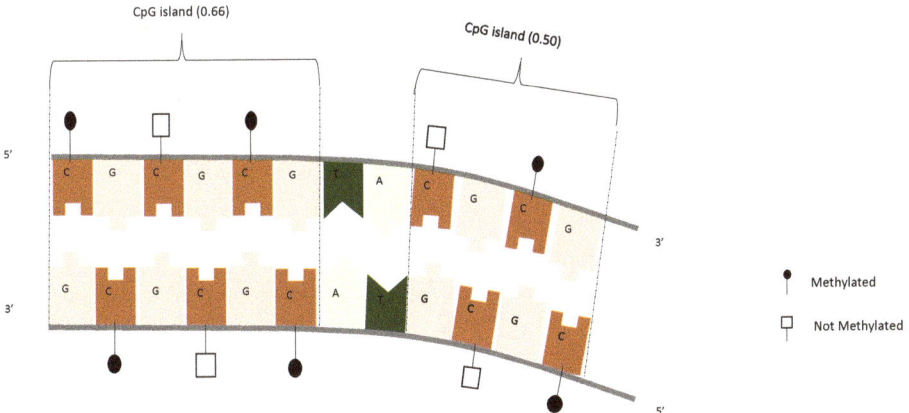

Figure 3. DNA methylation illustration.

Motivation and Aims

Biomarkers are an increasingly important field, particularly when they can be analyzed using non or minimally invasive techniques. In this regard, blood is a particularly interesting tissue as it can be cheaply and quickly obtained from a patient causing only minimal discomfort. Blood has a significant advantage over other tissues such as brain matter, which is much harder to obtain. DNA methylation data can be accurately and rapidly analyzed using technologies such as the Illumina machines. Shannon Entropy is a concept frequently used in machine learning. The motivation to use this approach for data selection is in trying to find techniques that might reduce the dimensionality of the data. Shannon Entropy is one of the few concepts in the existing literature directly related to the amount of information contained in the data, which seems to be a reasonable starting point when trying to reduce the dimensionality of the data while maintaining as much information as possible.

The aim of this article is to develop techniques to identify DNA methylation signatures applicable for the identification of multiple sclerosis patients.

2. Materials and Methods

The DNA methylation data for each individual was stored in a vector X^i.

$$X^i = \begin{Bmatrix} X_1^i \\ X_2^i \\ \vdots \\ X_m^i \end{Bmatrix} \qquad (1)$$

where m is the number of CpGs analyzed per patient. A numerical example would be:

$$X^2 = \begin{Bmatrix} 0.211 \\ 0.723 \\ \vdots \\ 0.983 \end{Bmatrix} \qquad (2)$$

Which represents all the CpG information available for patient number 2. In this example, the methylation level in the first and second CpGs are 21.1% and 72.3%, respectively. As there is a large number of cases analyzed it is more convenient to group the data in a matrix form.

$$X = \begin{pmatrix} X_1^1 & X_1^2 & \cdots & X_1^n \\ X_2^1 & X_2^2 & \cdots & X_2^n \\ \vdots & \vdots & & \vdots \\ X_m^1 & X_m^2 & \cdots & X_m^n \end{pmatrix} \qquad (3)$$

In this notation, there are n cases (including both patients and controls) with m CpGs associated with each case. The status of the individual analyzed (multiple sclerosis or control) was defined with a binary variable $\{0,1\}$ stored in a target vector T, with the value 0 indicating a healthy control case and the value 1 indicating a patient with multiple sclerosis.

$$T = \{0, 1, 0, \ldots, 1\} \qquad (4)$$

As there are n cases, there will be n entries for this vector. In this example, the first and third cases are control cases, and the second one a patient with MS. As a preliminary step, each CpG was individually linearly modeled against the classification vector T and only those with a p-value below 5% were included. The rest of the CpGs were discarded. The dimension of X was reduced from $(n \cdot m)$ to $(n \cdot l)$, where l is the number of CpGs with a p-value below 5%. p-value prefiltering was carried out in all the data. The Shannon Entropy (H) concept was then used to further filter the number of CpGs used. The Shannon Entropy approach step was carried out only for the training dataset. Shannon Entropy can be intuitively understood as the amount of information contained in some data and it is a concept borrowed from information theory. The mathematical expression for Shannon Entropy is as follows:

$$H = -\sum_i P_i \log_2(P_i) \qquad (5)$$

This concept is typically applied in discrete mathematics. The probabilities can be estimated empirically. In simple terms, more entropy translates into more information contained. After the initial filtering, the absolute value of the Shannon Entropy was estimated for each CpG.

$$H = \begin{Bmatrix} H_1 \\ H_2 \\ \vdots \\ H_l \end{Bmatrix} \qquad (6)$$

Only CpGs with an entropy value (H_i) bigger than certain predefined value (H_i^f) were considered. All the other CpGs were excluded from the analysis. In this way we obtained H^*.

$$H^* = \begin{Bmatrix} H_1^* \\ H_2^* \\ \cdot \\ \cdot \\ \cdot \\ H_q^* \end{Bmatrix} \qquad (7)$$

In this notation $q \leq l$. After selecting the CpGs, it is necessary to choose the classification algorithm that is used. A neural network with a hidden layer and an output layer was used. The hidden layer contained 50 artificial neurons, while the output layer contained a single artificial neuron. The 50 neurons in the hidden layer are of the sigmoid symmetric transfer function type. The neuron in the output layer is of the type sigmoid positive transfer function (both of these transfer functions are built-in in Matlab). All the neurons include a bias factor. The neural network was trained with the scaled conjugate backpropagation algorithm. Another four learning algorithms were tested (Levenberg–Marquardt, resilient backpropagation, one-step secant and gradient descent). As in the case of the transfer functions in the artificial neural networks, the learning algorithms are also built-in options in Matlab. Among all the learning algorithms, the best results were obtained using the scaled conjugate backpropagation approach. The data was divided into a training and a testing dataset. The testing dataset accounted for approximately 15% of the data. All the calculations were carried out in Matlab. Neural networks have been extensively used for modeling purposes and can accurately describe many complex underlying dynamics. An important step is to check that the classification error obtained using the above mentioned Shannon Entropy approach for CpG selection is more accurate than the one obtained when using the same number of randomly selected CpGs; in other words, controlling that the improvement in accuracy is not simply due to the reduction in the dimensionality of the data.

All the calculations were done in Matlab, the Shannon Entropy value was calculated using an existing Matlab function. The methylation data was analyzed using two decimals of precision in percentage terms. The analysis did not appear to be very sensitive to an increase to the third decimal place, but it started to have more impact thereafter (four or five decimal places in percentage terms). We believe that using two decimal places is a reasonable precision considering the likely accuracy of the experimental data.

A sensitivity analysis was also carried out. The underlying assumption was that CpGs with very little data variation would be less useful for classification purposes. In an extreme case, if the DNA methylation level for a given CpG was the same for all patients, then this information would not be useful for classification purposes. We did not assume that the CpGs with the most data variation (measured as the standard deviation) were necessarily the best choices, as other factors such as experimental noise (and potentially many others) can increase the variation of the data. However, it seemed reasonable to carry out a sensitivity analysis over reasonable values of the volatility of the DNA methylation data.

Data

DNA methylation data for 279 individuals were obtained from the GEO database (publicly available data) with the accession code GSE 106648 [43]. The database contained both individuals with multiple sclerosis (140) as well as control individuals (139). The age range was from 16 to 66 years old, and there were 77 male individuals. There were more females than male patients. This is consistent with the observation that MS tends to be more common among females than males; 138 of the individuals in the dataset were smokers. Age, gender and smoking status (Table 1) were used as inputs in the model. As in the case of DNA methylation, these factors were allocated to their corresponding training or testing dataset.

Table 1. Basic descriptive information of the patients.

Description	Amount
Male	77
Female	202
Smokers	138
Non-smokers	141
Age	16, 77

The DNA methylation data [43] was obtained from peripheral blood tissue using the Illumina Human Methylation 450 Beach Chip. There were 485,512 CpG DNA methylation data per patient.

3. Results

As can be seen in Figure 4, the average classification error using all the available data with a p-value below 5% was 55.4%, while the error obtained when using only the CpGs with the top 10% Shannon Entropy values (9499 CpGs) was 19.93%, which is a statistically significant improvement. Equivalently, the proposed approach (using Shannon Entropy as a filter) generated a successful classification rate of approximately 80.07%, while the direct approach (using all the data) generated a successful classification rate of approximately 44.6%. The direct approach likely generates poor classifications due to the issue of local minima, which is likely improved by the introduced Shannon Entropy filtering. The model accuracy was substantially improved while at the same time reducing the amount of input data required in the mode. After the two steps (p-value filtering and Shannon Entropy filtering), the amount of CpGs was reduced by approximately 98% compared to the total initial data available. These results were obtained by dividing the data into training and testing datasets, with the testing dataset not used during the training phase. The testing dataset contained approximately 15% of the total data. Unless explicitly mentioned, all the results shown below refer to the testing dataset results. All the models controlled for age, gender and smoking status of the patients. As it can be seen in Table 2, the average sensitivity and specificity obtained were 78.3% and 81.8%, respectively. An example showing a confusion matrix and ROC can be seen in Figures 5 and 6.

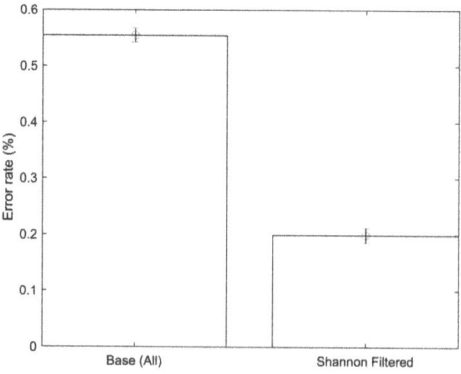

Figure 4. Error rate comparison between direct approach and Shannon Entropy filtered approach.

Table 2. Average classification forecasting accuracy.

Accuracy Measure	Percentage
Average successful classification	80.1%
Sensitivity	78.3%
Specificity	81.8%

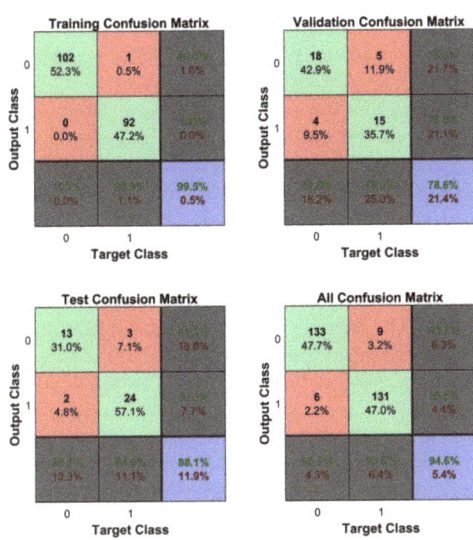

Figure 5. A sample confusion matrix (after *p*-value prefiltering and Shannon Entropy filtering).

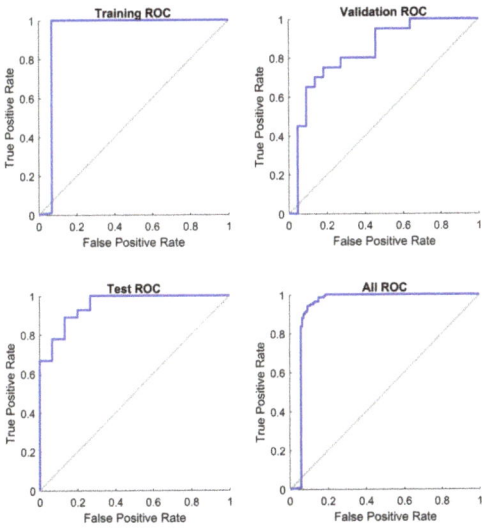

Figure 6. ROC (after *p*-value prefiltering and Shannon Entropy filtering).

In order to compare the results, two baseline values were obtained using the volatility (standard deviation) as an indicator. In the first baseline case, the top 2% most volatile CpGs were selected without any prefiltering (such as p-value). This was done in order to have a dimensionality comparable to the results obtained using the proposed approach (p-value prefiltering plus Shannon Entropy filtering). The classification success ratio using this technique was approximately 51.6%. A second base line level was obtained. In this case, p-value prefiltering was carried out followed by a selection of the most volatile CpGs. The threshold value for the volatility was selected in order to make the final dimension of the data, i.e., number of CpGs selected, approximately the same as the one obtained in the proposed approach (p-value plus Shannon filtering). The successful classification rate was 56.1%.

An important test to carry out is comparing the performance of the obtained CpGs by the Shannon Entropy approach (as inputs for the classification algorithm) to the results using a matrix of randomly selected CpGs. In this way, we account for the reduction in dimensionality of the data. Ten randomly selected sets of CpGs of the same size as the one obtained using the Shannon Entropy approach (9499) were selected. All the included CpGs in this random approach had p-values of less than 5%, i.e., this analysis was carried out after the initial linear filtering. Ten simulations were carried out for each of the ten different randomly selected sets of CpGs. The average value and the confidence interval can be seen in Figure 7. The Shannon Entropy approach generates classifications that are statistically significantly more accurate than a random selection of the same size.

As mentioned in the methods and materials section, a sensitivity analysis using the standard deviation of the DNA methylation data for each CpG was also carried out. In Figure 8, the results of selecting the CpGs with the highest volatility are shown. The range selected encompassed the top 5% to the top 50%, in 5% increments. For example, the first column shows the error rate (misclassifications) when using the top 5% of CpGs according to their standard deviation from the initial pool containing 9499 CpGs (after the initial filtering using Shannon Entropy filtering).

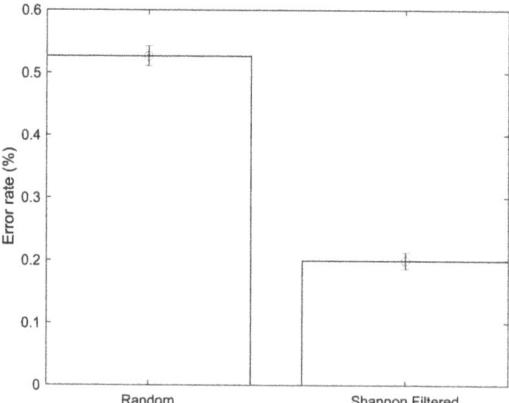

Figure 7. Error rate comparison between the Shannon Entropy filtered approach and random selection of the same size.

The intuition behind this approach is selecting CpGs with variation in the methylation values. As an extreme example, completely flat data (with standard deviation equal to zero) will arguably contain no value from a classification point of view. It is also acknowledged that some of that volatility might be caused by experimental and other sources of noise. The best results were obtained when using the top 15% most volatile CpGs with an average correct classification rate of 81.42%. However, the results were not statistically different (at a 5% significance) when compared with the results obtained by filtering for Shannon Entropy only (no filtering according to the standard deviation of the CpGs).

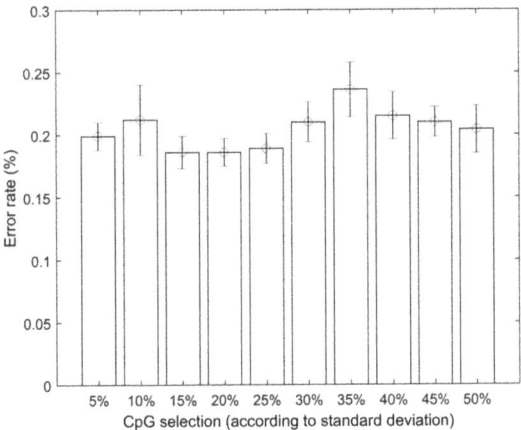

Figure 8. Sensitivity analysis according to the standard deviation of the value of the CpGs. Error rate as a function of the amount of CpGs selected according to their standard deviation.

4. Discussion

An innovative approach is shown for the selection of DNA methylation CpGs to be used in non-linear classification models. This approach is based on the concept of Shannon Entropy, which it is an idea borrowed from the information theory field. Shannon Entropy, in simple terms, can be understood as a measure of the amount of information contained in a set of data. The overall data was first filtered, discarding the CpG with p-values above 5%. A quality pre-check of the data was also carried out, excluding CpGs with missing data. The analyzed dataset appeared to be of good quality with no major data issues. Using the two steps approach of p-value prefiltering followed by the proposed Shannon Entropy filtering, the dataset was reduced from an original size of approximately 485,512 to a final size of 9499 CpGs, which represents a 98% reduction. The classification analysis, distinguishing between control and multiple sclerosis patients, using the entire dataset, did not generate accurate results. The error rate when using the Shannon Entropy approach was 19.93% (80.07% correct classification), which is a statistically significant improvement over the base case. These error rates were obtained using artificial neural networks as the classification algorithm. All the analyses were carried out controlling for age, gender and smoking status of the patients. It was also tested if the increase in accuracy was due simply to the reduction in the dimensionality of the data. In order to do this, several random CpG configurations of the same size (9499 CpGs) as the one obtained using the Shannon Entropy approach were tested. Their average error rate was 52.66%, which is statistically significantly higher than the results obtained using the Shannon Entropy. This suggests that the Shannon Entropy approach might be a reasonable approach to select potential CpGs relevant for the classification analysis. This type of tool might become rather useful in the future, as the amount of CpGs analyzed per person increases and the computational costs increase accordingly. Another interesting analysis is controlling for the volatility, i.e., the standard deviation, of the CpGs. A sensitivity analysis was carried out in this regard by selecting CpGs according to their standard deviation (in buckets of 5%), i.e., top 5%, top 10%, and so on. When carrying out this type of analysis, there were some improvements in the average accuracy, but these improvements were not statistically significant.

These results were consistent with other articles that found a relationship between DNA methylation in other tissues such as the hippocampus [44]. Using blood as the selected tissue [43] is better suited for clinical purposes. Having a simple test, such as one based on DNA methylation data, which can be applied to many different diseases in a rapid and inexpensive way, can be useful. Multiple sclerosis is a relatively difficult illness to diagnose. Using only clinical symptoms and imaging, such as MRI, is frequently requested when the presence of illness is suspected. From a clinical point of view, it might be practical to have techniques, such as DNA methylation levels in the blood, which can be identified, with a reasonable level of accuracy, the presence of MS with a simple blood test. The physician can use the results from the blood-based biomarker combined with the clinical assessment to decide if it is necessary to carry out further tests, such as imaging.

A very interesting area of future research is the temporal evolution of the DNA methylation in multiple sclerosis, given the diverse evolution of the illness, particularly the long periods of remission experienced by some patients. Further research is necessary to determine feasibility, but it might be possible to use this type of approach for early detection. As more data becomes available, it might be possible to distinguish between different types of illness progression using DNA methylation data. It is possible that differentiating between the different types of evolution might help in targeting therapies in a more precise way.

5. Conclusions

Technical improvements are making possible the generation of large amounts of epigenetic data, such as DNA CpG methylation data, that can be used for the detection of several different types of illnesses, such as multiple sclerosis (MS). Multiple sclerosis is a complex illness with genetic and environmental factors, and importantly, an uncertain evolution with some patients experiencing long periods of remission. In this paper, we present a technique based on the Shannon Entropy concept for the selection of CpGs as inputs for MS identification using non-linear techniques such as artificial neural networks. It was shown that using the proposed approach, the number of CpGs used decreased while the accuracy of the classifications significantly improved. As more DNA methylation data becomes available, it is important to have techniques to efficiently filter these large amounts of information. In this regard, borrowing concepts like Shannon Entropy from other disciplines, such as information theory, might be an interesting approach. Having more data is likely beneficial but not all the new data will be helpful for analysis with a large percentage potentially adding noise. Therefore, it is important to develop techniques to further facilitate quantitative data analysis.

In the future, as more DNA CpG methylation data becomes available, it might be possible to extend this type of analysis in order to identify patients with different types of MS evolution. Currently, MS has no cure, but it is a field of intense research. It is possible that differentiating between the different types of evolution might help in targeting therapies in a more precise way, and this is a very appealing area of future research.

Author Contributions: Conceptualization, G.A.P.; methodology, G.A.P. and J.C.V.; software, G.A.P.; validation, G.A.P. and J.C.V.; formal analysis, G.A.P. and J.C.V.; investigation, G.A.P. and J.C.V.; resources, G.A.P. and J.C.V.; data curation, G.A.P. and J.C.V.; writing—original draft preparation, G.A.P.; writing—review and editing, G.A.P. and J.C.V.; visualization, G.A.P. and J.C.V.; supervision, G.A.P. and J.C.V.; project administration, G.A.P. and J.C.V.; funding acquisition, G.A.P. and J.C.V. All authors have read and agreed to the published version of the manuscript.

Funding: This research received no external funding.

Institutional Review Board Statement: Not applicable.

Informed Consent Statement: Not applicable.

Data Availability Statement: The data is available in the GEO Database with accession code GSE 106648.

Conflicts of Interest: The authors declare no conflict of interest.

References

1. Sospedra, M.; Martin, R. Immunology of multiple sclerosis. *Annu. Rev. Immunol.* **2005**, *23*, 683–747. [CrossRef]
2. Dendrou, C.; Fugger, L.; Friese, M. Immunophatology of multiple sclerosis. *Nat. Rev. Immunol.* **2015**, *15*, 545–558. [CrossRef] [PubMed]
3. Lassmann, H. Multiple sclerosis phatology. *Cold Spring Harb. Perespect. Med.* **2018**, *18*. [CrossRef]
4. Frohman, E.; Racke, M.; Raine, C. Multiple sclerosis—The plaque abd its pathogenesis. *N. Engl. J. Med.* **2006**, *9*, 942–955. [CrossRef] [PubMed]
5. Goldenberg, M. Multiple sclerosis review. *Pharm. Ther.* **2012**, *37*, 175–184.
6. Dobson, R.; Giovannoni, G. Multiple sclerosis a review. *Eur. J. Neurol.* **2019**, *26*, 27–40. [CrossRef] [PubMed]
7. Ebers, G. Environmental factors and multiple sclerosis. *Lancet Neurol.* **2008**, *7*, 268–277. [CrossRef]
8. Dyment, D.; Ebers, G.; Sadovnick, D. Genetics of multiple sclerosis. *Lancet Neurol.* **2004**, *3*, 104–110. [CrossRef]
9. Rudick, R.; Cohen, J.; Weinstock-Guttman, B.; Kinkel, R.; Ransohoff, R. Management of multiple sclerosis. *N. Engl. J. Med.* **1997**, *22*, 1604–1611. [CrossRef]
10. Wu, G.; Alvarez, E. The immunopathophysiology of multiple sclerosis. *Neurol. Clin.* **2011**, *29*, 257–278. [CrossRef]
11. Krupp, L. Fatigue in multiple sclerosis. *Arch. Neurol.* **1988**, *45*, 435–437. [CrossRef]
12. Rudick, R.; Schiffer, R.; Schwetz, K.; Herdon, R. Multiple sclerosis: The problem of incorrect diagnosis. *Arch. Neurol.* **1986**, *43*, 578–583. [CrossRef]
13. Feinstein, A. The neuropsychiatry of multiple sclerosis. *Can. J. Psychiatry* **2004**, *49*, 157–163. [CrossRef]
14. Chiaravalloti, N.; DeLuca, J. Cognitive impairment in multiple sclerosis. *Lancent Neurol.* **2008**, *7*, 1139–1151. [CrossRef]
15. Heldner, M.; Kaufmann-Ezra, S.; Gutbrod, K.; Bernasconi, C.; Bigi, S.; Blatter, V.; Kamm, C. Behavioral changes in patients with multiple sclerosis. *Front. Neurol.* **2017**, *8*, 437. [CrossRef]
16. McFarlin, D.; McFarland, H. Multiple sclerosis. *N. Engl. J. Med.* **1982**, *307*, 1246–1251. [CrossRef]
17. Liu, D.; Wang, Y.; Jing, H.; Meng, Q.; Yang, J. Mendelian randomization integrating GWAS and mQTL data identified novel pleiotropic DNA methylation loci for neuropathology of Alzheimer's disease. *Neurobiol. Aging* **2021**, *97*, 18–27. [CrossRef]
18. Mastroeni, D.; Grover, A.; Whiteside, C.; Coleman, P. Epigenetic changes in alzheimer's disease: decremens in DNA methylation. *Neurobiol. Aging* **2010**, *31*, 2025–2037. [CrossRef]
19. Bollati, V.; Galimberti, D.; Pergoli, L.; Dalla Valle, E.; Barretta, F.; Cortini, F. DNA methylation in repetitive elementsand Alzheimer disease. *Brain Behav. Immunity* **2011**, *25*, 1078–1083. [CrossRef]
20. Blanch, M.; Mosquera, J.; Ansoleaga, B.; Ferrer, I.; Barrachina, M. Altered mitochondrial DNA methylation pattern in Alzheimer disease-related pathology and in Parkinson disease. *Am. J. Pathol.* **2016**, *186*, 385–397. [CrossRef]
21. Masliah, E.; Duamop, W.; Galasko, D.; Desplants, P. Distinctive patterns of DNA methylation associated with Parkinson disease: Identification pf concordant epigenetic changes in brain and peripherak blood leukocytes. *Epigenetics* **2013**, *8*, 1030–1038. [CrossRef]
22. Miranda-Morales, E.; Meier, K.; Sandoval-Carrillo, A.; Salas-Pacheco,J.; Vazquez-Cardenas, P.; Arias-Carrion, O. Implications of DNA methylation in Parkinson's disease. *Front. Mol. Neurosci.* **2017**, *10*, 225. [CrossRef]
23. Wulner, U.; Kaut, O.; Piston, D.; Schmitt, I. DNA methylation in Parkinson's disease. *J. Neurochem.* **2016**, *139*, 108–120. [CrossRef]
24. Chan, K.A.; Jiang, P.; Chan, C.W.; Sun, K.; Wong, J.; Hui, E.P.; Ng, S.S.; Chan, H.L. Noninvasive detection of cancer-associated genome-wide hypomethylation and copy number aberrations by plasma DNA bisulfite sequencing. *Proc. Natl. Acad. Sci. USA* **2013**, *110*, 18761–18768. [CrossRef]
25. Lehmann-Werman, R.; Neiman, D.; Zemmour, H.; Moss, J.; Magenheim, J.; Vaknin-Dembinsky A.; Rubertsson, S.; Nellgard, B.; Blennow, K.; Zetterberg, H.; et al. Identification of tissue specific cell death using methylation patterns of circulating DNA. *Proc. Natl. Acad. Sci. USA* **2016**, *29*, 1826–1834. [CrossRef]
26. Guo, S.; Diep, D.; Plongthongkum, N.; Fung, H.L.; Zhang, K.; Zhang, K. Identification of methylation haplotype blocks aids in deconvolution pf heterogeneous tissue samples and tumor tissue-of-origin mapping from plasma DNA. *Nat. Genet.* **2017**, *49*, 635–642. [CrossRef]
27. Chen, L.H.; Pan, C.; Diplas, B.H.; Xu, C.; Hansen, L.J.; Wu, Y.; Chen X.; Geng, Y.; Sun, T.; Sun, Y.; et al. The integrated genomic and epigenomic landscape of brainsteam glioma. *Nat. Genet.* **2020**, *11*, 3077.
28. Bell, C.; Christopher, G. Genome-wide DNA methylation analysis for diabetic nephropathy in type 1 diabetes melitus. *BMC Med. Genet.* **2010**, *3*, 33.
29. Bansal, A.; Pinney, S. DNA methylation and its role in the pathogenesis of diabetes. *Pediatr. Diabetes* **2017**, *18*, 167–177. [CrossRef]
30. Davegardh, C.; Garcia-Calzon, S.; Bacos, K.; Ling, C. DNA methylation in the pathogenesis of type 2 diabetes in humans. *Mol. Metab.* **2018**, *14*, 12–25. [CrossRef]
31. Rakyan, V.; Beyan, H.; Down, T.; Hawa, M.; Maslau, S.; Anden, D.; Leslie, R. Identification of type 1 diabetes-associated DNA methylation variable positions that precede disease diagnosis. *Epigenomics* **2015**, *7*, 451–460. [CrossRef] [PubMed]
32. Ronn, T.; Ling, C. DNA methylation as a diagnostic and therapeutic target in the battle agaisnt Type 2 diabetes. *PLoS Genet.* **2011**, *7*, 451–460.

33. Bos, S.; Page, C.; Andreassen, B.; Elboudwarej, E.; Gustavsen, M.; Briggs, F.; Barcellos, L. Genome-wide DNA methylation profiles indicate CD8+ T cell hypermethylation in multiple sclerosis. *PLoS ONE* **2015**, *10*, e0117403. [CrossRef] [PubMed]
34. Kukalova, O.; Kabilov, M.; Danilova, L.; Popova, E.; Baturina, O.; Tsareva, E. Whole-Genome DNA methylation analysis of peripheral blood mononuclear cells in multiple sclerosisi patients with different disease courses. *Acta Nat.* **2016**, *8*, 103–110.
35. Cruz, J.; Wishart, D. Applications of machine learning in cancer prediction and prognosis. *Cancer Inform.* **2006**, *2*, 59–77. [CrossRef]
36. Fan, Y.; Li, Y.; Bao, X.; Zhu, H.; Lu, L.; Yao, Y.; Li, Y.; Su, M.; Feng, F.; Feng, S.; et al. Development of Machine Learning Models for Predicting Postoperative Delayed Remission in Patients With Cushing's Disease. *J. Clin. Endocrinol. Metab.* **2021**, *106*, 217–231. [CrossRef]
37. Kourou, K.; Exarchos, T.; Exarchos, K.; Karamouzis, M.; Fotiadis, D. Machine learning applications in cancer prognosis and prediction. *Comput. Struct. Biotechnol.* **2015**, *13*, 8–17. [CrossRef]
38. Li, Y.; Chen, Z. Performance evaluation of machine learning methods for breast cancer prediction. *Appl. Comput. Math.* **2018**, *7*, 212–216. [CrossRef]
39. Park, C.; Ha, J.; Park, S. Prediction of Alzheimer's disease based on deep neural network by integrating gene expression and DNA methylation dataset. *Expert Syst. Appl.* **2020**, *140*, 112873. [CrossRef]
40. Alfonso Perez, G.; Caballero Villarraso, J. Alzheimer Identification through DNA Methylation and Artificial Intelligence Techniques. *Mathematics* **2021**, *9*, 2482. [CrossRef]
41. Spolnicka, M.; Pospiech, E.; Peplonska, B. DNA methylation in EVOVL2 amd C!orf132 correctly predicted chronologicalage of individuals from three disease groups. *Int. J. Leg. Med.* **2018**, *132*, 1–11. [CrossRef]
42. Shannon, C.E. A mathematical theory of communication. *Bell Syst. Tech. J.* **1948**, *27*, 379–423. [CrossRef]
43. Kular, L.; Liu, Y.; Ruhrmann, S.; Zheleznyakova, G.; Marabita, F.; Gomez-Cabrero, D.; James, T.; Ewing, E.; Linden, M.; Gornikiewicz, B.; et al. DNA methylation as a mediator of HLA-DRB1*15:01 and a protective variant in multiple sclerosis. *Nat. Commun.* **2018**, *9*, 2397. [CrossRef]
44. Chomyk, A.M.; Volsko, C.; Tripathi, A.; Deckard, S.A.; Trapp, B.D.; Fox, R.J.; Dutta, R. DNA methylation in demyelinated multiple sclerosis hippocampus. *Bell Syst. Tech. J. Sci. Rep.* **2017**, *18*. [CrossRef]

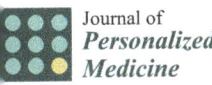

Journal of Personalized Medicine

Article

Polymorphisms and Gene-Gene Interaction in AGER/IL6 Pathway Might Be Associated with Diabetic Ischemic Heart Disease

Kuo Liu [1], Yunyi Xie [1], Qian Zhao [2], Wenjuan Peng [1], Chunyue Guo [1], Jie Zhang [1] and Ling Zhang [1,*]

1. Beijing Municipal Key Laboratory of Clinical Epidemiology, Department of Epidemiology and Health Statistics, School of Public Health, Capital Medical University, Beijing 100069, China; liukuo@ccmu.edu.cn (K.L.); yiyi95127@126.com (Y.X.); pengwenjuan0311@126.com (W.P.); angela460314@163.com (C.G.); zhangjie@ccmu.edu.cn (J.Z.)
2. Department of Biostatistics, FMD K & L, Fort Washington, PA 19034, USA; qiz39@pitt.edu
* Correspondence: zlilyepi@ccmu.edu.cn or zlily_epi@ccmu.edu.cn

Abstract: Background: Although the genetic susceptibility to diabetes and ischemic heart disease (IHD) has been well demonstrated, studies aimed at exploring gene variations associated with diabetic IHD are still limited; Methods: Our study included 204 IHD cases who had been diagnosed with diabetes before the diagnosis of IHD and 882 healthy controls. Logistic regression was used to find the association of candidate SNPs and polygenic risk score (PRS) with diabetic IHD. The diagnostic accuracy was represented with AUC. Generalized multifactor dimensionality reduction (GMDR) was used to illustrate gene-gene interactions; Results: For *IL6R* rs4845625, the CT and TT genotypes were associated with a lower risk of diabetic IHD than the CC genotype (OR = 0.619, $p = 0.033$; OR = 0.542, $p = 0.025$, respectively). Haplotypes in the *AGER* gene (rs184003-rs1035798-rs2070600-rs1800624) and *IL6R* gene (rs7529229-rs4845625-rs4129267-rs7514452-rs4072391) were both significantly associated with diabetic IHD. PRS was associated with the disease (OR = 1.100, $p = 0.005$) after adjusting for covariates, and the AUC were 0.763 ($p < 0.001$). The GMDR analysis suggested that rs184003 and rs4845625 were the best interaction model after permutation testing ($p = 0.001$) with a cross-validation consistency of 10/10; Conclusions: SNPs and haplotypes in the *AGER* and *IL6R* genes and the interaction of rs184003 and rs4845625 were significantly associated with diabetic IHD.

Keywords: diabetic complication; gene-gene interaction; *AGER*; *IL6R*

1. Introduction

Ischemic heart disease (IHD) remains the leading global cause of death and lost life years in adults, and it is also the leading cause of mortality in people with type 2 diabetes mellitus (T2DM). Approximately 68% of deaths in type 2 diabetic patients are caused by cardiac complications [1,2]. It has been demonstrated that the advanced glycation end products (AGER)/interleukin-6 (IL-6) pathway plays an important role in the physiological mechanism of diabetic cardiovascular complications [3–5]; however, whether gene polymorphisms in this pathway can influence the disease susceptibility are still unknown.

Several single nucleotide polymorphisms (SNPs) in the *AGER* gene have been reported to be associated with diabetes or its complications [6–8]. A meta-analysis including 27 original articles showed that *AGER* genetic polymorphisms with CAD were potentiated in patients with diabetes mellitus disease, but the association was not consistently significant [9–11]. A Mendelian randomization study also showed that the C allele in rs2228145 was associated with a lower risk of coronary heart disease [12], but a meta-analysis of three GWA scans with 4107 type 2 diabetes cases and 5187 controls in Caucasians found no evidence that *IL6R* variants were associated with type 2 diabetes [13]. Due to the different effects of the *IL6R* gene on diabetes and coronary heart disease, further research is still needed to demonstrate the association between *IL6R* variants and diabetic macrovascular complications. Gene-gene interactions can explain the missing heritability of cardiometabolic disease and better reflect the complex pathophysiological process of disease [14]. However, few studies have focused on the influence of the gene-gene interactions among several SNPs on CVD susceptibility until now [15–17]. Machine learning methods may effectively reduce Type I and II errors and increase robustness, of which the generalized multifactor dimensionality reduction (GMDR) method has remained popular in detecting the interaction effect since its appearance [18,19].

The current study aimed to illustrate the association of *AGER* and *IL6R* gene polymorphisms with the risk for diabetic ischemic heart disease (IHD) and to assess the modulatory effect of gene-gene interactions between these variants on disease risk. SNPs that were previously reported to be associated with cardiometabolic disease, inflammatory disease, or located in miRNA binding sites were selected for the analysis (see Supplementary Materials Table S1).

2. Materials and Methods

2.1. Study Design and Population

A total of 204 diabetic ischemic heart disease cases and 882 healthy controls were enrolled from communities in Beijing. All subjects gave written informed consent. This study was approved by the Ethics Committee of Capital Medical University (No: 2016SY24).

The inclusion criteria for the cases were as follows: (1) Self-reported or physician-diagnosed diabetes according to the American Diabetes Association Criteria [20]; (2) Ischemic heart disease defined by clinical history, including acute myocardial infarction, angina pectoris, non-ST-elevation acute coronary syndromes, and/or ischemic electrocardiographic alterations; (3) T2DM was diagnosed earlier than ischemic heart disease for at least one year; and (4) Medical records or copies should be provided to verify the diagnosis of diseases.

The exclusion criteria for the cases were as follows: (1) Other diabetic complications: including diabetic nephropathy, diabetic foot, diabetic retinopathy, and diabetic neuropathy; (2) Ischemic cerebrovascular disease or cerebral hemorrhage; (3) Pregnant or lactating women; and (4) Critical physical disability or mental disorder and could not cooperate with the survey.

The inclusion criteria for the controls were as follows: (1) Subjects had not been diagnosed with T2DM before, and fasting blood glucose was less than 5.6 mmol/L in the current survey; (2) Subjects did not have ischemic heart disease, ischemic stroke, or cerebral hemorrhage; (3) Subjects did not have chronic kidney disease; and (4) Subjects were not in the acute phase of infection.

The exclusion criteria for the controls were as follows: (1) Pregnant or lactating women; and (2) Critical physical disability or mental disorder and could not cooperate with the survey.

2.2. Measurements

Lifestyle risk factors were obtained from a structured questionnaire. Smoking status was categorized as "currently smoking" and "past/never smoking". Current smoking was defined as at least 1 cigarette per day, lasting for more than 1 year. Those who had never smoked before or had not smoked for at least 3 months were defined as past/never smoking. Alcohol drinking was categorized as "current alcohol drinking" and "past/never alcohol drinking". Current drinking was defined as drinking at least once per week and still drinking at that frequency in the previous month. Those who never drank alcohol or had not consumed alcohol for at least one month were defined as never/past alcohol drinking.

Blood pressure (BP) was measured in the morning before participants used antihypertensive medication. Participants were asked to rest for at least 30 min before BP measurement if they had just smoked or had caffeinated products. BP (mmHg) was measured three times at sitting positions by a mercury sphygmomanometer. The average of the last two measurements was used for data analysis.

2.3. Serum Markers

After overnight fasting, all participants underwent fasting blood sampling. Fasting blood samples were collected and restored in a 2% EDTA vacutainer for each participant. After centrifugation, the plasma and blood cell samples were separated into two cryovials. Fasting plasma glucose (FPG), total cholesterol (TC), triglycerides (TG), high-density lipoprotein cholesterol (HDLC), and low-density lipoprotein cholesterol (LDLC) were tested using the Beckman Coulter chemistry analyzer AU5800 in the clinical laboratory of Beijing Hepingli Hospital.

Venous blood samples were obtained and stored in a 4 °C refrigerator. All biochemical analyses were performed within 8 h. Serum glucose and biochemical determinations were measured by an enzymatic method using a chemistry analyzer (Beckman LX20, Beckman, Brea, CA, USA) at the central laboratory of the hospital. Highly sensitive C-reactive protein was assessed using a Beckman Coulter chemistry analyzer AU5800 and white blood cell counts were obtained using an AcT5diff cell counter (Beckman Coulter®).

2.4. Genotyping

Important functional SNPs and previously reported susceptible SNPs were selected as candidate SNPs. Five SNPs (rs1035798, rs1800624, rs1800625, rs184003, and rs2070600) in the *AGER* gene and seven SNPs (rs2228144, rs4072391, rs4129267, rs4537545, rs4845625, rs7514452, and rs7529229) in the *IL6R* gene were selected in the current study.

Genomic DNA was extracted from 1 mL of peripheral blood cells using a TIANGEN DNA kit (TIANGEN Biotech, China, DP319-01) according to the manufacturer's protocol. The primers were designed by AssayDesigner3.1 software and they were synthesized by Shanghai Thermo Fisher Scientific Co., Ltd., in China. Detailed information on the primers is shown in Supplementary Materials Table S1. A Sequenom MassARRAY® matrix-assisted laser desorption/ionization-time of flight mass spectrometry (MALDI-TOF MS) platform (Sequenom Inc., San Diego, CA, USA) was used to genotype SNPs.

2.5. Definition of Diseases and Recommendation Level of Their Risk Factors

T2DM was defined as FPG $\geq$ 7.0 mmol/L or self-reported physician-diagnosed diabetes and/or the use of antidiabetic agents, according to the American Diabetes Association Criteria [21]. Ischemic heart disease (IHD) includes non-fatal acute myocardial infarction [22], angina pectoris [23], acute coronary syndromes [24], and/or ischemic electrocardiographic alterations. Ischemic heart disease in T2DM patients was defined as diabetic ischemic heart disease. Hypertension was defined as systolic blood pressure (SBP) $\geq$ 140 mmHg and/or diastolic blood pressure (DBP) $\geq$ 90 mmHg and/or on current antihypertensive medication. Participants with TG $\geq$ 2.3 mmol/L, TC $\geq$ 6.2 mmol/L, LDLC $\geq$ 4.1 mmol/L, or HDLC $\leq$ 1.0 mmol/L were defined as having dyslipidemia according to the criteria of the 2016 Chinese guidelines for the management of dyslipidemia in adult [25]. The acute phase of infection was defined by hsCRP > 10 mg/L or white blood cell counts > 10.0×10^9. Kidney disease was defined as self-report of diagnosed chronic kidney disease or GFR $\leq$ 90 mL/min over 3 months. The CKD-EPI equations were used to estimate the glomerular filtration rate [26].

2.6. Statistical Analysis

Each continuous variable was tested for normality by the Shapiro-Wilk test. The continuous variables with a normal distribution are expressed as the means ± standard deviations (SD), and the mean difference between groups was tested by Student's *t*-test. The continuous variables that were non-normally distributed are displayed as the median (interquartile range), and the difference between groups was tested by the Mann-Whitney U test. The categorical variables are expressed as numbers (percentages). The polygenic risk score (PRS) was calculated by summing the number of risk alleles of all candidate SNPs. Logistic regression was used to evaluate the association of diabetic ischemic heart disease with candidate SNPs and PRS, and the diagnostic accuracy was quantified with the area under the ROC curve (AUC). SPSS 25.0 software (SPSS Inc., Chicago, IL, USA) was used for all abovementioned statistical analyses. The generalized multifactor dimensionality reduction (GMDR) method was used to estimate the gene-gene interactions. For the adjustment for multiple testing, a permutation test with 1000 replications was performed. Haplotypes were identified and visualized by Haploview software. The association between haplotypes and diabetic ischemic heart disease and Hardy-Weinberg equilibrium (HWE) was demonstrated by using Plink software (version 1.07). All the SNPs were in HWE ($p > 0.05$). We also performed subgroup analysis by considering FPG and ICVD risk scores. The "10-year ICVD Risk Assessment Form" applicable to the "Cardiovascular Disease Prevention Guidelines in China" was used to estimate ICVD risk score [27]. A two-sided $p \leq 0.05$ was considered statistically significant.

3. Results

3.1. General Characteristics of the Studied Participants

A total of 882 healthy controls and 204 diabetic ischemic heart disease cases were included in the current study. The levels of AGEs, TG, FPG, and DBP were significantly higher in the ischemic heart disease cases than in the controls ($p < 0.001$). Serum IL-6 was also higher in the case group, but the difference was not statistically significant. The levels of TC, LDLC, HDLC, and SBP were significantly higher in the controls than in the cases ($p < 0.001$). According to the recommendation of the "2017 Guidelines for the prevention and treatment of type 2 diabetes in China", the percentages of SBP, DBP, HDLC, LDLC, TG, and TC in the ideal range were significantly higher in the control group than in the case group ($p < 0.001$), see Supplementary Materials Table S2. In people with diabetic ischemic heart disease, the proportion of current smokers or alcohol drinkers was significantly lower than in the controls ($p < 0.001$). The details are shown in Table 1.

Table 1. Demographic and biochemical characteristics of the participants.

	Controls	T2DM + IHD	p Value
Age (years) [1]	64.00 ± 11.25	65 ± 11.00	0.126
Male (n, %)	488 (55.3)	119 (58.3)	0.436
SBP (mmHg) [1]	136.00 (24.00)	130.00 (19.50)	<0.001 **
DBP (mmHg) [1]	79.00 (14.00)	80 (12.00)	0.001 **
BMI (kg/m^2) [1]	25.64 (4.46)	25.36 (3.53)	0.578
TC (mmol/L) [1]	5.12 (1.41)	4.68 (1.53)	<0.001 **
HDLC (mmol/L) [1]	1.34 (0.48)	1.22 (0.45)	<0.001 **
LDLC (mmol/L) [1]	3.02 (1.17)	2.68 (1.04)	<0.001 **
TG (mmol/L) [1]	1.40 (0.90)	2.35 (1.57)	<0.001 **
FPG (mmol/L) [1]	5.60 (0.93)	7.07 (3.53)	<0.001 **
Current smoking (n, %)	194 (22.0)	18 (8.8)	<0.001 **
Current drinking (n, %)	295 (33.5)	32 (15.7)	<0.001 **
AGEs (mmol/L) [1]	31.05 (15.94)	38.07 (16.82)	<0.001 **
IL-6 (mmol/L) [1]	133.08 (49.32)	136.83 (40.18)	0.353

[1] Variables, which have non-normal distribution, were displayed as median (interquartile range), and were tested by Mann-Whitney U test. T2DM: type 2 diabetes, IHD: ischemic heart disease, BMI: body mass index, SBP: systolic blood pressure, DBP: diastolic blood pressure, FPG: fasting plasma glucose, TG: triglyceride, TC: total cholesterol, LDL-C: low density lipoprotein cholesterol, HDL-C: high density lipoprotein cholesterol, AGEs: advanced glycation end products, IL-6: interleukin 6. ** $p < 0.01$.

3.2. Association of AGER and IL6R Polymorphisms with Diabetic Ischemic Heart Disease

All polymorphisms were in Hardy-Weinberg equilibrium (all p-values were greater than 0.05). For AGER rs184003, participants with the GT and TT genotypes had a significantly higher risk of diabetic ischemic heart disease than those with the CC genotype (OR = 1.435, $p = 0.039$; OR = 2.525, $p = 0.030$, respectively). The T allele was associated with an increased risk of diabetic ischemic heart disease by 50% in additive and dominant models ($p = 0.005$; $p = 0.012$, respectively). For *AGER* rs2070600, the T allele was associated with about a 30% lower risk of diabetic ischemic heart disease in the additive and dominant models ($p = 0.025$; $p = 0.030$, respectively). However, after adjusting for potential confounders, the association between the above two SNPs and disease was null. The details are shown in Table 2.

Table 2. Associations of rs184003, rs2070600, and rs4845625 with the risk of diabetic cardiovascular disease.

	Genotype	Crude OR [1] (95%CI)	Crude p Value	Adjusted OR¤ (95%CI)	Adjusted p Value
rs184003	GG	Ref	Ref	Ref	Ref
	GT	1.435 (1.019, 2.020)	0.039 *	1.223 (0.797, 1.878)	0.357
	TT	2.525 (1.092, 5.837)	0.030 *	1.651 (0.580, 4.702)	0.348
	additive	1.491 (1.125, 1.976)	0.005 **	1.247 (0.880, 1.767)	0.215
	dominant	1.518 (1.093, 2.017)	0.012 *	1.265 (0.839, 1.905)	0.261
	recessive	2.282 (0.993, 5.241)	0.046	1.571 (0.555, 4.449)	0.395
rs2070600	CC	Ref	Ref	Ref	Ref
	CT	0.713 (0.496, 1.024)	0.067	0.843 (0.550, 1.294)	0.435
	TT	0.536 (0.237, 1.211)	0.134	0.611 (0.206, 1.807)	0.373
	additive	0.721 (0.542, 0.960)	0.025 *	0.819 (0.578, 1.162)	0.264
	dominant	0.684 (0.485, 0.964)	0.030 *	1.399 (0.914, 2.140)	0.122
	recessive	0.587 (0.261, 1.320)	0.198	2.204 (0.493, 9.851)	0.301
rs4845625	CC	Ref	Ref	Ref	Ref
	CT	0.692 (0.483, 0.991)	0.045 *	0.619 (0.398, 0.961)	0.033
	TT	0.503 (0.318, 0.795)	0.003 **	0.542 (0.318, 0.924)	0.025
	additive	0.707 (0.563, 0.888)	0.003 **	0.732 (0.557, 0.961)	0.025
	dominant	0.632 (0.448, 0.889)	0.008 **	0.594 (0.392, 0.902)	0.014
	recessive	0.644 (0.434, 0.955)	0.028	0.757 (0.481, 1.191)	0.229

[1] No variables were adjusted in logistic regression model ¤ Dyslipidemia, hypertension, smoking, and drinking were adjusted in the logistic regression model. Adjusted p-values shown in the table are adjusted only by covariates. * $p < 0.05$, ** $p < 0.01$.

For *IL6R* rs4845625, participants with the CT and TT genotypes had a significantly lower risk of diabetic ischemic heart disease than those with the CC genotype (OR = 0.692, $p = 0.045$; OR = 0.503, $p = 0.003$, respectively). The T allele significantly decreased the risk of diabetic ischemic heart disease in additive and dominant models (OR = 0.707, $p = 0.003$; OR = 0.632, $p = 0.008$, respectively). The association between rs4845625 and disease was still significant after adjusting for potential confounders. The details are shown in Table 2. The association between other SNPs and disease were shown in Supplementary Materials Table S3. The polygenic risk score was also associated with an increased risk of diabetic ischemic heart disease by 10% (OR = 1.101, 95% CI: 1.042–1.162, $p = 0.001$). After adjusting for dyslipidemia, hypertension, smoking, and drinking status, PRS was consistently associated with the disease (OR = 1.100, 95% CI: 1.029–1.176, $p = 0.005$).

Compared with models containing only traditional risk factors (AUC = 0.756; 95% CI: 0.714–0.798; $p < 0.001$), the diagnostic accuracy of models containing traditional risk factors together with *IL6R* and *AGER* polymorphisms (AUC = 0.759; 95% CI: 0.716–0.801; $p < 0.001$) and traditional risk factors together with PRS (AUC = 0.763; 95% CI: 0.72–0.80; $p < 0.001$) had slightly higher diagnostic accuracies. However, models containing genetic markers did not improve the diagnostic accuracy significantly ($p > 0.05$). The details were shown in Figure 1.

3.3. Association between Haplotypes and Diabetic Ischemic Heart Disease

Four out of five SNPs in the *AGER* gene (Block 1: rs184003-rs1035798-rs2070600-rs1800624) and five out of seven SNPs in the *IL6R* gene (Block 2: rs7529229-rs4845625-rs4129267-rs7514452-rs4072391) showed linkage disequilibrium (see Figure 2). These two blocks were both significantly associated with diabetic ischemic heart disease (Block 1: $p = 0.008$; Block 2: $p = 0.007$). Four haplotypes were constructed in block 1, and two of them were associated with diabetic ischemic heart disease (C-G-T-A: $p = 0.018$; A-G-C-A:

$p = 0.004$). Four haplotypes were constructed in block 2, and two of them were associated with diabetic ischemic heart disease (T-C-C-T-C: $p = 0.033$; T-T-C-T-C: $p = 0.001$). The details of the haplotype analysis are shown in Table 3.

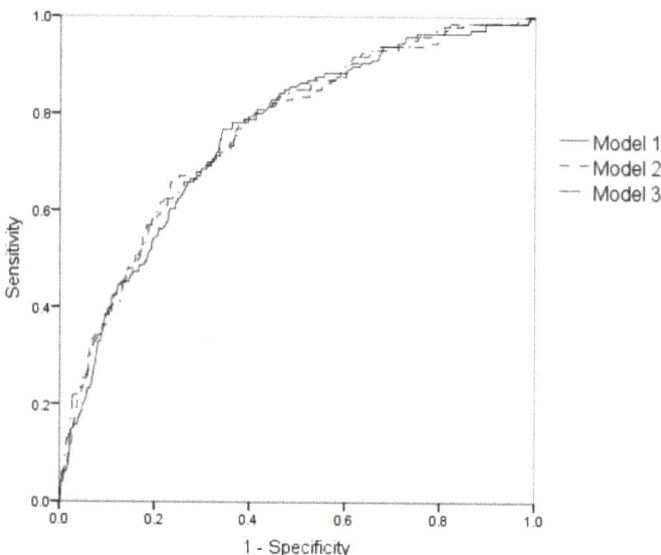

Figure 1. ROC curve of different statistical models. Models were built by logistic regression, variables contained in each model were as follows: Model 1: Age, sex, hyperlipidaemia, hypertension, smoking, and alcohol drinking behavior. Model 2: Variables in model 1 and rs184003 and rs4845625. Model 3: Variables in model 1 and PRS.

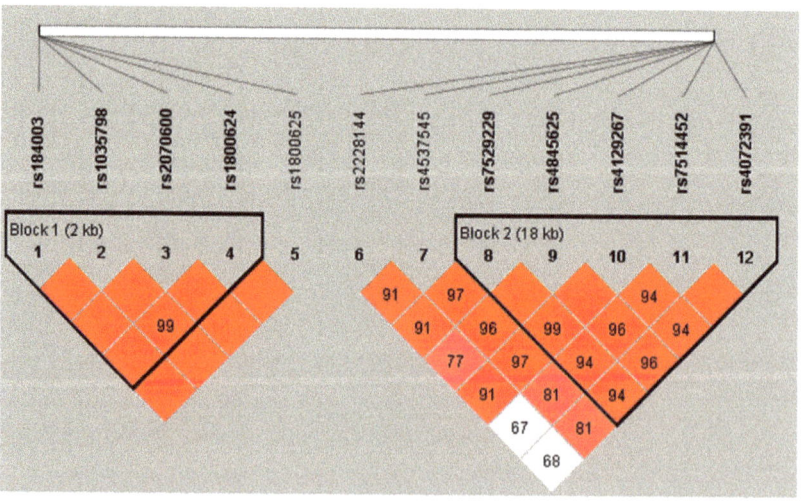

Figure 2. Haplotypes in *AGER* gene and *IL6R* gene. Two haplotypes were identified by haploview software. *AGER* gene: rs184003-rs1035798-rs2070600-rs180062; *IL6R* gene: rs7529229-rs4845625-rs4129267-rs7514452-rs4072391.

Table 3. Haplotype analysis for blocks in *AGER* and *IL6R* genes.

	Haplotypes	F_U [1]	F_A¤	Chi-Square	OR (95%CI)	p Value
Block 1 [2]	Omnibus test	-	-	11.750		0.008 **
	C-A-C-T	0.162	0.170	0.162	1.049 (0.830, 1.327)	0.687
	C-G-T-A	0.202	0.150	5.575	0.743 (0.580, 0.951)	0.018 *
	A-G-C-A	0.140	0.197	8.229	1.407 (1.114, 1.777)	0.004 **
	C-G-C-A	0.497	0.482	0.247	0.970 (0.859, 1.094)	0.620
Block 2 [3]	Omnibus test	-	-	11.99		0.007 **
	T-T-C-C-T	0.093	0.100	0.227	1.075 (0.798, 1.449)	0.634
	C-C-T-T-C	0.387	0.431	2.639	1.114 (0.978, 1.268)	0.104
	T-C-C-T-C	0.095	0.131	4.551	1.379 (1.026, 1.853)	0.033 *
	T-T-C-T-C	0.426	0.338	10.32	0.793 (0.689, 0.914)	0.001 **

[1] F_U: minor allele frequency in controls; ¤ F_A: minor allele frequency in cases; [2] Block1: rs184003-rs1035798-rs2070600-rs1800624; [3] Block2: rs7529229-rs4845625-rs4129267-rs7514452-rs4072391; * $p < 0.05$; ** $p < 0.01$.

3.4. The Effect of Gene-Gene Interactions on Diabetic Ischemic Heart Disease

GMDR analysis was performed to assess the effect of gene-gene interactions on diabetic ischemic heart disease risk after adjustment for dyslipidemia, hypertension, smoking, and drinking. The GMDR analysis suggested that rs184003 in the *AGER* gene and rs4845625 in the *IL6R* gene were the best models in terms of statistical significance after permutation testing ($p = 0.001$). The two-locus models had a cross-validation consistency of 10/10 and a testing accuracy of 0.597. Logistic regression was subsequently used to obtain the odds ratios (ORs) and 95% confidence intervals (CIs) for the interaction between rs184003 and rs4845625. In the additive model, the joint effect of rs184003 and rs4845625 was associated with an increased risk of diabetic ischemic heart disease by 38% (OR = 1.38, 95% CI: 1.13–1.69, $p = 0.002$). The GeneMANIA was subsequently used to construct a gene network and predict gene function. As shown in Figure 3, *IL6R* and *AGER* have physical interactions with each other.

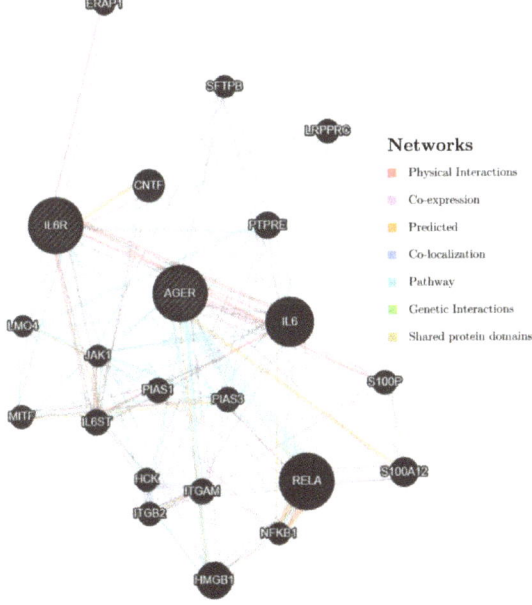

Figure 3. The gene network between *AGER* and *IL6R*. According to the gene network constructed by GeneMANIA, *IL6R* and *AGER* have physical interactions with each other.

3.5. Sensitivity Analysis and Subgroup Analysis

The results of sensitivity analysis showed that both *AGER* and *IL6R* polymorphisms were still significantly associated with disease after the adjustment of blood glucose or other potential confounding factors. The interaction between rs4845625 and rs184003 turned to be null after the adjustment of FPG (OR = 1.166, 95% CI: 0.893–1.521, p = 0.259). Details were shown in Supplementary Materials Table S4.

Subgroup analysis was performed by considering FPG and ICVD risk scores. The results of subgroup analysis showed that rs184003 was significantly associated with disease in higher FPG subgroup (OR = 0.496, 95% CI: 0.288–0.856, p = 0.012), and rs4845625 was significantly associated with diabetic IHD in normal ICVD risk score group (OR = 0.389, 95% CI: 0.197–0.768, p = 0.007). Details were shown in Supplementary Materials Table S5. Subsequently, we found that *AGER* and *IL6R* polymorphisms were not associated with FPG and ICVD risk score, see Supplementary Materials Table S6.

4. Discussion

Individuals with T2DM have an increased risk of CVD, which cannot be fully explained by elevated glucose [28]. Genetic risk factors contribute greatly to the pathogenesis of diabetic macrovascular complications, but their role has not yet been fully illustrated. In the present community-based case-control study, rs4845625 in the *IL6R* gene and the interaction of rs184003 in the *AGER* gene and rs4845625 in *IL6R* were significantly associated with diabetic ischemic heart disease. The polygenic risk score calculated by summing the number of risk alleles of the SNPs located in the above two genes was also associated with an elevated risk of diabetic ischemic heart disease.

AGER is a multiligand cell surface receptor. Advanced glycation end products (AGEs), which are produced after high glucose exposure, can bind to AGER. Their interaction has been implicated in the pathogenesis of atherosclerosis. In addition, HMGB1 (high-mobility group protein 1) and neutrophil-derived S100 calcium-binding family members (S100A8/A9/A11/A12 and S100B) are ligands of AGER. After ligand binding, pro-inflammatory and pro-coagulant pathways are activated. Rs2070600 was found to be significantly associated with diabetic ischemic heart disease in the current study. However, after adjustments for covariates, the associations became null. Rs2070600 is located in the ligand-binding V domain of the *AGER* gene, often referred to as Gly82Ser [29]. Genome-wide association studies (GWAS) showed that rs2070600 was strongly and dose-dependently correlated with sRAGE levels in whites and blacks from the Atherosclerosis Risk in Communities Study and a Chinese population [30,31]. Interestingly, although soluble RAGE levels were found to be associated with diabetic complications in many studies, the association between rs2070600 and ischemic heart disease or other diabetic complications was not consistent. In the Atherosclerosis Risk in Communities Study, rs2070600 was not significantly associated with incident coronary heart disease or diabetes in either whites or blacks with a median follow-up of 20 years [30]. Chinese researchers [32] found a significant association between rs2070600 and coronary arterial disease in 175 cases and 170 controls. A meta-analysis found that the discrepancy may be attributable to ethnicity, and subjects with the rs2070600 risk allele were at higher risk of coronary arterial disease (CAD) in the Chinese population than in the non-Chinese population [11]. However, our study found that the association between rs2070600 and diabetic ischemic heart disease was null. Another study also found that rs2070600 was associated with the circulating levels of esRAGE but not with CAD in Chinese patients with T2DM [33]. These results might indicate that the association between rs2070600 and CAD may also be different in the general population and T2DM patients.

Only a few studies have demonstrated the association between rs184003 and ischemic heart disease. In the current study, we also found that the haplotypes C-G-T-A and A-G-C-A in the *AGER* gene (rs184003-rs1035798-rs2070600-rs1800624) were significantly associated with diabetic ischemic heart disease. Additionally, the association between haplotypes and potential confounders were null (Supplementary Materials Table S7). A hospital-based case-control study involving 1142 patients diagnosed with CAD and 1106 age- and sex-matched controls in a Chinese population was better powered and designed. In this study, the T allele in rs184003 and haplotypes in the *AGER* gene (rs1800625-rs1800624-rs2070600-rs184003, C-T-G-G and T-A-G-T) were also found to be associated with an increased risk of CAD [34]. In addition to the significant association with CAD, the result of a meta-analysis also showed that the homogeneity of the rs184003 polymorphism with the T allele conferred an increased risk of diabetes mellitus in East Asians (OR = 1.21; 95% CI: 1.04–1.40; $I^2 = 0$) [35]. A previous study conducted in a Chinese population involving 200 gastric cancer patients and 207 cancer-free controls showed that subjects carrying the rs184003 T variant allele had an increased ability to produce soluble RAGE (sRAGE) [36]. Given that the T allele in rs184003 was associated with a higher risk of both diabetes and CAD, sRAGE might act on the common pathogenetic pathways of cardiovascular and metabolic diseases. Soluble RAGE levels were found to be significantly associated with CAD and diabetes [37–39] in many studies, and the association between haplotypes in the *AGER* gene and diabetic ischemic heart disease in the current study indicated that sRAGE levels could serve as a marker of diabetic ischemic disease. A recent review demonstrated that RAGE signaling contributed to vascular calcification in diabetic and nondiabetic subjects, presumably on account of the generation of RAGE ligands such as AGEs and other proinflammatory/pro-oxidative ligands [40]. The current study also found that the level of AGEs was elevated in the diabetic ischemic disease group, which supports the above hypothesis. To our knowledge, few studies have illustrated the relationship between rs184003 and diabetic macrovascular complications. Although the findings suggest potential benefits with RAGE antagonism both in the causes and consequences of diabetes and its macrovascular complications, more research is still needed to validate our results.

Mendelian randomization analysis illustrated that IL6R signaling might have a causal role in the development of coronary heart disease [12]. A previous meta-analysis demonstrated that the C allele in rs7529229 *IL6R* was associated with a lower risk of coronary heart disease [12,41]. Although the meta-analysis included a large sample size and better designed original studies, the populations of the studies were all Caucasian, so the evidence from Asian populations was still insufficient. In the current study, the association between rs7529229 and diabetic ischemic heart disease was null in the Chinese population. Chen et al. also did not find a significant effect of rs7529229 on coronary stenosis or acute myocardial infarction in the Chinese Han population with a sample size of 187 patients and 231 controls [42]. However, according to the sample size, allele frequency, and OR reported in the above study, the statistical power was relatively low and might lead to false negative results. Thus, studies with larger sample sizes are still needed to replicate the above findings. Likewise, He et al. conducted a hospital-based case-only study in 402 patients with left main coronary artery disease (LMCAD) and 804 patients with more peripheral coronary artery disease (MPCAD) in a Chinese population, and the results showed that rs7529229 CC or TC/CC genotypes were associated with an increased risk of LMCAD compared with MPCAD [43]. The haplotype T-T-C-T-C (rs7529229-rs4845625-rs4129267-rs7514452-rs4072391) in the *IL6R* gene and rs4845625 were associated with diabetic ischemic heart disease in our study, and the association held after adjusting for potential confounders. In addition, haplotypes T-T-C-C-T were significantly associated with TC (Supplementary Materials Table S8). Rs4845625 was found to be significantly associated with hypertriglyceridemia in the Japanese population [44], and the T allele was associated with a lower serum concentration of creatinine and increased EGFR [45]. Hypertriglyceridemia and chronic kidney disease (CKD) have common pathways, such as endothelial dysfunction, dyslipidemia, and inflammation, leading to metabolic cardiovascular disease [20]. Although few studies have focused on the association between rs4845625 and diabetic heart disease, its association with triglycerides and kidney function might indicate the potential mechanisms of rs4645625 in diabetic ischemic heart disease.

In response to hyperglycemia, AGER is activated by S100A8/A9 on hepatic Kupffer cells, leading to the secretion of IL-6. IL-6 subsequently binds to its receptor (IL6R) on hepatocytes to enhance the production of thrombopoietin, thereby regulating platelet production and resulting in diabetes-induced thrombocytosis [46]. In the current study, we found that the gene-gene interactions between *AGER* and *IL6R* increased the risk of diabetic ischemic heart disease. We subsequently used GeneMANIA to construct a gene network and predict gene function. *IL6R* and *AGER* have physical interactions with each other, and several pathways, including NF-kB/RelA and JAK/STAT, are involved in these interactions (Figure 3). The function of *AGER* and *IL6R* polymorphisms were listed in Supplementary Materials Table S9. These interactions illustrated that the interaction of SNPs in *IL6R* and *AGER* was not only a statistical interaction but also a biological interaction. To our knowledge, this is the first study aimed at identifying the interaction of the *AGER* and *IL6R* genes, and our results provide genetic evidence on the physiological mechanism of diabetic macrovascular complications. Whether the main effect and gene-gene interactions in these two genes could be used to predict the risk of diabetic macrovascular complications still needs to be validated by cohort studies in the future. Although we found a significant interaction between the *AGER* gene and the *IL6R* gene, the association between circulating IL-6 and diabetic ischemic heart disease was null. This result indicated that *IL6R* polymorphisms still need to be further demonstrated. The most common hypothesis is that IL-6 in hematopoietic cells, but not circulating IL-6, were more likely to affect TPO production and macrovascular complications [46,47].

The results of the sensitivity analysis showed that both *AGER* and *IL6R* polymorphisms were still significantly associated with disease after the adjustment of different risk factors, respectively. In the current study, SBP, TC, and LDLC levels and the proportion of people with smoking and drinking habits were significantly lower in the cases than in the controls, which is not consistent with other studies. According to the "2017 Guidelines for the prevention and treatment of type 2 diabetes in China", diabetes patients have more stringent standards on blood pressure (BP) and blood lipids than the healthy population, and diabetes patients with ischemic heart disease should quit smoking and drinking [48]. Diabetes patients might change their lifestyles and medication to maintain their BP or blood lipids at a lower level. Due to the case-control study design of the current study, we were not able to collect lifestyle risk factors and blood samples before the incidence of diabetic ischemic heart disease. However, the percentages of SBP, DBP, HDLC, LDLC, TG, and TC in the ideal range were significantly higher in the control group than in the case group ($p < 0.001$, Supplementary Materials Table S2). Due to the above limitation of our study, more longitudinal studies are still needed to demonstrate whether genetic variants will increase the incidence of diabetic macrovascular complications. In addition, we did not collect any information about diabetic ketoacidosis in the current study. Since diabetic ketoacidosis predisposes individuals to ischemic heart disease, our study might induce bias to a certain extent. Moreover, medication information was not included in the investigation. Given that some antidiabetic medications, such as SGLT-2 inhibitors [49], will reduce the risk of ischemic heart disease in diabetes patients, future studies considering antidiabetic medication are still needed to validate the genetic effect on diabetic macrovascular complications. Since we did not recruit participants who only have diabetes or only have ICH, we performed subgroup analysis by considering FPG and ICVD risk scores. The ICVD risk scores were simple used as a tool to reflect the cumulative risk factors of ICVD in order to rule out the possibility of candidate SNPs that affect IHD. The subgroup analysis helps to rule out the possibility that diabetes or the ICVD risk score are confounders of the current study. Future research, including T2DM group without complications and ischemic heart disease (IHD) group without diabetes, would provide additional information in clarifying the roles of the *AGER* gene and *IL6R* gene.

5. Conclusions

Haplotypes in the *AGER* gene (C-G-T-A and A-G-C-A) were risk factors for diabetic ischemic disease, and rs4845625 and haplotypes in the *IL6R* gene (T allele and T-T-C-T-C) were associated with a lower risk of diabetic ischemic heart disease. The gene-gene interactions between rs184003 in *AGER* and rs4845625 in *IL6R* were associated with a higher risk of diabetic ischemic heart disease.

Supplementary Materials: The following supporting information can be downloaded at: https://www.mdpi.com/article/10.3390/jpm12030392/s1, Table S1: General information of the candidate SNPs and their primer sequences; Table S2: Recommendation cutoffs and proportions according to cutoffs in healthy people and ischemic heart disease patients with diabetes; Table S3: Associations of gene polymorphisms with the risk of diabetic cardiovascular disease; Table S4: Sensitivity analysis for the association between AGER and IL6R gene polymorphisms and diabetic ischemic heart disease; Table S5: Subgroup analysis for the association between candidate SNPs and diabetic IHD; Table S6: The association between candidate SNPs and FPG or ICVD risk scores; Table S7: The association of traits and haplotypes constituted by rs184003-rs1035798-rs2070600-rs1800624; Table S8: The association of traits and haplotypes constituted by rs7529229-rs4845625-rs4129267-rs7514452-rs4072391; Table S9: The function of AGER and IL6R polymorphisms. References [50–66] are cited in the supplementary materials.

Author Contributions: K.L. designed the study and wrote the manuscript, Y.X. analyzed data and visualized the interaction diagram. Q.Z. provided the statistical plan and helped to revise the manuscript. W.P. contributed to the verification of diabetic ischemic heart diseases in case group. C.G. and J.Z. contributed to the management of blood sample and DNA extraction. L.Z. contributed to the collection of controls and participated in the study design. All authors have read and agreed to the published version of the manuscript.

Funding: This study was funded by National Science Foundation of China, grant number 81602908, and National key research and development program of China, grant number 2016YFC0900600/2016YFC0900603.

Institutional Review Board Statement: This study was approved by the Ethics Committee of Capital Medical University (No:2016SY24).

Informed Consent Statement: Informed consent was obtained from all subjects involved in the study.

Data Availability Statement: Research could contact communication author to access data.

Acknowledgments: The authors thank all the participants and community health workers for their participation in this research effort.

Conflicts of Interest: The authors declare no conflict of interest.

References

1. Shah, A.D.; Langenberg, C.; Rapsomaniki, E.; Denaxas, S.; Pujades-Rodriguez, M.; Gale, C.P.; Deanfield, J.; Smeeth, L.; Timmis, A.; Hemingway, H. Type 2 diabetes and incidence of cardiovascular diseases: A cohort study in 1.9 million people. *Lancet Diabetes Endocrinol.* **2015**, *3*, 105–113. [CrossRef]
2. GBD 2015 Mortality and Causes of Death Collaborators. Global, regional, and national life expectancy, all-cause mortality, and cause-specific mortality for 249 causes of death, 1980–2015: A systematic analysis for the Global Burden of Disease Study 2015. *Lancet* **2016**, *388*, 1459–1544. [CrossRef]
3. Maugeri, N.; Malato, S.; Femia, E.A.; Pugliano, M.; Campana, L.; Lunghi, F.; Rovere-Querini, P.; Lussana, F.; Podda, G.; Cattaneo, M.; et al. Clearance of circulating activated platelets in polycythemia vera and essential thrombocythemia. *Blood* **2011**, *118*, 3359–3366. [CrossRef] [PubMed]
4. Zegeye, M.M.; Lindkvist, M.; Falker, K.; Kumawat, A.K.; Paramel, G.; Grenegard, M.; Sirsjö, A.; Ljungberg, L.U. Activation of the JAK/STAT3 and PI3K/AKT pathways are crucial for IL-6 trans-signaling-mediated pro-inflammatory response in human vascular endothelial cells. *Cell Commun. Signal.* **2018**, *16*, 55. [CrossRef]
5. Grozovsky, R.; Giannini, S.; Falet, H.; Hoffmeister, K.M. Novel mechanisms of platelet clearance and thrombopoietin regulation. *Curr. Opin. Hematol.* **2015**, *22*, 445–451. [CrossRef]
6. Serveaux-Dancer, M.; Jabaudon, M.; Creveaux, I.; Belville, C.; Blondonnet, R.; Gross, C. Pathological Implications of Receptor for Advanced Glycation End-Product (AGER) Gene Polymorphism. *Dis. Markers* **2019**, *2019*, 2067353. [CrossRef]
7. Li, J.; Cai, W.; Zhang, W.; Zhu, W.F.; Liu, Y.; Yue, L.X.; Zhu, L.Y.; Xiao, J.R.; Liu, J.Y.; Xu, J.X. Polymorphism 2184A/G in the AGER gene is not associated with diabetic retinopathy in Han Chinese patients with type 2 diabetes. *J. Int. Med. Res.* **2016**, *44*, 520–528. [CrossRef]
8. Fan, W.Y.; Gu, H.; Yang, X.F.; She, C.Y.; Liu, X.P.; Liu, N.P. Association of candidate gene polymorphisms with diabetic retinopathy in Chinese patients with type 2 diabetes. *Int. J. Ophthalmol.* **2020**, *13*, 301–308. [CrossRef]

9. Peng, F.; Hu, D.; Jia, N.; Li, X.; Li, Y.; Chu, S.; Zhu, D.; Shen, W.; Lin, J.; Niu, W. Association of four genetic polymorphisms of AGER and its circulating forms with coronary artery disease: A meta-analysis. *PLoS ONE* **2013**, *8*, e70834. [CrossRef]
10. Lu, W.; Feng, B. The -374A allele of the RAGE gene as a potential protective factor for vascular complications in type 2 diabetes: A meta-analysis. *Tohoku J. Exp. Med.* **2010**, *220*, 291–297. [CrossRef]
11. Ma, W.Q.; Qu, Q.R.; Zhao, Y.; Liu, N.F. Association of RAGE gene Gly82Ser polymorphism with coronary artery disease and ischemic stroke: A systematic review and meta-analysis. *Medicine* **2016**, *95*, e5593. [CrossRef] [PubMed]
12. Interleukin-6 Receptor Mendelian Randomisation Analysis (IL6R MR) Consortium; Swerdlow, D.I.; Holmes, M.V.; Kuchenbaecker, K.B.; Engmann, J.E.; Shah, T.; Sofat, R.; Guo, Y.; Chung, C.; Peasey, A.; et al. The interleukin-6 receptor as a target for prevention of coronary heart disease: A mendelian randomisation analysis. *Lancet* **2012**, *379*, 1214–1224. [PubMed]
13. Rafiq, S.; Melzer, D.; Weedon, M.N.; Lango, H.; Saxena, R.; Scott, L.J.; DIAGRAM Consortium; Palmer, C.N.; Morris, A.D.; McCarthy, M.I.; et al. Gene variants influencing measures of inflammation or predisposing to autoimmune and inflammatory diseases are not associated with the risk of type 2 diabetes. *Diabetologia* **2008**, *51*, 2205–2213. [CrossRef] [PubMed]
14. Manolio, T.A.; Collins, F.S.; Cox, N.J.; Goldstein, D.B.; Hindorff, L.A.; Hunter, D.J.; McCarthy, M.I.; Ramos, E.M.; Cardon, L.R.; Chakravarti, A.; et al. Finding the missing heritability of complex diseases. *Nature* **2009**, *461*, 747–753. [CrossRef]
15. Peng, D.Q.; Zhao, S.P.; Nie, S.; Li, J. Gene-gene interaction of PPARgamma and ApoE affects coronary heart disease risk. *Int. J. Cardiol.* **2003**, *92*, 257–263. [CrossRef]
16. Carty, C.L.; Heagerty, P.; Heckbert, S.R.; Enquobahrie, D.A.; Jarvik, G.P.; Davis, S.; Tracy, R.P.; Reiner, A.P. Association of genetic variation in serum amyloid-A with cardiovascular disease and interactions with IL6, IL1RN, IL1beta and TNF genes in the Cardiovascular Health Study. *J. Atheroscler. Thromb.* **2009**, *16*, 419–430. [CrossRef]
17. Carty, C.L.; Heagerty, P.; Heckbert, S.R.; Jarvik, G.P.; Lange, L.A.; Cushman, M.; Tracy, R.P.; Reiner, A.P. Interaction between fibrinogen and IL-6 genetic variants and associations with cardiovascular disease risk in the Cardiovascular Health Study. *Ann. Hum. Genet.* **2010**, *74*, 1–10. [CrossRef]
18. Zhu, Z.; Tong, X.; Zhu, Z.; Liang, M.; Cui, W.; Su, K.; Li, M.D.; Zhu, J. Development of GMDR-GPU for gene-gene interaction analysis and its application to WTCCC GWAS data for type 2 diabetes. *PLoS ONE* **2013**, *8*, e61943. [CrossRef]
19. Xu, H.M.; Xu, L.F.; Hou, T.T.; Luo, L.F.; Chen, G.B.; Sun, X.W.; Lou, X.Y. GMDR: Versatile Software for Detecting Gene-Gene and Gene-Environment Interactions Underlying Complex Traits. *Curr. Genom.* **2016**, *17*, 396–402. [CrossRef]
20. Gajjala, P.R.; Sanati, M.; Jankowski, J. Cellular and Molecular Mechanisms of Chronic Kidney Disease with Diabetes Mellitus and Cardiovascular Diseases as Its Comorbidities. *Front. Immunol.* **2015**, *6*, 340. [CrossRef]
21. American Diabetes Association. Diagnosis and classification of diabetes mellitus. *Diabetes Care* **2014**, *37*, S81–S90. [CrossRef] [PubMed]
22. Thygesen, K.; Alpert, J.S.; Jaffe, A.S.; Chaitman, B.R.; Bax, J.J.; Morrow, D.A.; White, H.D.; Executive Group on behalf of the Joint European Society of Cardiology (ESC)/American College of Cardiology (ACC)/American Heart Association (AHA)/World Heart Federation (WHF) Task Force for the Universal Definition of Myocardial Infarction. Fourth Universal Definition of Myocardial Infarction. *J. Am. Coll. Cardiol.* **2018**, *72*, 2231–2264. [CrossRef]
23. Luepker, R.V.; Apple, F.S.; Christenson, R.H.; Crow, R.S.; Fortmann, S.P.; Goff, D.; Goldberg, R.J.; Hand, M.M.; Jaffe, A.S.; Julian, D.G.; et al. Case definitions for acute coronary heart disease in epidemiology and clinical research studies: A statement from the AHA Council on Epidemiology and Prevention; AHA Statistics Committee; World Heart Federation Council on Epidemiology and Prevention; the European Society of Cardiology Working Group on Epidemiology and Prevention; Centers for Disease Control and Prevention; and the National Heart, Lung, and Blood Institute. *Circulation* **2003**, *108*, 2543–2549.
24. Amsterdam, E.A.; Wenger, N.K.; Brindis, R.G.; Casey, D.E., Jr.; Ganiats, T.G.; Holmes, D.R., Jr.; Jaffe, A.S.; Jneid, H.; Kelly, R.F.; Kontos, M.C.; et al. 2014 AHA/ACC Guideline for the Management of Patients with Non-ST-Elevation Acute Coronary Syndromes: A report of the American College of Cardiology/American Heart Association Task Force on Practice Guidelines. *J. Am. Coll. Cardiol.* **2014**, *64*, e139–e228. [CrossRef] [PubMed]
25. Liu, L.S. Joint committee for guideline revision. 2016 Chinese guidelines for the management of dyslipidemia in adults. *J. Geriatr. Cardiol.* **2018**, *15*, 1–29.
26. Stevens, L.A.; Schmid, C.H.; Greene, T.; Zhang, Y.L.; Beck, G.J.; Froissart, M.; Hamm, L.L.; Lewis, J.B.; Mauer, M.; Navis, G.J.; et al. Comparative performance of the CKD Epidemiology Collaboration (CKD-EPI) and the Modification of Diet in Renal Disease (MDRD) Study equations for estimating GFR levels above 60 mL/min/1.73 m^2. *Am. J. Kidney Dis.* **2010**, *56*, 486–495. [CrossRef] [PubMed]
27. Zhang, M.; Huang, Z.J.; Li, Y.C.; Wang, L.M.; Jiang, Y.; Zhao, W.H. Prediction of 10-year risk for ischemic cardiovascular disease in adults aged ≥35 years in China. *Zhonghua Liu Xing Bing Xue Za Zhi* **2016**, *37*, 689–693. [PubMed]
28. Kirkman, M.S.; Mahmud, H.; Korytkowski, M.T. Intensive Blood Glucose Control and Vascular Outcomes in Patients with Type 2 Diabetes Mellitus. *Endocrinol. Metab. Clin. N. Am.* **2018**, *47*, 81–96. [CrossRef] [PubMed]
29. Lu, W.; Feng, B.; Xie, G.; Liu, F. Association of AGER gene G82S polymorphism with the severity of coronary artery disease in Chinese Han population. *Clin. Endocrinol.* **2011**, *75*, 470–474. [CrossRef]
30. Maruthur, N.M.; Li, M.; Halushka, M.K.; Astor, B.C.; Pankow, J.S.; Boerwinkle, E.; Coresh, J.; Selvin, E.; Kao, W.H. Genetics of Plasma Soluble Receptor for Advanced Glycation End-Products and Cardiovascular Outcomes in a Community-based Population: Results from the Atherosclerosis Risk in Communities Study. *PLoS ONE* **2015**, *10*, e0128452.

31. Lim, S.C.; Dorajoo, R.; Zhang, X.; Wang, L.; Ang, S.F.; Tan, C.S.H.; Yeoh, L.Y.; Ng, X.W.; Li, N.; Su, C.; et al. Genetic variants in the receptor for advanced glycation end products (RAGE) gene were associated with circulating soluble RAGE level but not with renal function among Asians with type 2 diabetes: A genome-wide association study. *Nephrol. Dial. Transpl.* **2017**, *32*, 1697–1704. [CrossRef] [PubMed]
32. Gao, J.; Shao, Y.; Lai, W.; Ren, H.; Xu, D. Association of polymorphisms in the RAGE gene with serum CRP levels and coronary artery disease in the Chinese Han population. *J. Hum. Genet.* **2010**, *55*, 668–675. [CrossRef] [PubMed]
33. Peng, W.H.; Lu, L.; Wang, L.J.; Yan, X.X.; Chen, Q.J.; Zhang, Q.; Zhang, R.Y.; Shen, W.F. RAGE gene polymorphisms are associated with circulating levels of endogenous secretory RAGE but not with coronary artery disease in Chinese patients with type 2 diabetes mellitus. *Arch. Med. Res.* **2009**, *40*, 393–398. [CrossRef] [PubMed]
34. Yu, X.; Liu, J.; Zhu, H.; Xia, Y.; Gao, L.; Li, Z.; Jia, N.; Shen, W.; Yang, Y.; Niu, W. An interactive association of advanced glycation end-product receptor gene four common polymorphisms with coronary artery disease in northeastern Han Chinese. *PLoS ONE* **2013**, *8*, e76966.
35. Niu, W.; Qi, Y.; Wu, Z.; Liu, Y.; Zhu, D.; Jin, W. A meta-analysis of receptor for advanced glycation end products gene: Four well-evaluated polymorphisms with diabetes mellitus. *Mol. Cell Endocrinol.* **2012**, *358*, 9–17. [CrossRef]
36. Li, T.; Qin, W.; Liu, Y.; Li, S.; Qin, X.; Liu, Z. Effect of RAGE gene polymorphisms and circulating sRAGE levels on susceptibility to gastric cancer: A case-control study. *Cancer Cell Int.* **2017**, *17*, 19. [CrossRef]
37. Ligthart, S.; Sedaghat, S.; Ikram, M.A.; Hofman, A.; Franco, O.H.; Dehghan, A. EN-RAGE: A novel inflammatory marker for incident coronary heart disease. *Arterioscler. Thromb. Vasc. Biol.* **2014**, *34*, 2695–2699. [CrossRef]
38. Reichert, S.; Triebert, U.; Santos, A.N.; Hofmann, B.; Schaller, H.G.; Schlitt, A.; Schulz, S. Soluble form of receptor for advanced glycation end products and incidence of new cardiovascular events among patients with cardiovascular disease. *Atherosclerosis* **2017**, *266*, 234–239. [CrossRef]
39. Heier, M.; Margeirsdottir, H.D.; Gaarder, M.; Stensæth, K.H.; Brunborg, C.; Torjesen, P.A.; Seljeflot, I.; Hanssen, K.F.; Dahl-Jørgensen, K. Soluble RAGE and atherosclerosis in youth with type 1 diabetes: A 5-year follow-up study. *Cardiovasc. Diabetol.* **2015**, *14*, 126. [CrossRef]
40. Egaña-Gorroño, L.; López-Díez, R.; Yepuri, G.; Ramirez, L.S.; Reverdatto, S.; Gugger, P.F.; Shekhtman, A.; Ramasamy, R.; Schmidt, A.M. Receptor for Advanced Glycation End Products (RAGE) and Mechanisms and Therapeutic Opportunities in Diabetes and Cardiovascular Disease: Insights from Human Subjects and Animal Models. *Front. Cardiovasc. Med.* **2020**, *7*, 37. [CrossRef]
41. IL6R Genetics Consortium Emerging Risk Factors Collaboration; Sarwar, N.; Butterworth, A.S.; Freitag, D.F.; Gregson, J.; Willeit, P.; Gorman, D.N.; Gao, P.; Saleheen, D.; Rendon, A.; et al. Interleukin-6 receptor pathways in coronary heart disease: A collaborative meta-analysis of 82 studies. *Lancet* **2012**, *379*, 1205–1213.
42. Chen, Z.; Qian, Q.; Tang, C.; Ding, J.; Feng, Y.; Ma, G. Association of two variants in the interleukin-6 receptor gene and premature coronary heart disease in a Chinese Han population. *Mol. Biol. Rep.* **2013**, *40*, 1021–1026. [CrossRef] [PubMed]
43. He, F.; Teng, X.; Gu, H.; Liu, H.; Zhou, Z.; Zhao, Y.; Hu, S.; Zheng, Z. Interleukin-6 receptor rs7529229 T/C polymorphism is associated with left main coronary artery disease phenotype in a Chinese population. *Int. J. Mol. Sci.* **2014**, *15*, 5623–5633. [CrossRef] [PubMed]
44. Abe, S.; Tokoro, F.; Matsuoka, R.; Arai, M.; Noda, T.; Watanabe, S.; Horibe, H.; Fujimaki, T.; Oguri, M.; Kato, K.; et al. Association of genetic variants with dyslipidemia. *Mol. Med. Rep.* **2015**, *12*, 5429–5436. [CrossRef]
45. Horibe, H.; Fujimaki, T.; Oguri, M.; Kato, K.; Matsuoka, R.; Abe, S.; Tokoro, F.; Arai, M.; Noda, T.; Watanabe, S.; et al. Association of a polymorphism of the interleukin 6 receptor gene with chronic kidney disease in Japanese individuals. *Nephrology* **2015**, *20*, 273–278. [CrossRef] [PubMed]
46. Kraakman, M.J.; Lee, M.K.; Al-Sharea, A.; Dragoljevic, D.; Barrett, T.J.; Montenont, E.; Basu, D.; Heywood, S.; Kammoun, H.L.; Flynn, M.; et al. Neutrophil-derived S100 calcium-binding proteins A8/A9 promote reticulated thrombocytosis and atherogenesis in diabetes. *J. Clin. Investig.* **2017**, *127*, 2133–2147. [CrossRef] [PubMed]
47. Qu, D.; Liu, J.; Lau, C.W.; Huang, Y. IL-6 in diabetes and cardiovascular complications. *Br. J. Pharmacol.* **2014**, *171*, 3595–3603. [CrossRef]
48. Society, C.D. Guidelines for the prevention and control of type 2 diabetes in China (2017 Edition). *Chin. J. Pract. Int. Med.* **2018**, *38*, 292–344.
49. Scheen, A.J. Cardiovascular Effects of New Oral Glucose-Lowering Agents: DPP-4 and SGLT-2 Inhibitors. *Circ. Res.* **2018**, *122*, 1439–1459. [CrossRef]
50. Olsson, S.; Jood, K. Genetic variation in the receptor for advanced glycation end-products (RAGE) gene and ischaemic stroke. *Eur. J. Neurol.* **2013**, *20*, 991–993. [CrossRef]
51. Wang, Z.T.; Wang, L.Y.; Wang, L.; Cheng, S.; Fan, R.; Zhou, J.; Zhong, J. Association between RAGE gene polymorphisms and ulcerative colitis susceptibility: A case-control study in a Chinese Han population. *Genet. Mol. Res.* **2015**, *14*, 19242. [CrossRef]
52. Kang, P.; Tian, C.; Jia, C. Association of RAGE gene polymorphisms with type 2 diabetes mellitus, diabetic retinopathy and diabetic nephropathy. *Gene* **2012**, *500*, 1–9. [CrossRef] [PubMed]
53. Niu, H.; Niu, W.; Yu, T.; Dong, F.; Huang, K.; Duan, R.; Qumu, S.; Lu, M.; Li, Y.; Yang, T.; et al. Association of RAGE gene multiple variants with the risk for COPD and asthma in northern Han Chinese. *Aging* **2019**, *11*, 3220–3237. [CrossRef] [PubMed]

54. Wadén, J.M.; Dahlström, E.H.; Elonen, N.; Thorn, L.M.; Wadén, J.; Sandholm, N.; Forsblom, C.; Groop, P.H.; FinnDiane Study Group. Soluble receptor for AGE in diabetic nephropathy and its progression in Finnish individuals with type 1 diabetes. *Diabetologia* **2019**, *62*, 1268–1274. [CrossRef] [PubMed]
55. Kim, D.H.; Yoo, S.D.; Chon, J.; Yun, D.H.; Kim, H.S.; Park, H.J.; Kim, S.K.; Chung, J.H.; Kang, J.K.; Lee, S.A. Interleukin-6 Receptor Polymorphisms Contribute to the Neurological Status of Korean Patients with Ischemic Stroke. *J. Korean Med. Sci.* **2016**, *31*, 430–434. [CrossRef] [PubMed]
56. He, F.; Yang, R.; Li, X.Y.; Ye, C.; He, B.C.; Lin, T.; Xu, X.Q.; Zheng, L.L.; Luo, W.T.; Cai, L. Single nucleotide polymorphisms of the NF-κB and STAT3 signaling pathway genes predict lung cancer prognosis in a Chinese Han population. *Cancer Genet.* **2015**, *208*, 310–318. [CrossRef]
57. Key, K.V.; Mudd-Martin, G.; Moser, D.K.; Rayens, M.K.; Morford, L.A. Inflammatory Genotype Moderates the Association Between Anxiety and Systemic Inflammation in Adults at Risk for Cardiovascular Disease. *J. Cardiovasc. Nurs.* **2022**, *37*, 64–72. [CrossRef]
58. Arguinano, A.A.; Naderi, E.; Ndiaye, N.C.; Stathopoulou, M.; Dadé, S.; Alizadeh, B.; Visvikis-Siest, S. IL6R haplotype rs4845625*T/rs4537545*C is a risk factor for simultaneously high CRP, LDL and ApoB levels. *Genes Immun.* **2017**, *18*, 163–169. [CrossRef]
59. Tabassum, R.; Mahendran, Y.; Dwivedi, O.P.; Chauhan, G.; Ghosh, S.; Marwaha, R.K.; Tandon, N.; Bharadwaj, D. Common variants of IL6, LEPR, and PBEF1 are associated with obesity in Indian children. *Diabetes* **2012**, *61*, 626–631. [CrossRef]
60. Van Dongen, J.; Jansen, R.; Smit, D.; Hottenga, J.J.; Mbarek, H.; Willemsen, G.; Kluft, C.; Penninx, B.W.; Ferreira, M.A.; Boomsma, D.I.; et al. The contribution of the functional IL6R polymorphism rs2228145, eQTLs and other genome-wide SNPs to the heritability of plasma sIL-6R levels. *Behav. Genet.* **2014**, *44*, 368–382. [CrossRef]
61. Walston, J.D.; Matteini, A.M.; Nievergelt, C.; Lange, L.A.; Fallin, D.M.; Barzilai, N.; Ziv, E.; Pawlikowska, L.; Kwok, P.; Cummings, S.R.; et al. Inflammation and stress-related candidate genes, plasma interleukin-6 levels, and longevity in older adults. *Exp. Gerontol.* **2009**, *44*, 350–355. [CrossRef] [PubMed]
62. Naitza, S.; Porcu, E.; Steri, M.; Taub, D.D.; Mulas, A.; Xiao, X.; Strait, J.; Dei, M.; Lai, S.; Busonero, F.; et al. A genome-wide association scan on the levels of markers of inflammation in Sardinians reveals associations that underpin its complex regulation. *PLoS Genet.* **2012**, *8*, e1002480. [CrossRef] [PubMed]
63. Rafiq, S.; Frayling, T.M.; Murray, A.; Hurst, A.; Stevens, K.; Weedon, M.N.; Henley, W.; Ferrucci, L.; Bandinelli, S.; Corsi, A.M.; et al. A common variant of the interleukin 6 receptor (IL-6r) gene increases IL-6r and IL-6 levels, without other inflammatory effects. *Genes Immun.* **2007**, *8*, 552–559. [CrossRef] [PubMed]
64. Webb, T.R.; Erdmann, J.; Stirrups, K.E.; Stitziel, N.O.; Masca, N.G.; Jansen, H.; Kanoni, S.; Nelson, C.P.; Ferrario, P.G.; König, I.R.; et al. Systematic Evaluation of Pleiotropy Identifies 6 Further Loci Associated with Coronary Artery Disease. *J. Am. Coll. Cardiol.* **2017**, *69*, 823–836. [CrossRef]
65. Christiansen, M.K.; Larsen, S.B.; Nyegaard, M.; Neergaard-Petersen, S.; Ajjan, R.; Würtz, M.; Grove, E.L.; Hvas, A.M.; Jensen, H.K.; Kristensen, S.D. Coronary artery disease-associated genetic variants and biomarkers of inflammation. *PLoS ONE* **2017**, *12*, e0180365.
66. Gigante, B.; Strawbridge, R.J.; Velasquez, I.M.; Golabkesh, Z.; Silveira, A.; Goel, A.; Baldassarre, D.; Veglia, F.; Tremoli, E.; Clarke, R.; et al. Analysis of the role of interleukin 6 receptor haplotypes in the regulation of circulating levels of inflammatory biomarkers and risk of coronary heart disease. *PLoS ONE* **2015**, *10*, e0119980.

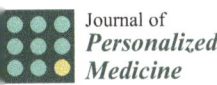

Journal of Personalized Medicine

Review

Artificial Intelligence in Cardiovascular Atherosclerosis Imaging

Jia Zhang [1,†], Ruijuan Han [2,†], Guo Shao [3], Bin Lv [4] and Kai Sun [3,*]

1. Hohhot Health Committee, Hohhot 010000, China; zhangjia4717@163.com
2. The People's Hospital of Longgang District, Shenzhen 518172, China; ruijuanhan@163.com
3. The Third People's Hospital of Longgang District, Shenzhen 518100, China; shao.guo.china@gmail.com
4. Fuwai Hospital, National Center for Cardiovascular Diseases, Beijing 100037, China; blu@vip.sina.com
* Correspondence: henrysk@163.com
† These authors contributed equally to this work.

Abstract: At present, artificial intelligence (AI) has already been applied in cardiovascular imaging (e.g., image segmentation, automated measurements, and eventually, automated diagnosis) and it has been propelled to the forefront of cardiovascular medical imaging research. In this review, we presented the current status of artificial intelligence applied to image analysis of coronary atherosclerotic plaques, covering multiple areas from plaque component analysis (e.g., identification of plaque properties, identification of vulnerable plaque, detection of myocardial function, and risk prediction) to risk prediction. Additionally, we discuss the current evidence, strengths, limitations, and future directions for AI in cardiac imaging of atherosclerotic plaques, as well as lessons that can be learned from other areas. The continuous development of computer science and technology may further promote the development of this field.

Keywords: artificial intelligence; atherosclerosis; plaque characterization

1. Introduction

Although modern medical care has increasingly advanced, cardiovascular disease (CVDs) that has an increasing incidence worldwide still poses a serious threat to the quality of human life and health. According to the latest report, CVDs remains the main cause of premature death in most countries, especially low- and middle-income countries [1], which suggests that treatment and prevention of CVDs still need to be improved [2]. Coronary atherosclerosis underlies CAD and major adverse cardiac events (MACEs). Detection of these atherosclerotic plaques, identification of components, and assessment of their risk are essential for the management of patients with cardiovascular disease. Over the past two decades, various medical imaging techniques, including the invasive measurements such as optical coherence tomography (OCT), intravascular ultrasound (IVUS), and noninvasive measurements, such as computed tomography (CT), magnetic resonance imaging (MRI), and ultrasonography (US) have been developed for the assessment of coronary atherosclerosis [3].

With the continuous development of imaging technology and the popularization of imaging examination, massive image datasets have been generated. Meanwhile, big data are a major driver in the development of precision medicine clinicians and researchers alike have more opportunities than ever before to engage in the development and evaluation of novel image analysis algorithms, with the ultimate goal of creating new tools to optimize patient care [4,5]. Artificial intelligence (AI) is regarded as an exciting research topic in multifarious fields, as major advances in AI have occurred in recent years [6]. The application of artificial intelligence to the medical imaging field allows the identification of the information that improve clinical work efficiency. Additionally, AI has recently been propelled to the forefront of cardiovascular medical imaging research [7,8].

The aim of this paper was to focus on research that applied AI for coronary atherosclerotic plaques so as to summarize imaging methods (e.g., OCT, IVUS, CT) and different fields of coronary atherosclerotic plaques (e.g., identification of plaque properties, identification of vulnerable plaque, detection of myocardial function and risk prediction). Finally, we pointed out some current existing problems and future directions.

2. Application of AI in Coronary Atherosclerotic Plaque

2.1. Overview of Artificial Intelligence

Previous articles have described in detail AI algorithms for cardiovascular imaging [5,9–11]. To facilitate understanding of this review, this section provides a short introduction to some terminology. The concept of AI, which instructed machines to have intelligence similar to humans through learning so as to perform specific intelligent tasks [12], discover patterns, and make decisions based on data, was born in the 1950s. Machine learning (ML) is a branch of AI, in which machines or algorithms extract information independently from big data to make predictions without explicit programming [13]. The predictive pattern of ML is similar to traditional regression statistical methods. Still, ML makes predictions based on information obtained from a broad range of big data rather than a limited set of risk factors. Deep learning (DL) is the most advanced branch of ML that most commonly uses a multilayer artificial neural network and a multilayer machine learning model. The distribution characteristics of data are extracted by combining the low-level local image features and converting them to high-level features, and thus developing a model simulating the human brain through a neural network. Nowadays, DL is being used more and more for dealing with large and complex datasets [14]. ML and DL can be classified into two varieties according to whether the labels are clear or not; these two varieties are namely supervised and unsupervised learning. When the label of input data is clear, the supervised learning mode can be selected. When the label of input data is not clear or is lost, the unsupervised mode can be selected to capture and classify the data automatically [15].

2.2. Coronary Atherosclerotic Plaque

Coronary atherosclerosis is a common physiological disorder characterized by the formation of fatty streaks proliferation of intimal smooth muscle cells, which eventually leads to coronary artery stenosis [16]. Atherosclerosis (AS) is a complex process that involves interactions between monocyte-derived macrophages, endothelial cells, lymphocyte, and smooth muscle cells [17,18]. The vast majority of CVDs and MACEs usually occurs following the buildup of plaque inside the coronary arteries that supply oxygen-rich blood to the heart muscle. Atherosclerotic lesions start with adaptive thickening of intima characterized by aggregation of intimal smooth muscle cells, which can gradually develop into pathological intima thickening, and are characterized by the presence of cell-free lipid pools. The presence of a necrotic core is the characteristic manifestation of the fibrous aneurysm, where fibrocalcific plaque tends to form following the further development of necrotic core [19]. With complex pathological environmental components, there are notable differences among different evolution stages and compositions of coronary atherosclerotic plaques with regard to outcome [20]. Detection of these atherosclerotic plaques, identification of components, and assessment of their risk are essential for the management of patients with cardiovascular disease.

2.3. Characterization of Coronary Atherosclerotic Plaques

Different components of coronary atherosclerotic plaques correspond to different mechanisms, leading to different outcomes [21]. Therefore, accurate identification of plaque components is essential for follow-up treatment. Several previous studies have automatically identified plaque components.

In the field of noninvasive examinations, Zreik [22] and Rajendra [23] have developed training models to identify plaque calcification in the CCTA automatically. The former uses a multi-task recurrent convolutional neural network (RCNN) to develop an ML model to characterize atherosclerotic plaque properties and coronary stenosis automatically. CCTA images of 81, 17, and 65 patients were used for model training, validation, and testing. The accuracy of this model for plaque characterization (calcification, no calcification, mixing, no plaque) was 0.77 [22]. The latter achieved higher accuracy. He compared the efficacy of different ML algorithms and probabilistic neural networks (PNN), obtaining the best accuracy of 0.89 [23].

Masuda and colleagues proposed a model combining ML with a histogram to detect the characteristics of coronary atherosclerotic plaques (fibrous plaques, fatty plaques) in CCTA. The model shows a significantly higher area under the curve than the traditional method (area under curve 0.92 and 95%, confidence interval 0.86–0.92 vs. 0.83 and 0.75–0.92, $p = 0.001$) [24]. Yamak et al. trained a supervised model using organic phantom plaques fabricated from low-density polyethylene (LDPE) and high-density polyethylene (HDPE). Plaque images from a dual-energy CT scan were used as training data, and the model has shown the ability to identify lipid and calcified plaque by validation analysis in coronary scan images of three patients [25].

In the field of invasive examinations, Kim [26] and Sheet [27] attempted to identify plaque components in IVUS images automatically. Kim extracted six image texture features from IVUS images, after which a three-level network classification model was used to classify the coronary plaque into fibrous tissue (FT), fibro-fatty tissue (FFT), necrotic cor (NC), and dense calcium (DC) based on the image texture. The method achieved relatively high sensitivity (82.0%) and specificity (87.1%) in distinguishing between FT/FFT and NC/DC groups [26]. Sheet et al. developed a novel machine-learning-based technique called Stochastic Driven Histology (SDH), which can automatically characterize image components in IVUS images. Validation analysis revealed that SDH is highly consistent with traditional histology in characterizing calcification, fibrotic tissues, and lipids, with 99%, 97%, and 99% accuracy, respectively [27].

There were many studies directed at OCT. Shalev [28] and Xu [29] used a support vector machine (SVM) to identify plaque components in OCT. Shalev trained and validated the model using frozen microscopic data, and the accuracy of calcified plaque recognition achieved 0.97. Xu used a linear SVM classifier to detect unhealthy objects. On this basis, Zhou [30] used more data and improved models to identify lipid plaques and mixed plaques, reaching an accuracy of 91.5% and 78.1%, respectively. Kolluru's [31] model also trained on frozen images to classify plaques in OCT into four categories, fiber, lipid, calcium, and others. OCT images were paired with frozen images to extract features, after which five-fold cross-validation was performed on the training dataset to optimize classifier parameters. The model achieved an accuracy value that exceeded 90% in all categories. Rico-Jimenez [32] proposed an A-line modeling method to characterize plaques in OCT, which can automatically identify fibrotic plaques and lipid-containing plaques with 85% accuracy. Wilson et al. [33] developed a of convolutional neural network (CNN) in identifying plaque properties in OCT images using line-based modeling methods, learning that CNN can significantly outperform in this task. After that, they proposed a method based on the SegNet deep learning network, proving that the performance of the model was significantly improved compared with the previous method [34]. Athanasiou [35] and Ughi [36] used random forest (RF) classifier to classify atherosclerotic plaques (calcium, lipid pools, fibrous tissue, and mixed plaques) with an accuracy of 80.41% and 81.5%, respectively.

2.4. Detection of Coronary Atherosclerotic Plaque

After years of research, a variety of medical imaging techniques have now been used to analyze atherosclerotic plaques. These techniques can detect anatomical and functional abnormalities caused by atherosclerosis, provide detailed information about plaque composition, and even evaluate the risk of atherosclerotic plaques. These methods provide a reference for measuring the severity of coronary atherosclerosis in daily clinical practice and cardiovascular research and have an important role in the diagnosis and treatment of related patients [37].

Mainstream noninvasive measurements of coronary atherosclerotic plaques include CT and MRI. The CT can be used to characterize luminal stenosis, assess the component load of plaques and vascular remodeling. As a noninvasive test, it can detect asymptomatic patients with high-risk plaques and stratify the risk of cardiovascular disease [34]. At the same time, CCTA detection of high-risk plaque can identify high-risk patients with MACE events and can be used as an independent predictor of the acute coronary syndrome (ACS) [38]. However, due to the constraints of spatial resolution and radiation dose, CT cannot identify subtle lesions [39]. MRI provides good contrast resolution of soft tissues. In addition to showing the vascular cavity and vascular wall structure, it can also clearly show the plaque load and the progress of plaque bleeding. However, its low spatial resolution and long imaging time make it unsuitable for the diagnosis of active vascular such as coronary arteries. Additionally, there are contraindications in the examination of patients with pacemakers or metals [40], so it is less used for clinical diagnosis of coronary plaque.

Mainstream invasive measurements of coronary atherosclerotic plaques include OCT and IVUS, which are intravascular techniques that provide a cross-sectional view of the coronary artery. IVUS has special advantages in detecting vulnerable plaques as it can clearly distinguish the properties and composition of different plaques [41]. Yet, IVUS is invasive and expensive, so it is not suitable for a wide population-based screening. OCT provides a greater resolution than IVUS, which clearly shows thin fiber caps; however, some large lipid cores and extravascular elastic layers cannot be observed due to weak tissue penetration [42].

Existing imaging tools can analyze coronary atherosclerotic plaques based on their morphology and structure, but modern precision medicine requires a more detailed analysis of plaque. A large amount of data in the image is inevitably overlooked due to the limitations of the naked eye. Additionally, the methods mentioned above produce large amounts of image data. Working long hours increases the possibility of missed diagnosis or misdiagnosis risks made by radiologist due to the subtle variations in the image that can be easily ignored. Therefore, new imaging diagnosis approaches are urgently required to improve diagnosis efficiency and accuracy by using existing medical imaging data with the ultimate goal of Precision Medicine.

3. Application of AI in Coronary Atherosclerotic Plaque Analysis
3.1. Identification of Vulnerable Plaques

Vulnerable plaque rupture is the most common cause of acute coronary syndrome (ACS), which is the most dangerous type of CAD [43]. Pathological features of most vulnerable plaques are characterized by a large necrotic core covered with a thin fibrous cap, as well as abundant inflammatory cells and small amounts of smooth muscle cells [44]. The identification of vulnerable plaques is important for predicting acute cardiovascular events [45].

Numerous studies have focused on the field of CCTA. Kolossvary et al. extracted 4400 radiological features from CCTA images of 60 patients by using radiomics and found that 916 features (20.6%) were associated with napkin-ring sign (NRS), of which 440 (9.9%) multiple radiographic features (short-run low-gray-level emphasis, long-run low-gray-level emphasis, the surface ratio of component 2 to the total surface) were more sensitive to high-risk plaques than plaque volume and other conventional quantitative parameters [36]. Then, they performed coronary CT angiography on 21 vitro coronary arteries in the hearts of 7 male donors (average age, 52.3 ± 5.3). Training radiomics-based ML models were used for the diagnosis of advanced atherosclerotic lesions on 333 cross-sections of 95 plaques and evaluation of an additional 112 cross-sections. The results showed that the model was superior to several traditional methods (plaque attenuation pattern scheme in CT angiography cross-sections, histogram-based measurements area of low attenuation (<30 HU), average Hounsfield units of the plaque cross sections) [46]. Recently, they conducted research on

44 plaques of 25 patients. CTA, OCT, IVUS, and NaF 18-PET examinations were performed in all patients. The study found that radiomics outperformed traditional CTA parameters in detecting IVUS low-attenuating plaques, OCT validated thin-cap fibroatheroma (TVFA), and naf18-pet positive lesions (AUC: 0.59 vs. 0.72, 0.66 vs. 0.80, 0.65 vs. 0.87) [43]. They conducted a series of studies, which confirmed the feasibility of using radiomics to detect vulnerable plaques in CCTA, but with similar problems: the studies were based on a single center, using the same scanning and reconstruction parameters, with the small sample size, which may limit the extensive use.

Madani formulated the training model to predict the maximum von Mises stress, which could indicate the risk of plaque rupture, and provide new ideas for the detection of high-risk plaques in the clinical field [44].

Bae [47] and Jun [48] used ML to predict OCT-TCFA in IVUS and compare the accuracy of several different algorithms (SVM, ANN, RF, CNN, etc.). The overall prediction accuracy of the OCT-TFCA exceeds 80%. Sheet et al. collected 13 isolated hearts, using a machine learning framework to identify real necrotic areas of plaques in the IVUS, which is a marker of vulnerable plaques. The speckled appearance of these regions is similar to that of real shaded or severe signal loss regions. Compared with a traditional method such as histological, the sensitivity and specificity of the method were 96.15% and 77.78% [26].

Concerning OCT, Wang et al. [49] proposed a computer-aided method for quantification of fibrous cap (FC) thickness to indicate vulnerable plaques. Liu [50] proposed an automatic detection system of vulnerable plaque for IVOCT images based on a deep convolutional neural network (DCNN). The system is mainly composed of four modules: pre-processing, deep convolutional neural networks (DCNNs), post-processing, and ensemble. The method was intensively evaluated in 300 IVOCT images. The accuracy of the system reached 88.84%, which was a great improvement compared with the previous detection methods.

Fractional flow reserve (FFR) derived from coronary CTA(CT-FFR) is a promising noninvasive maker of coronary physiology and identification of high-risk plaques. Lee, J.M. [51] investigated the utility of noninvasive hemodynamic assessment in the identification of high-risk plaques that caused subsequent acute coronary syndrome (ACS). In this study, the process of deep learning-based CT-FFR is as follows: (1) coronary models, including all epicardial coronary arteries, were constructed by the extraction of vessel centerlines, identification of coronary plaques, and segmentation of lumen boundary along the coronary trees. (2) The flow and pressure in the coronary model were computed by solving the Navier–Stokes equations, using computational fluid dynamics (CFD) methods with assumptions of a rigid wall and a Newtonian fluid [52]. (3) Boundary conditions for hyperemia were derived from myocardial mass, vessel sizes at each outlet, and the response of the microcirculation to adenosine. (4) Combine physiological parameters and fluid mechanics principles with anatomical models to calculate the blood flow and blood pressure of the coronary arteries in the state of maximum hyperemia, and then computed the CT-FFR, change in CT-FFR across the lesion (ΔCT-FFR), wall shear stress (WSS) [53]. Additionally, axial plaque stress [54]. The results showed lower CT-FFR and higher ΔCT-FFR, WSS, and axial plaque stress in culprit lesions compared with non-culprit lesions (all p values < 0.01), indicating noninvasive hemodynamic assessment enhanced the identification of high-risk plaques that subsequently caused ACS. This study suggests that the integration of noninvasive hemodynamic assessment would enhance the prediction ability for ACS risk and may help provide optimal treatment for those high-risk patients.

Since the recent machine learning algorithm with pixel-level coarse coronary segmentation was insufficient for surface model reconstruction, a new CT-FFR technique with a "Coarse-to-Fine Subpixel" algorithm for lumen contour was proposed to achieve more precise reconstructions. This technique computed subpixel level lumen contour generating the artery centerline after the first coarse coronary segmentation on a pixel level. The new technology would lead to more precise lumen boundary and vessel reconstructions and provide a high diagnostic performance in identifying hemodynamically significant stenosis, "gray zone" lesions, high-risk plaques, and severely calcified lesions.

3.2. Assessment of Myocardium

At present, the gold standard for the diagnosis of myocardial specific ischemia is the fractional flow reserve (FFR), which can guide interventional therapy and improve the prognosis of patients with CAD [55]. The study showed that the characteristics of coronary plaque can also characterize myocardial ischemia [56]. Dey et al. [57] combined quantitative stenosis, plaque burden, and myocardial quality into a comprehensive risk score to predict the impairment of MFR through enhanced integrated machine learning algorithms. The experiment demonstrated that arterial non-calcified plaque (NCP) load and the approach combined CTA quantitative stenosis and the above comprehensive score significantly improved the identification of vascular dysfunction in the downstream compared with stenosis. Next, they explored the possibility of effectively combining CTA clinical data, quantitative stenosis, and plaque indicators with AI to predict specific ischemia. A total of 254 patients were enrolled, and quantitative plaque analysis was used to predict lesion-specific ischemia, with a final AUC of 0.84 [58]. Other experts tried to combine AI-based plaque analysis tools with CT-FFR to improve the prediction of myocardial ischemia. Teams of Gaur [59], von Knebel Doeberitz [60], and Kawasaki [61] used FFR as the gold standard and proposed machine-learning-based approaches combining CCTA plaque analysis and CT-FFR. Their results showed that the predictive ability of local ischemia was 0.90, 0.93 and 0.835, respectively, which was superior to that of traditional CCTA narrow grading.

3.3. Risk Prediction

The risk assessment of cardiovascular disease depends on a variety of factors, such as sex, age, weight, smoking, drinking, and so on [62]. Moreover, the risk level of patients with diabetes [63], elevated cholesterol, or blood pressure [64] also tend to differ. Different morphologies of plaques in medical imaging are significant for cardiovascular risk stratification [65,66]. Therefore, another important application of AI algorithms in the medical field is the prediction of cardiovascular disease risk.

In the field of IVUS, Araki presented a model to assess the risk of coronary heart disease by combining the IVUS grayscale plaque morphology and carotid B-mode ultrasound carotid intima-media thickness (cIMT) based on SMV, which is a marker of subclinical atherosclerosis [67]. The team then added plaque major component analysis to the model, proposed an SVM framework based on plaque morphology and major component (PAC) to assess coronary plaque risk, AUC = 0.98 [64]. The same team established an ML model by merging the plaques texture-based with the wall-based measurement features (coronary calcium area, coronary vessel area, coronary lumen area, coronary atheroma area, coronary wall thickness, and coronary wall thickness variability), which improved the accuracy of risk assessment by about 6% compared with the plaques texture-based information [68]. Cao [69] proposed a neural network-based method to determine the critical point of a vulnerability index, which distinguishes the fragile plaque from the stable plaque, AUC = 0.7143. Zhang [70] reported a machine learning approach for predicting the location and type of high-risk coronary plaque in patients treated with statins therapy.

Considering the studies of risk predicting focuses on CCTA in the field of noninvasive examination, van Assen [71] used ML to automatically extract plaque information so as to predict MACEs, AUC = 0.924. Van Rosendael [72] trained the ML model using coronary artery stenosis and plaque component information to predict mortality in patients with CAD, AUC = 0.771, beyond other conventional risk scores. Johnson [73] evaluated the prognosis of 6892 CCTA patients by ML, reporting that the AUC for all-cause death, CAD death, coronary heart disease death, and nonfatal myocardial infarction was 0.77, 0.72, 0.85, and 0.79, respectively. Motwani et al. [74] further added clinical risk factors to predict 5-year all-cause mortality in patients with CAD. They evaluated 25 clinical and 44 CCTA parameters, and ML showed higher AUC than other models (segment stenosis score, segment involvement score, modified Duke Index, Framingham risk score). Han [75] and Kigka [76] used ML to predict the rapid development of coronary plaque, which was thought to be associated with cardiovascular events [77,78], revealing the prediction accuracy of 0.81 and 0.84, respectively. Table 1 displays the application of AI in coronary atherosclerotic plaque analysis.

Table 1. Application of AI in coronary atherosclerotic plaque analysis.

Authors	Vascular Segments	Year	The Method Applied	Outcomes	Advantages	Disadvantages
Athanasiou	Plaques	2011	OCT	Random forest (RF), accuracy of 80.41%	Random forest (RF) classifier to classify atherosclerotic plaques (calcium, lipid pools, fibrous tissue, and mixed plaques)	Invasive
Wang	Vulnerable plaques	2012	Fibrous cap (FC)	Proposed a computer-aided method for quantification of fibrous cap (FC) thickness to indicate vulnerable plaques	A method for quantification of fibrous cap (FC) thickness	Invasive
Sheet D	Coronary plaque	2013	IVUS	Validation analysis revealed that SDH is highly consistent with traditional histology in characterizing calcification, fibrotic tissues, and lipids, with 99%, 97%, 99% accuracy, respectively	Developed a novel machine-learning-based technique called Stochastic Driven Histology (SDH), which can automatically characterize image components in IVUS images	Invasive, the small number of observation
Ughi	Plaques	2013	OCT	Random forest (RF), accuracy of 81.5%%	Random forest (RF) classifier to classify atherosclerotic plaques (calcium, lipid pools, fibrous tissue, and mixed plaques)	Invasive
Yamak D	Coronary plaque	2014	Non-calcified coronary atherosclerotic plaque. Characterization by Dual Energy Computed Tomography	Learning approaches were explored as a more advanced mathematical analysis to use additional information provided by DECT	Three models (ANN, RF and SVM)	The small number of observations is the other limitation of this study
Xu M	Atherosclerotic heart disease	2014	OCT	A linear SVM classifier to detect unhealthy objects	The system classifies the image from healthy and unhealthy subjects automatically by utilizing texture features	Invasive
Gaur	Coronary	2016	Coronary CTA stenosis, plaque volumes, FFRCT, and FFR were assessed	Redictive ability of local ischemia was 0.90	Coronary atherosclerotic plaque and FFRCT assessment improve the discrimination of ischaemia	Did not confirm plaque findings by intravascular ultrasound
Shalev R	Coronary plaque	2016	OCT	Rained and validated the model using frozen microscopic data, and the accuracy of calcified plaque recognition achieved 0.97	Regions for extraction of sub-images (SI's) were selected by experts to include calcium, fibrous, or lipid tissues	Invasive

Table 1. Cont.

Authors	Vascular Segments	Year	The Method Applied	Outcomes	Advantages	Disadvantages
Rico-Jimenez	Aining plaques	2016	OCT	An A-line modeling method to characterize plaques in OCT, which can automatically identify fibrotic plaques and lipid-containing plaques with 85% accuracy	Automatically identify fibrotic plaques and lipid-containing plaques	Invasive
Kolossváry M	Coronary vulnerable plaques	2017	Features are superior to conventional quantitative computed tomographic metrics to identify coronary plaques with napkin-ring sign	Radiomics and found that 916 features (20.6%) were associated with napkin-ring sign (NRS), of which 440 (9.9%) multiple radiographic features (short-run low-gray-level emphasis, long-run low-gray-level emphasis	High-risk plaques, napkin-ring sign	The true prevalence of the NRS is considerably smaller compared with non-NRS plaques in a real population
Kim G	Coronary plaque	2018	Plaque components were classifed into FT, FFT, NC, or DC using an intensity-based multi-level classifcation model	The classifers had classifcation accuracies of 85.1%, 71.9%, and 77.2%, respectively	Three diferent nets. Net 1 diferentiated low-intensity components into FT/FFT and NC/DC groups. Then, net 2 subsequently divided FT/FFT into FT or FFT, NC or DC via net 3	Invasive, it did not acquire signifcant classifcation results compared with VH
Kolluru	Classify plaques in OCT	2018	OCT	The model achieved an accuracy value that exceeded 90% in all categories.	Model also trained on frozen images to classify plaques in OCT into four categories, fiber, lipid, calcium, and others	Invasive
Wilson	Plaques	2018	OCT	Convolutional neural network (CNN) in identifying plaque properties in OCT images using line-based modeling methods, learning that CNN can significantly outperform in this task	A method based on the SegNet deep learning network	Invasive
Zreik M	Coronary artery plaque	2019	A recurrent CNN for automatic detection and classification of coronary crtery plaque and stenosis in coronary CT angiography	For detection and characterization of coronary plaque, the method was achieved an accuracy of 0.77	Three-dimensional convolutional neural network and neural networkautomatic detection and classification of coronary artery plaque and stenosis are feasible	Coronary artery bifurcations were not manually annotated and the network was not trained to detect these as a separate class
Rajendra	Coronary artery plaque	2019	Seven features are extracted from the Gabor coefficients: energy, and Kapur, Max, Rényi, Shannon, Vajda, and Yager entropies	The features acquired were also ranked according to F-value and input to several classifiers, an accuracy, positive predictive value, sensitivity, and specificity of 89.09%, 91.70%, 91.83% and 83.70% were obtained	Automated plaque classification using computed tomography angiography and Gabor transformationscan be helpful in the automated classification of plaques present in CTA images	The database was limited to only 73 patients. Furthermore, no quantitative calcium score was calculated

Table 1. Cont.

Authors	Vascular Segments	Year	The Method Applied	Outcomes	Advantages	Disadvantages
Masuda T	Coronary artery plaque	2019	Recorded the coronary CT number and 7 histogram parameters (minimum and mean value, standard deviation (SD), maximum value, skewness, kurtosis, and entropy) of the plaque CT number	Coronary CT number (0.19) followed by the minimum value (0.17), kurtosis (0.17), entropy (0.14), skewness (0.11), the mean value (0.11), the standard deviation (0.06), and the maximum value (0.05), and energy (0.00)	The machine learning was superior the conventional cut-off method for coronary plaque characterization using the plaque CT number on CCTA images	A small single-protocol study and only the performance of the machine learning algorithm was evaluated
Kolossváry M.	Coronary vulnerable plaques	2019	Diagnosis of advanced atherosclerotic lesions on 333 cross-sections of 95 plaques and evaluation of an additional 112 cross-sections	The results showed that the model was superior to several traditional methods.	Radiomics-based ML models outperformed expert visual assessment and histogram-based methods in the identification of advanced atheroscle radiomics-based machine learning rotic lesion	Limited spatial resolution of coronary CT angiography
Kolossváry M.	Coronaryvuinerable plaques	2019	Radiomics outperformed traditional CTA parameters in detecting IVUS low-attenuating plaques, OCT validated thin-cap fibroatheroma (TVFA) and naf18-pet	CTA, IVUS, OCT, positive lesions (AUC: 0.59 vs. 0.72, 0.66 vs. 0.80, 0.65 vs. 0.87)	Coronary CTA radiomics showed a good diagnostic accuracy to identify IVUS-attenuated plaques and excellent diagnostic accuracy to identify OCT-TCFA	Our results of the general populations are limited, multicenter longitudinal studies are warranted
von Knebel	Coronary	2019	ICA, CT-FFR	Redictive ability of local ischemia was 0.93	CCTA-derived plaque markers and CT-FFR have discriminatory power to differentiate between hemodynamically significant and non-significant coronary lesions	Did not systematically correlate our findings on CCTA with an invasive reference standard
Kawasaki	Coronary	2019	CT-FFR	rRdictive ability of local ischemia was 0.835	CCTA features and functional CT-FFR was helpful for detecting lesion-specific ischemia	Did not evaluate the influence of CT image quality on the CT-FFR measurements
Liu	Vulnerable plaques	2019	IVOCT images based on a deep convolutional neural network (DCNN).	Automatic detection system of vulnerable plaque for IVOCT images based on a deep convolutional neural network (DCNN). The accuracy of the system reached 88.84%	Intravascular optical coherence tomography (IVOCT)	Invasive

4. Limitations

There are still limitations in this field. In the research of ML used in coronary atherosclerotic plaques analysis, more prominent problems are the following two points: first, in almost all studies, data derived from a single research center or an old public dataset make it difficult to cover patients with different conditions and scanning parameters, making the training model difficult to satisfy the complex scenarios of clinical. Larger, rich public datasets should be established in the future for higher-quality research. Second, most of the research in this field takes the diagnostic opinion of artificial experts as the standard, lacking validation of the gold standard of pathology; therefore, the individual bias of experts may affect the accuracy of the final model. Future research on artificial intelligence for coronary atherosclerotic plaque analysis should be based on more big data; additionally, multicenter research is necessary to provide better algorithmic models.

5. Conclusions

In summary, artificial intelligence has the potential to expand and improve medical technologies for better patient care, by reducing the analysis time and provide automated recommendations to physicians regarding diagnosis and downstream treatment decision making. A proposed workflow for the incorporation of machine learning and deep learning analysis of imaging modalities in clinical practice. The workflow brings in a promising algorithm, based on a recurrent convolutional neural network, for automatic detection and characterization of coronary artery plaque, as well as detection and characterization of the anatomical significance of coronary artery stenosis. The areas of AI-based cardiovascular imaging covered range from imaging analysis (e.g., image segmentation, automated measurements, and eventually, automated diagnosis) to diagnostic imaging, including identifying plaques, assessing plaque vulnerability, myocardial hemodynamic evaluation, such as deep learning-based CT-FFR, and carrying out risk prognosis assessments. Specifically, the ability of the AI algorithms to make more accurate diagnoses is useful for physicians to detect diseases earlier in their course to plan for the right treatment action (Figure 1). With the development of computer technology, bioengineering, and medical imaging technology, the future of AI in cardiovascular imaging is bright as the collaboration between investigators and clinicians will have great benefits.

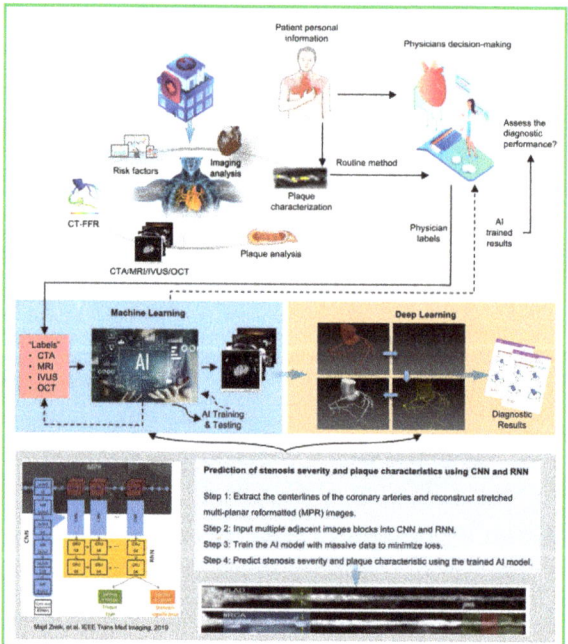

Figure 1. AI in cardiovascular atherosclerosis imaging. A proposed workflow for the incorporation of machine learning and deep learning analysis of imaging modalities in clinical practice. AI analysis can reduce the analysis time and provide automated recommendations to physicians regarding diagnosis and downstream treatment decision making. The workflow brings in a promising algorithm, based on a recurrent convolutional neural network, for the automatic detection and characterization of coronary artery plaque, as well as the detection and characterization of the anatomical significance of coronary artery stenosis.

Author Contributions: Study design: K.S. and B.L.; Paper writing: J.Z.; Paper quality assurance: R.H., G.S. and K.S. All authors have read and agreed to the published version of the manuscript.

Funding: The study was funded by the Economic and Technological Development Special Fund Medical and Health Technology Plan Project of Shenzhen Longgang District (No: LGKCYLWS2021000032).

Conflicts of Interest: The authors declare no conflict of interest.

Abbreviations

AI	Artificial intelligence
MACEs	Major adverse cardiac events
CVDs	Cardiovascular disease
CAD	Coronary artery disease
OCT	Optical coherence tomography
CT	Computed tomography
MRI	Magnetic resonance imaging
IVUS	Intravascular ultrasound
AS	Atherosclerosis
ACS	Acute coronary syndrome
ML	Machine learning
DL	Deep learning
ROI	Region of interest

References

1. Mattiuzzi, C.; Lippi, G. Cancer statistics: A comparison between World Health Organization (WHO) and Global Burden of Disease (GBD). *Eur. J. Public Health* **2020**, *30*, 1026–1027. [CrossRef] [PubMed]
2. Walli-Attaei, M.; Joseph, P.; Rosengren, A.; Chow, C.K.; Rangarajan, S.; Lear, S.A.; AlHabib, K.F.; Davletov, K.; Dans, A.; Lanas, F.; et al. Variations between women and men in risk factors, treatments, cardiovascular disease incidence, and death in 27 high-income, middle-income, and low-income countries (PURE): A prospective cohort study. *Lancet* **2020**, *396*, 97–109. [CrossRef]
3. Plana, J.C.; Thavendiranathan, P.; Bucciarelli-Ducci, C.; Lancellotti, P. Multi-Modality Imaging in the Assessment of Cardiovascular Toxicity in the Cancer Patient. *JACC Cardiovasc. Imaging* **2018**, *11*, 1173–1186. [CrossRef] [PubMed]
4. Williams, A.M.; Liu, Y.; Regner, K.R.; Jotterand, F.; Liu, P.; Liang, M. Artificial intelligence, physiological genomics, and precision medicine. *Physiol. Genom.* **2018**, *50*, 237–243. [CrossRef] [PubMed]
5. Henglin, M.; Stein, G.; Hushcha, P.V.; Snoek, J.; Wiltschko, A.B.; Cheng, S. Machine Learning Approaches in Cardiovascular Imaging. *Circ. Cardiovasc. Imaging* **2017**, *10*, e005614. [CrossRef]
6. Jordan, M.I.; Mitchell, T.M. Machine learning: Trends, perspectives, and prospects. *Science* **2015**, *349*, 255–260. [CrossRef]
7. Nicol, E.D.; Norgaard, B.L.; Blanke, P.; Ahmadi, A.; Weir-McCall, J.; Horvat, P.M.; Han, K.; Bax, J.J.; Leipsic, J. The Future of Cardiovascular Computed Tomography: Advanced Analytics and Clinical Insights. *JACC Cardiovasc. Imaging* **2019**, *12*, 1058–1072. [CrossRef]
8. Dey, D.; Slomka, P.J.; Leeson, P.; Comaniciu, D.; Shrestha, S.; Sengupta, P.P.; Marwick, T.H. Artificial Intelligence in Cardiovascular Imaging: JACC State-of-the-Art Review. *J. Am. Coll. Cardiol.* **2019**, *73*, 1317–1335. [CrossRef]
9. Al'Aref, S.J.; Anchouche, K.; Singh, G.; Slomka, P.J.; Kolli, K.K.; Kumar, A.; Pandey, M.; Maliakal, G.; Van Rosendael, A.R.; Beecy, A.N.; et al. Clinical applications of machine learning in cardiovascular disease and its relevance to cardiac imaging. *Eur. Heart J.* **2019**, *40*, 1975–1986. [CrossRef]
10. Johnson, K.; Soto, J.T.; Glicksberg, B.; Shameer, K.; Miotto, R.; Ali, M.; Ashley, E.; Dudley, J.T. Artificial Intelligence in Cardiology. *J. Am. Coll. Cardiol.* **2018**, *71*, 2668–2679. [CrossRef]
11. Ching, T.; Himmelstein, D.S.; Beaulieu-Jones, B.K.; Kalinin, A.A.; Do, B.T.; Way, G.P.; Ferrero, E.; Agapow, P.M.; Zietz, M.; Hoffman, M.M.; et al. Opportunities and obstacles for deep learning in biology and medicine. *J. R. Soc. Interface* **2018**, *15*, 20170387. [CrossRef] [PubMed]
12. Lancet, T. Artificial intelligence in health care: Within touching distance. *Lancet* **2017**, *390*, 2739. [CrossRef]
13. Tearney, G.J.; Regar, E.; Akasaka, T.; Adriaenssens, T.; Barlis, P.; Bezerra, H.G.; Bouma, B.; Bruining, N.; Cho, J.M.; Chowdhary, S.; et al. Consensus standards for acquisition, measurement, and reporting of intravascular optical coherence tomography studies: A report from the International Working Group for Intravascular Optical Coherence Tomography Standardization and Validation. *J. Am. Coll. Cardiol.* **2012**, *59*, 1058–1072. [CrossRef] [PubMed]
14. Camacho, D.; Collins, K.M.; Powers, R.K.; Costello, J.C.; Collins, J.J. Next-Generation Machine Learning for Biological Networks. *Cell* **2018**, *173*, 1581–1592. [CrossRef]

15. Sohail, A.; Arif, F. Supervised and unsupervised algorithms for bioinformatics and data science. *Prog. Biophys. Mol. Biol.* **2020**, *151*, 14–22. [CrossRef] [PubMed]
16. Ross, R. The pathogenesis of atherosclerosis: A perspective for the 1990s. *Nature* **1993**, *362*, 801–809. [CrossRef]
17. Weissberg, P.L.; Bennett, M.R. Atherosclerosis—An inflammatory disease. *N. Engl. J. Med.* **1999**, *340*, 1928–1929.
18. Libby, P.; Ridker, P.M.; Hansson, G.K. Progress and challenges in translating the biology of atherosclerosis. *Nature* **2011**, *473*, 317–325. [CrossRef]
19. Bentzon, J.F.; Otsuka, F.; Virmani, R.; Falk, E. Mechanisms of plaque formation and rupture. *Circ. Res.* **2014**, *114*, 1852–1866. [CrossRef]
20. Otsuka, F.; Yasuda, S.; Noguchi, T.; Ishibashi-Ueda, H. Pathology of coronary atherosclerosis and thrombosis. *Cardiovasc. Diagn. Ther.* **2016**, *6*, 396–408. [CrossRef]
21. Kriszbacher, I.; Koppan, M.; Bodis, J. Inflammation, atherosclerosis, and coronary artery disease. *N. Engl. J. Med.* **2005**, *353*, 429–430. [PubMed]
22. Zreik, M.; Van Hamersvelt, R.W.; Wolterink, J.M.; Leiner, T.; Viergever, M.A.; Isgum, I. AA Recurrent CNN for Automatic Detection and Classification of Coronary Artery Plaque and Stenosis in Coronary CT Angiography. *IEEE Trans. Med. Imaging* **2019**, *38*, 1588–1598. [CrossRef] [PubMed]
23. Acharya, U.R.; Meiburger, K.M.; Koh, J.E.W.; Vicnesh, J.; Ciaccio, E.J.; Lih, O.S.; Tan, S.K.; Aman, R.R.A.R.; Molinari, F.; Ng, K.H. Automated plaque classification using computed tomography angiography and Gabor transformations. *Artif. Intell. Med.* **2019**, *100*, 101724. [CrossRef] [PubMed]
24. Kolluru, C.; Prabhu, D.; Gharaibeh, Y.; Bezerra, H.; Guagliumi, G.; Wilson, D. Deep neural networks for A-line-based plaque classification in coronary intravascular optical coherence tomography images. *J. Med. Imaging* **2018**, *5*, 044504. [CrossRef]
25. Yamak, D.; Panse, P.; Pavlicek, W.; Boltz, T.; Akay, M. Non-calcified coronary atherosclerotic plaque characterization by dual energy computed tomography. *IEEE J. Biomed. Health Inform.* **2014**, *18*, 939–945. [CrossRef]
26. Kim, G.Y.; Lee, J.H.; Na Hwang, Y.; Kim, S.M. A novel intensity-based multi-level classification approach for coronary plaque characterization in intravascular ultrasound images. *Biomed. Eng. Online* **2018**, *17*, 151. [CrossRef] [PubMed]
27. Sheet, D.; Karamalis, A.; Eslami, A.; Noël, P.; Chatterjee, J.; Ray, A.K.; Laine, A.F.; Carlier, S.G.; Navab, N.; Katouzian, A. Joint learning of ultrasonic backscattering statistical physics and signal confidence primal for characterizing atherosclerotic plaques using intravascular ultrasound. *Med. Image Anal.* **2014**, *18*, 103–117. [CrossRef] [PubMed]
28. Shalev, R.; Bezerra, H.G.; Ray, S.; Prabhu, D.; Wilson, D.L. Classification of calcium in intravascular OCT images for the purpose of intervention planning. In Proceedings of the Medical Imaging 2016: Image-Guided Procedures, Robotic Interventions, and Modeling, San Diego, CA, USA, 27 February–3 March 2016; Volume 9786, p. 978605. [CrossRef]
29. Xu, M.; Cheng, J.; Wong, D.W.K.; Taruya, A.; Tanaka, A.; Liu, J. Automatic atherosclerotic heart disease detection in intracoronary optical coherence tomography images. In Proceedings of the 2014 36th Annual International Conference of the IEEE Engineering in Medicine and Biology Society, Chicago, IL, USA, 26 February–30 August 2014; pp. 174–177. [CrossRef]
30. Zhou, P.; Zhu, T.; He, C.; Li, Z.-Y. Automatic classification of atherosclerotic tissue in intravascular optical coherence tomography images. *J. Opt. Soc. Am. A Opt. Image Sci. Vis.* **2017**, *34*, 1152–1159. [CrossRef]
31. Kolluru, C.; Prabhu, D.; Gharaibeh, Y.; Wu, H.; Wilson, D.L. Voxel-based plaque classification in coronary intravascular optical coherence tomography images using decision trees. In Proceedings of the Medical Imaging 2018: Computer-Aided Diagnosis, Houston, TX, USA, 10–15 February 2018; Volume 10575, p. 105752Y. [CrossRef]
32. Rico-Jimenez, J.J.; Campos-Delgado, D.U.; Villiger, M.; Otsuka, K.; Bouma, B.E.; Jo, J.A. Automatic classification of atherosclerotic plaques imaged with intravascular OCT. *Biomed. Opt. Express* **2016**, *7*, 4069–4085. [CrossRef] [PubMed]
33. Lee, J.; Prabhu, D.; Kolluru, C.; Gharaibeh, Y.; Zimin, V.N.; Bezerra, H.G.; Wilson, D.L. Automated plaque characterization using deep learning on coronary intravascular optical coherence tomographic images. *Biomed. Opt. Express* **2019**, *10*, 6497–6515. [CrossRef] [PubMed]
34. Stocker, T.J.; Deseive, S.; Leipsic, J.; Hadamitzky, M.; Chen, M.Y.; Rubinshtein, R.; Heckner, M.; Bax, J.J.; Fang, X.M.; Grove, E.L.; et al. Reduction in radiation exposure in cardiovascular computed tomography imaging: Results from the PROspective multicenter registry on radiaTion dose Estimates of cardiac CT anglOgraphy iN daily practice in 2017 (PROTECTION VI). *Eur. Heart J.* **2018**, *39*, 3715–3723. [CrossRef] [PubMed]
35. Athanasiou, L.S.; Exarchos, T.P.; Naka, K.K.; Michalis, L.K.; Prati, F.; Fotiadis, D.I. Atherosclerotic plaque characterization in Optical Coherence Tomography images. In Proceedings of the 2011 Annual International Conference of the IEEE Engineering in Medicine and Biology Society, Boston, MA, USA, 30 August–3 September 2011; pp. 4485–4488. [CrossRef] [PubMed]
36. Kolossváry, M.; Karády, J.; Szilveszter, B.; Kitslaar, P.; Hoffmann, U.; Merkely, B.; Maurovich-Horvat, P. Radiomic Features Are Superior to Conventional Quantitative Computed Tomographic Metrics to Identify Coronary Plaques with Napkin-Ring Sign. *Circ. Cardiovasc. Imaging* **2017**, *10*, e006843. [CrossRef]
37. Tarkin, J.; Dweck, M.; Evans, N.R.; Takx, R.A.; Brown, A.J.; Tawakol, A.; Fayad, Z.A.; Rudd, J.H. Imaging Atherosclerosis. *Circ. Res.* **2016**, *118*, 750–769. [CrossRef]
38. Puchner, S.B.; Liu, T.; Mayrhofer, T.; Truong, Q.A.; Lee, H.; Fleg, J.L.; Nagurney, J.T.; Udelson, J.E.; Hoffmann, U.; Ferencik, M. High-risk plaque detected on coronary CT angiography predicts acute coronary syndromes independent of significant stenosis in acute chest pain: Results from the ROMICAT-II trial. *J. Am. Coll. Cardiol.* **2014**, *64*, 684–692. [CrossRef]

39. Wang, J.; Fleischmann, D. Improving Spatial Resolution at CT: Development, Benefits, and Pitfalls. *Radiology* **2018**, *289*, 261–262. [CrossRef]
40. Nordbeck, P.; Ertl, G.; Ritter, O. Magnetic resonance imaging safety in pacemaker and implantable cardioverter defibrillator patients: How far have we come? *Eur. Heart J.* **2015**, *36*, 1505–1511. [CrossRef]
41. Peters, R.J.; Kok, W.E.; Havenith, M.G.; Rijsterborgh, H.; van der Wal, A.; Visser, C.A. Histopathologic validation of intracoronary ultrasound imaging. *J. Am. Soc. Echocardiogr. Off. Publ. Am. Soc. Echocardiogr.* **1994**, *7*, 230–241. [CrossRef]
42. Pighi, M.; Gratta, A.; Marin, F.; Bellamoli, M.; Lunardi, M.; Fezzi, S.; Zivelonghi, C.; Pesarini, G.; Tomai, F.; Ribichini, F. Cardiac allograft vasculopathy: Pathogenesis, diagnosis and therapy. *Transplant Rev. (Orlando)* **2020**, *34*, 100569. [CrossRef] [PubMed]
43. Schaar, J.A.; Muller, J.E.; Falk, E.; Virmani, R.; Fuster, V.; Serruys, P.W.; Colombo, A.; Stefanadis, C.; Casscells, S.W.; Moreno, P.R.; et al. Terminology for high-risk and vulnerable coronary artery plaques. Report of a meeting on the vulnerable plaque, 17–18 June 2003, Santorini, Greece. *Eur. Heart J.* **2004**, *25*, 1077–1082. [CrossRef] [PubMed]
44. Virmani, R.; Kolodgie, F.D.; Burke, A.P.; Farb, A.; Schwartz, S.M. Lessons from sudden coronary death: A comprehensive morphological classification scheme for atherosclerotic lesions. *Arterioscler. Thromb. Vasc. Biol.* **2000**, *20*, 1262–1275. [CrossRef] [PubMed]
45. Jia, H.; Abtahian, F.; Aguirre, A.D.; Lee, S.; Chia, S.; Lowe, H.; Kato, K.; Yonetsu, T.; Vergallo, R.; Hu, S.; et al. In vivo diagnosis of plaque erosion and calcified nodule in patients with acute coronary syndrome by intravascular optical coherence tomography. *J. Am. Coll. Cardiol.* **2013**, *62*, 1748–1758. [CrossRef] [PubMed]
46. Kolossváry, M.; Karády, J.; Kikuchi, Y.; Ivanov, A.; Schlett, C.L.; Lu, M.T.; Foldyna, B.; Merkely, B.; Aerts, H.J.; Hoffmann, U.; et al. Radiomics versus Visual and Histogram-based Assessment to Identify Atheromatous Lesions at Coronary CT Angiography: An ex Vivo Study. *Radiology* **2019**, *293*, 89–96. [CrossRef] [PubMed]
47. Kolossváry, M.; Park, J.; Bang, J.-I.; Zhang, J.; Lee, J.M.; Paeng, J.C.; Merkely, B.; Narula, J.; Kubo, T.; Akasaka, T.; et al. Identification of invasive and radionuclide imaging markers of coronary plaque vulnerability using radiomic analysis of coronary computed tomography angiography. *Eur. Heart J. Cardiovasc. Imaging* **2019**, *20*, 1250–1258. [CrossRef] [PubMed]
48. Sheet, D.; Karamalis, A.; Eslami, A.; Noël, P.; Virmani, R.; Nakano, M.; Chatterjee, J.; Ray, A.K.; Laine, A.F.; Carlier, S.; et al. Hunting for necrosis in the shadows of intravascular ultrasound. *Comput. Med. Imaging Graph. Off. J. Comput. Med. Imaging Soc.* **2014**, *38*, 104–112. [CrossRef]
49. Wang, Z.; Chamié, D.; Bezerra, H.G.; Yamamoto, H.; Kanovsky, J.; Wilson, D.L.; Costa, M.A.; Rollins, A.M. Volumetric quantification of fibrous caps using intravascular optical coherence tomography. *Biomed. Opt. Express* **2012**, *3*, 1413–1426. [CrossRef]
50. Liu, R.; Zhang, Y.; Zheng, Y.; Liu, Y.; Zhao, Y.; Yi, L. Automated Detection of Vulnerable Plaque for Intravascular Optical Coherence Tomography Images. *Cardiovasc. Eng. Technol.* **2019**, *10*, 590–603. [CrossRef]
51. Lee, J.M.; Choi, G.; Koo, B.-K.; Hwang, D.; Park, J.; Zhang, J.; Kim, K.-J.; Tong, Y.; Kim, H.J.; Grady, L.; et al. Identification of High-Risk Plaques Destined to Cause Acute Coronary Syndrome Using Coronary Computed Tomographic Angiography and Computational Fluid Dynamics. *JACC Cardiovasc. Imaging* **2019**, *12*, 1032–1043. [CrossRef]
52. Park, J.B.; Choi, G.; Chun, E.J.; Kim, H.J.; Park, J.; Jung, J.H.; Lee, M.-H.; Otake, H.; Doh, J.H.; Nam, C.W.; et al. Computational fluid dynamic measures of wall shear stress are related to coronary lesion characteristics. *Heart* **2016**, *102*, 1655–1661. [CrossRef] [PubMed]
53. Samady, H.; Eshtehardi, P.; McDaniel, M.C.; Suo, J.; Dhawan, S.S.; Maynard, C.; Timmins, L.H.; Quyyumi, A.A.; Giddens, D.P. Coronary artery wall shear stress is associated with progression and transformation of atherosclerotic plaque and arterial remodeling in patients with coronary artery disease. *Circulation* **2011**, *124*, 779–788. [CrossRef]
54. Choi, G.; Lee, J.M.; Kim, H.J.; Park, J.B.; Sankaran, S.; Otake, H.; Doh, J.H.; Nam, C.W.; Shin, E.S.; Taylor, C.A.; et al. Coronary Artery Axial Plaque Stress and its Relationship with Lesion Geometry: Application of Computational Fluid Dynamics to Coronary CT Angiography. *JACC Cardiovasc. Imaging* **2015**, *8*, 1156–1166. [CrossRef] [PubMed]
55. Tonino, P.A.; De Bruyne, B.; Pijls, N.H.; Siebert, U.; Ikeno, F.; van't Veer, M.; Klauss, V.; Manoharan, G.; Engstrøm, T.; Oldroyd, K.G.; et al. Fractional flow reserve versus angiography for guiding percutaneous coronary intervention. *N. Engl. J. Med.* **2009**, *360*, 213–224. [CrossRef] [PubMed]
56. van Nunen, L.X.; Zimmermann, F.M.; Tonino, P.A.L.; Barbato, E.; Baumbach, A.; Engstrøm, T.; Klauss, V.; MacCarthy, P.A.; Manoharan, G.; Oldroyd, K.G.; et al. Fractional flow reserve versus angiography for guidance of PCI in patients with multivessel coronary artery disease (FAME): 5-year follow-up of a randomised controlled trial. *Lancet* **2015**, *386*, 1853–1860. [CrossRef]
57. Nakazato, R.; Shalev, A.; Doh, J.H.; Koo, B.K.; Gransar, H.; Gomez, M.J.; Leipsic, J.; Park, H.B.; Berman, D.S.; Min, J.K. Aggregate plaque volume by coronary computed tomography angiography is superior and incremental to luminal narrowing for diagnosis of ischemic lesions of intermediate stenosis severity. *J. Am. Coll. Cardiol.* **2013**, *62*, 460–467. [CrossRef]
58. Dey, D.; Zamudio, M.D.; Schuhbaeck, A.; Orozco, L.E.J.; Otaki, Y.; Gransar, H.; Li, D.; Germano, G.; Achenbach, S.; Berman, D.S.; et al. Relationship Between Quantitative Adverse Plaque Features from Coronary Computed Tomography Angiography and Downstream Impaired Myocardial Flow Reserve by 13N-Ammonia Positron Emission Tomography: A Pilot Study. *Circ. Cardiovasc. Imaging* **2015**, *8*, e003255. [CrossRef]
59. Dey, D.; Gaur, S.; Ovrehus, K.A.; Slomka, P.J.; Betancur, J.; Goeller, M.; Hell, M.M.; Gransar, H.; Berman, D.S.; Achenbach, S.; et al. Integrated prediction of lesion-specific ischaemia from quantitative coronary CT angiography using machine learning: A multicentre study. *Eur. Radiol.* **2018**, *28*, 2655–2664. [CrossRef]

60. Gaur, S.; Øvrehus, K.A.; Dey, D.; Leipsic, J.; Bøtker, H.E.; Jensen, J.M.; Narula, J.; Ahmadi, A.; Achenbach, S.; Ko, B.S.; et al. Coronary plaque quantification and fractional flow reserve by coronary computed tomography angiography identify ischaemia-causing lesions. *Eur. Heart J.* **2016**, *37*, 1220–1227. [CrossRef]
61. von Knebel Doeberitz, P.L.; De Cecco, C.N.; Schoepf, U.J.; Duguay, T.M.; Albrecht, M.H.; Van Assen, M.; Bauer, M.J.; Savage, R.H.; Pannell, J.T.; De Santis, D.; et al. Coronary CT angiography-derived plaque quantification with artificial intelligence CT fractional flow reserve for the identification of lesion-specific ischemia. *Eur. Radiol.* **2019**, *29*, 2378–2387. [CrossRef]
62. Kawasaki, T.; Kidoh, M.; Kido, T.; Sueta, D.; Fujimoto, S.; Kumamaru, K.K.; Uetani, T.; Tanabe, Y.; Ueda, T.; Sakabe, D.; et al. Evaluation of Significant Coronary Artery Disease Based on CT Fractional Flow Reserve and Plaque Characteristics Using Random Forest Analysis in Machine Learning. *Acad. Radiol.* **2020**, *27*, 1700–1708. [CrossRef] [PubMed]
63. Virani, S.S.; Alonso, A.; Benjamin, E.J.; Bittencourt, M.S.; Callaway, C.W.; Carson, A.P.; Chamberlain, A.M.; Chang, A.R.; Cheng, S.; Delling, F.N.; et al. Heart Disease and Stroke Statistics-2020 Update: A Report from the American Heart Association. *Circulation* **2020**, *141*, e139–e596. [CrossRef] [PubMed]
64. Sarwar, N.; Gao, P.; Seshasai, S.R.; Gobin, R.; Kaptoge, S.; Di Angelantonio, E.; Ingelsson, E.; Lawlor, D.A.; Selvin, E.; Stampfer, M.; et al. Diabetes mellitus, fasting blood glucose concentration, and risk of vascular disease: A collaborative meta-analysis of 102 prospective studies. *Lancet* **2010**, *375*, 2215–2222. [CrossRef] [PubMed]
65. Cho, I.; Al'Aref, S.J.; Berger, A.; Hartaigh, B.Ó.; Gransar, H.; Valenti, V.; Lin, F.Y.; Achenbach, S.; Berman, D.S.; Budoff, M.J.; et al. Prognostic value of coronary computed tomographic angiography findings in asymptomatic individuals: A 6-year follow-up from the prospective multicentre international CONFIRM study. *Eur. Heart J.* **2018**, *39*, 934–941. [CrossRef] [PubMed]
66. Williams, M.C.; Hunter, A.; Shah, A.S.V.; Assi, V.; Lewis, S.; Smith, J.; Berry, C.; Boon, N.A.; Clark, E.; Flather, M.; et al. Use of Coronary Computed Tomographic Angiography to Guide Management of Patients with Coronary Disease. *J. Am. Coll. Cardiol.* **2016**, *67*, 1759–1768. [CrossRef]
67. Araki, T.; Ikeda, N.; Shukla, D.; Londhe, N.D.; Shrivastava, V.; Banchhor, S.K.; Saba, L.; Nicolaides, A.; Shafique, S.; Laird, J.R.; et al. A new method for IVUS-based coronary artery disease risk stratification: A link between coronary & carotid ultrasound plaque burdens. *Comput. Methods Programs Biomed.* **2016**, *124*, 161–179. [CrossRef]
68. Araki, T.; Ikeda, N.; Shukla, D.; Jain, P.K.; Londhe, N.D.; Shrivastava, V.K.; Banchhor, S.K.; Saba, L.; Nicolaides, A.; Shafique, S.; et al. PCA-based polling strategy in machine learning framework for coronary artery disease risk assessment in intravascular ultrasound: A link between carotid and coronary grayscale plaque morphology. *Comput. Methods Programs Biomed.* **2016**, *128*, 137–158. [CrossRef]
69. Banchhor, S.K.; Londhe, N.D.; Araki, T.; Saba, L.; Radeva, P.; Laird, J.R.; Suri, J.S. Wall-based measurement features provides an improved IVUS coronary artery risk assessment when fused with plaque texture-based features during machine learning paradigm. *Comput. Biol. Med.* **2017**, *91*, 198–212. [CrossRef]
70. Cao, Y.; Xiao, X.; Liu, Z.; Yang, M.; Sun, D.; Guo, W.; Cui, L.; Zhang, P. Detecting vulnerable plaque with vulnerability index based on convolutional neural networks. *Comput. Med. Imaging Graph. Off. J. Comput. Med. Imaging Soc.* **2020**, *81*, 101711. [CrossRef]
71. Zhang, L.; Wahle, A.; Chen, Z.; Lopez, J.J.; Kovarnik, T.; Sonka, M. Predicting Locations of High-Risk Plaques in Coronary Arteries in Patients Receiving Statin Therapy. *IEEE Trans. Med. Imaging* **2018**, *37*, 151–161. [CrossRef]
72. van Assen, M.; Varga-Szemes, A.; Schoepf, U.J.; Duguay, T.M.; Hudson, H.T.; Egorova, S.; Johnson, K.; Pierre, S.S.; Zaki, B.; Oudkerk, M.; et al. Automated plaque analysis for the prognostication of major adverse cardiac events. *Eur. J. Radiol.* **2019**, *116*, 76–83. [CrossRef]
73. van Rosendael, A.R.; Maliakal, G.; Kolli, K.K.; Beecy, A.; Al'Aref, S.J.; Dwivedi, A.; Singh, G.; Panday, M.; Kumar, A.; Ma, X.; et al. Maximization of the usage of coronary CTA derived plaque information using a machine learning based algorithm to improve risk stratification; insights from the CONFIRM registry. *J. Cardiovasc. Comput. Tomogr.* **2018**, *12*, 204–209. [CrossRef] [PubMed]
74. Johnson, K.M.; Johnson, H.E.; Zhao, Y.; Dowe, D.A.; Staib, L.H. Scoring of Coronary Artery Disease Characteristics on Coronary CT Angiograms by Using Machine Learning. *Radiology* **2019**, *292*, 354–362. [CrossRef] [PubMed]
75. Motwani, M.; Dey, D.; Berman, D.S.; Germano, G.; Achenbach, S.; Al-Mallah, M.; Andreini, D.; Budoff, M.J.; Cademartiri, F.; Callister, T.Q.; et al. Machine learning for prediction of all-cause mortality in patients with suspected coronary artery disease: A 5-year multicentre prospective registry analysis. *Eur. Heart J.* **2017**, *38*, 500–507. [CrossRef] [PubMed]
76. Han, D.; Kolli, K.K.; Al'Aref, S.J.; Baskaran, L.; van Rosendael, A.R.; Gransar, H.; Andreini, D.; Budoff, M.J.; Cademartiri, F.; Chinnaiyan, K.; et al. Machine Learning Framework to Identify Individuals at Risk of Rapid Progression of Coronary Atherosclerosis: From the PARADIGM Registry. *J. Am. Heart Assoc.* **2020**, *9*, e013958. [CrossRef]
77. Kigka, V.I.; Sakellarios, A.I.; Tsompou, P.; Kyriakidis, S.; Siogkas, P.; Andrikos, I.; Michalis, L.K.; Fotiadis, D.I. Site specific prediction of atherosclerotic plaque progression using computational biomechanics and machine learning. In Proceedings of the 2019 41st Annual International Conference of the IEEE Engineering in Medicine and Biology Society (EMBC), Berlin, Germany, 23–27 July 2019; pp. 6998–7001. [CrossRef]
78. Falk, E.; Nakano, M.; Bentzon, J.F.; Finn, A.V.; Virmani, R. Update on acute coronary syndromes: The pathologists' view. *Eur. Heart J.* **2013**, *34*, 719–728. [CrossRef]

Predicting the 2-Year Risk of Progression from Prediabetes to Diabetes Using Machine Learning among Chinese Elderly Adults

Qing Liu [1], Qing Zhou [1], Yifeng He [2], Jingui Zou [2], Yan Guo [3] and Yaqiong Yan [3,*]

1. Department of Epidemiology, School of Public Health, Wuhan University, Wuhan 430071, China; liuqing@whu.edu.cn (Q.L.); zhouqing@whu.edu.cn (Q.Z.)
2. School of Geodesy and Geomatics, Wuhan University, Wuhan 430079, China; heyifeng@whu.edu.cn (Y.H.); jgzou@sgg.whu.edu.cn (J.Z.)
3. Wuhan Center for Disease Control and Prevention, Wuhan 430015, China; swallow315@whcdc.org
* Correspondence: yanyyq@whcdc.org

Abstract: Identifying people with a high risk of developing diabetes among those with prediabetes may facilitate the implementation of a targeted lifestyle and pharmacological interventions. We aimed to establish machine learning models based on demographic and clinical characteristics to predict the risk of incident diabetes. We used data from the free medical examination service project for elderly people who were 65 years or older to develop logistic regression (LR), decision tree (DT), random forest (RF), and extreme gradient boosting (XGBoost) machine learning models for the follow-up results of 2019 and 2020 and performed internal validation. The receiver operating characteristic (ROC), sensitivity, specificity, accuracy, and F1 score were used to select the model with better performance. The average annual progression rate to diabetes in prediabetic elderly people was 14.21%. Each model was trained using eight features and one outcome variable from 9607 prediabetic individuals, and the performance of the models was assessed in 2402 prediabetes patients. The predictive ability of four models in the first year was better than in the second year. The XGBoost model performed relatively efficiently (ROC: 0.6742 for 2019 and 0.6707 for 2020). We established and compared four machine learning models to predict the risk of progression from prediabetes to diabetes. Although there was little difference in the performance of the four models, the XGBoost model had a relatively good ROC value, which might perform well in future exploration in this field.

Keywords: machine learning; prediabetes; incident diabetes; predictive models

1. Introduction

Diabetes is one of the significant public problems worldwide, resulting in 536.6 million adults with diabetes, 541.0 million adults with impaired glucose tolerance (IGT), and 319.0 million adults with impaired fasting glucose (IFG) [1]. Prediabetes is often used to refer to the latter two states and is more commonly observed in the elderly [2]. Due to the growing economic burden and mortality caused by diabetes, the prevention of diabetes is imminent. Unlike incurable diabetes, the majority of prediabetes patients, especially the elderly, may revert to normoglycaemia or remain stable. Only a fraction of patients with prediabetes progress to diabetes [3], and this proportion can be further reduced by lifestyle and pharmacological interventions [4]. So, identifying people with a high risk of developing diabetes among prediabetic patients may facilitate the implementation of targeted interventions and avoid the burden of prevention for people at low risk.

Machine learning has been identified as a powerful tool for application in the medical field [5]. According to electronic health records, Neves et al. [6] predicted the outcome of diabetes by applying Bayesian Networks. Lama et al. [7] used a random forest (RF)

classifier to train a model for predicting whether an individual develops prediabetes or type 2 diabetes. Meng et al. [8] developed three multiple prediction models with logistic regression (LR), artificial neural networks, and decision tree (DT) for predicting diabetes or prediabetes. However, most machine learning models in the field of diabetes research are aimed at the onset and complications. Prediction models of progression from prediabetes to diabetes are limited, and they may not be reliable to generalize to Chinese people due to ethnicity differences [9].

Thus, the purpose of this study is to train machine learning models for predicting patients with prediabetes progress to diabetes based on demographic information and laboratory results. We select LR, DT, RF, and extreme gradient boosting (XGBoost) to build predictive models and optimize their hyperparameters by 10-fold cross-validation. Accuracy, sensitivity, specificity, and receiver operating characteristic (ROC) are also used to estimate the performance of these predictive models.

2. Materials and Methods

2.1. Study Design and Participants

We conducted a retrospective cohort study of participants who attended free health screening service in Wuhan, China, between 2018 and 2020. This project has provided annual physical examinations to adults older than 65 years, which covered 31.3% of the elderly population in Wuhan (388,420/1,242,470, in 2018).

We restricted our study to 26705 participants with prediabetes at baseline whose fasting plasma glucose (FPG) $\geq$ 6.1 mmol/L [10] and did not meet the criteria of diabetes as defined below. Those who had missing outcomes or were lost to follow-up were excluded (Figure 1). Available data included demographics, lifestyle, medical history, anthropometric indices, and laboratory results. Ethical approval was obtained from the Ethics Committee of Wuhan Center for Disease Control and Prevention (#WHCDCIRB-K-2018023).

2.2. Data Collection

Demographic characteristics included age, gender, marital status, and education level. Lifestyle included smoking, drinking, and exercise. An anthropometric examination was conducted by well-trained community physicians. Height and weight were measured with subjects wearing light clothes without shoes. The body mass index (BMI) was calculated as the individual's body weight (kg) divided by the square of height (m). Waist circumference (WC) was measured at the midpoint between the last rib and iliac crest. Blood pressure was measured three times by an electronic sphygmomanometer when participants were in a sitting position after 5 minutes of rest. Blood samples were drawn from individuals after at least 8 hours of fasting for laboratory tests. Exercise was defined as those who had more than three times of physical activity for 30 min per week. Smoking was defined as those who reported smoking at least once per month. Drinking was defined as those who drink alcohol more than once a month.

2.3. Definition of Outcome

An individual was regarded to reach the outcome of diabetes when FPG $\geq$ 7.0 mmol/L according to the American Diabetes Association diagnostic criteria [11] or a self-reported diagnosis by health care professionals during the follow-up.

2.4. Feature Selection

To reduce the computational complexity and generalization error of the model, it was important to determine which variables were most relevant. We selected the least absolute shrinkage and selection operator (LASSO) regression analysis to screen the candidate features. Finally, 8 features that included education, BMI, WC, FPG, total cholesterol (TC), triglyceride (TG), high density lipoprotein cholesterol (HDL-C), and Alanine aminotransferase (ALT) were selected to develop a machine learning model.

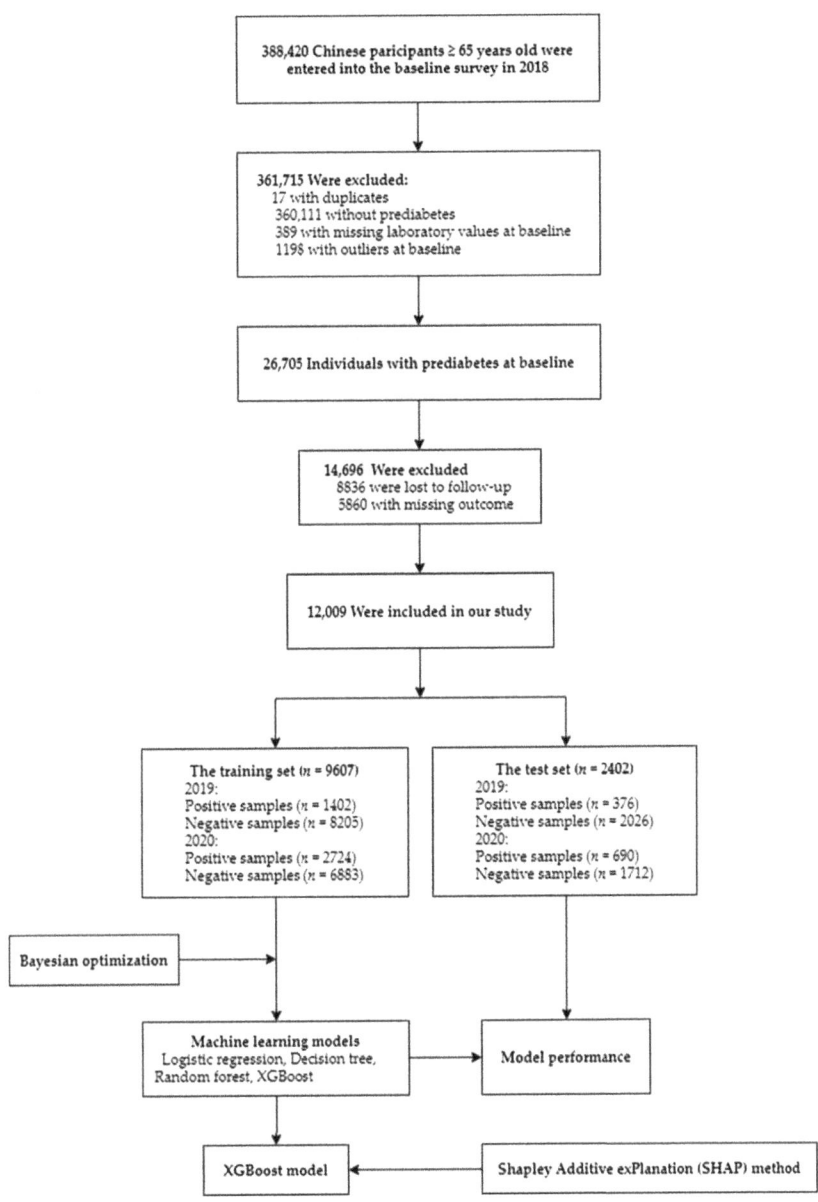

Figure 1. Flowchart of study participants.

2.5. Machine Learning Model Development and Evaluation

The processed data were randomly divided into a training set and a test set in a 4:1 ratio. In order to explore the differences in predictive ability and risk factors between 1-year and 2-year risk of diabetes onset, we constructed machine learning models for two forecast periods. Four machine learning algorithms, including LR, DT, RF, and XGBoost were used to develop models on the training set. LR is a linear model for classification, which predicts a probability value of occurrence of the objective using a sigmoid function and is widely used in biomedicine [12]. A decision tree is a flowchart-like tree structure, where each attribute can represent one internal node in a generated decision tree and has as many branches as its number of different value classes. Moreover, the final leaves of a decision tree represent the decision attribute [13]. Random forest is a supervised learning algorithm that randomly extracts multiple samples from the training set using a bootstrap algorithm and then generates multiple decision trees [14]. The classification results of new instances are determined by taking a majority vote over all the decision trees. XGBoost is an ensemble machine learning algorithm based on decision tree, which was first proposed by Chen and Guestrin [15]. As an optimized implementation of gradient boosting [16], XGBoost shows excellent performance in regression and classification tasks.

Hyperparameters of each model are important for model performance. We performed a 10-fold cross-validation for automated Bayesian optimization with 500 iterations to obtain optimized hyperparameters of each model.

All the machine learning models were assessed for their risk discrimination performance ROC curves on the test set. Multiple indicators containing sensitivity, specificity, accuracy, and F1 score were used to evaluate the predictive ability of four models. We further applied the Shapley Additive exPlanation (SHAP) algorithm to the training set for the model explanation.

2.6. Statistical Analysis

Analysis of statistical description was performed by SAS (version 9.4). Data were expressed as means ± standard deviation (normally distributed) or median (interquartile range) (non-normally distributed). Categorical variables were shown as frequency and percentages. A comparison among groups was conducted by one-way ANOVA, Wilcoxon rank-sum test, or Chi-square test according to the data types. P values were two-tailed and were considered to be significant when they were < 0.05. All model development and optimization were achieved by Python (version 3.11).

3. Results

3.1. Baseline Characteristics of Data Sets Used for the Analysis

The baseline characteristics between the groups of participants with incident diabetes at different time points are presented in Table 1. Within the free health screening project, 12009 elderly prediabetic subjects who met the inclusion criteria were included in our study. All the participants had complete information on demographics, lifestyles, medical history, and laboratory tests. During the two-year follow-up, a total of 3414 individuals progressed to diabetes from prediabetes, and their average annual rate of diabetes progression was 14.21%.

At baseline, the majority of the study population had primary school and lower education levels. The distribution of education was shown in the following categories: primary school and lower: 7456 (62.09%); middle school: 2424 (20.18%); high school:1134 (9.44%); and university and higher: 995 (8.29%). The mean BMI was 24.69 ± 3.42 kg/m^2. The mean WC was 86.02 ± 9.72 cm. The mean FPG was 6.44 ± 0.25 mmol/L. The mean TC was 5.04 ± 1.05 mmol/L. The median TG was 1.34 (0.97). The mean HDL-C was 1.38 ± 0.42 mmol/L, and the median ALT was 18.20 (11.00).

3.2. Performance Comparison between Different Machine Learning Models

Four different machine learning models using LR, DT, RF, and XGBoost were constructed for two forecast periods: 1 and 2 years.

Table 1. Baseline characteristics between the groups of participants with incident diabetes at different time points.

Variables	2019 Without DM (n = 10,231)	2019 DM (n = 1778)	p Value	2020 Without DM (n = 8595)	2020 DM (n = 3414)	p Value
Age (years)	72.06 ± 5.10	72.17 ± 5.22	0.393	72.08 ± 5.13	72.06 ± 5.10	0.813
Gender, n (%)			<0.001			0.018
Male	4536 (83.36)	873 (26.14)		3813 (70.49)	1596 (29.51)	
Female	5695 (86.29)	905 (13.71)		4782 (72.45)	1818 (27.55)	
Education, n (%)			<0.001			<0.001
≤Primary school	6485 (86.98)	971 (13.02)		5529 (74.16)	1927 (25.84)	
Middle school	1990 (82.10)	434 (17.90)		1615 (66.63)	809 (33.37)	
High school	931 (82.10)	203 (17.90)		764 (67.37)	370 (32.63)	
≥University	825 (82.91)	170 (17.09)		687 (69.05)	308 (9.02)	
Marital status, n (%)			0.383			0.897
Married	7762 (84.96)	1374 (15.04)		6541 (71.60)	2595 (28.40)	
Divorced	57 (87.69)	8 (12.31)		44 (67.69)	21 (32.31)	
Widowed	2331 (85.76)	387 (14.24)		1947 (71.63)	771 (28.37)	
Unmarried	81 (90.00)	9 (10.00)		63 (70.00)	27 (30.00)	
Hypertension, n (%)			<0.001			<0.001
No	4893 (87.02)	730 (12.98)		4153 (73.86)	1470 (26.14)	
Yes	5338 (85.39)	1048 (16.41)		4442 (69.56)	1944 (30.44)	
Myocardial infarction, n (%)			0.463			0.298
No	10,177 (85.18)	1771 (14.82)		8555 (71.60)	3393 (28.40)	
Yes	54 (88.52)	7 (11.48)		40 (65.57)	21 (34.43)	
Coronary heart disease, n (%)			0.841			0.144
No	9632 (85.22)	1670 (14.78)		8106 (71.72)	3196 (28.28)	
Yes	599 (84.72)	108 (15.28)		489 (69.17)	218 (30.83)	
Angina pectoris, n (%)			0.828			0.437
No	10,187 (85.19)	1771 (14.81)		8556 (71.55)	3402 (28.45)	
Yes	44 (86.27)	7 (13.73)		39 (76.47)	12 (23.53)	
Fatty liver, n (%)			0.315			0.055
No	9979 (85.25)	1727 (14.75)		8393 (71.70)	3313 (28.30)	
Yes	252 (83.17)	51 (16.83)		202 (66.67)	101 (33.33)	
Exercise, n (%)			0.587			0.455
No	3942 (85.42)	673 (14.58)		3321 (71.96)	1294 (28.04)	
Yes	6289 (85.06)	1105 (14.94)		5274 (71.33)	2120 (28.67)	
Smoking, n (%)			0.705			0.883
No	8804 (85.15)	1536 (14.85)		7403 (71.60)	2937 (28.40)	
Yes	1427 (85.50)	242 (14.50)		1192 (71.42)	477 (28.58)	
Drinking, n (%)			0.295			0.212
No	8544 (85.35)	1467 (14.65)		7188 (71.80)	2823 (28.20)	
Yes	1687 (84.43)	311 (15.57)		1407 (70.42)	591 (29.58)	
BMI (kg/m^2)	24.56 ± 3.41	25.48 ± 3.31	<0.001	24.44 ± 3.42	25.34 ± 3.33	<0.001
WC (cm)	85.57 ± 9.73	88.65 ± 9.23	<0.001	85.20 ± 9.68	88.10 ± 9.52	<0.001
SBP (mmHg)	139.17 ± 19.48	140.30 ± 18.70	0.023	138.96 ± 19.52	140.28 ± 18.96	<0.001
DBP (mmHg)	80.99 ± 11.09	81.57 ± 10.64	0.041	80.86 ± 11.11	81.60 ± 10.79	0.001
FPG (mmol/L)	6.42 ± 0.24	6.54 ± 0.26	<0.001	6.40 ± 0.24	6.52 ± 0.26	<0.001
TC (mmol/L)	5.05 ± 1.05	4.99 ± 1.03	0.021	5.06 ± 1.05	5.00 ± 1.03	0.007
TG (mmol/L)	1.32 (0.96)	1.50 (1.06)	<0.001	1.30 (0.93)	1.48 (1.05)	<0.001
HDL-C (mmol/L)	1.39 ± 0.40	1.34 ± 0.51	<0.001	1.40 ± 0.40	1.33 ± 0.44	<0.001
LDL-C (mmol/L)	2.80 ± 0.92	2.76 ± 1.02	0.147	2.78 ± 0.93	2.81 ± 0.95	0.231
ALT (U/L)	18.00 (11.00)	19.10 (12.00)	<0.001	18.00 (10.90)	19.00 (12.00)	<0.001
AST (U/L)	22.00 (8.30)	22.00 (9.90)	0.797	22.00 (8.30)	22.30 (9.50)	0.034
TBil (μmol/L)	12.80 (6.80)	13.10 (6.20)	0.131	12.80 (6.90)	12.90 (6.50)	0.931
Scr (μmol/L)	77.50 (29.00)	76.90 (29.00)	0.107	78.00 (28.00)	76.00 (29.00)	<0.001
BUN (mmol/L)	5.80 (2.26)	5.70 (2.05)	0.002	5.83 (2.29)	5.67 (2.07)	<0.001
SUA (μmol/L)	332.93 ± 99.46	347.54 ± 95.61	<0.001	333.43 ± 99.44	344.32 ± 97.40	<0.001

Data are shown as means ± standard deviation for normally distributed variables, median (interquartile range) for non-normally distributed variables, and percentages for categorical variables. DM: Diabetes mellitus; BMI: Body mass index; WC: Waist circumference; SBP: Systolic blood pressure; DBP: Diastolic blood pressure; FPG: Fasting plasma glucose; TC: Total cholesterol; TG: Triglyceride; HDL-C: High density lipoprotein cholesterol; LDL-C: Low density lipoprotein cholesterol; ALT: Alanine aminotransferase; AST: Aspartate aminotransferase; TBil: Total bilirubin; Scr: Serum creatinine; BUN: Blood urea nitrogen; SUA: Serum uric acid.

3.2.1. 1-Year Forecast Period

Among these 12009 participants, 1778 (14.81%) had developed diabetes within 1 year after baseline. The performance of the four machine learning models is displayed in Figure 2a and Table 2. All the models obtained the optimal hyperparameters using Bayesian optimization except LR (with default hyperparameters). The XGBoost model performed relatively well (ROC: 0.6742), followed by the RF model (ROC: 0.6697), and the DT model ranked last (ROC: 0.6530). Due to the imbalance ratio reaching 5.75, we identified the optimal threshold using an ROC curve. The XGBoost model showed good sensitivity (0.6569) but relatively poor specificity (0.5972) and accuracy (0.6066). The F1 score of XGBoost ranked second among these models. The confusion matrix of XGBoost is presented in Figure 3a.

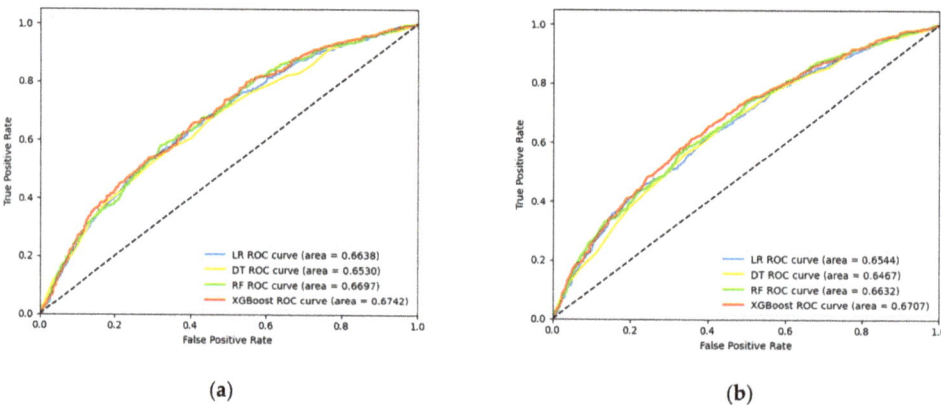

(a) (b)

Figure 2. Receiver operating characteristic (ROC) curves derived for prediction horizon of 1 and 2 years using the four models based logistic regression (LR), decision tree (DT), random forest (RF), and extreme gradient boosting (XGBoost): (a) 1-year forecast period; (b) 2-year forecast period.

Table 2. Performance of four machine learning models for two forecast periods.

Metrics	Machine Learning Models			
	LR	DT	RF	XGBoost
	1-year forecast period			
Sensitivity	0.5559	0.5213	0.5824	0.6569
Specificity	0.6876	0.7004	0.6807	0.5972
Accuracy	0.6669	0.6724	0.6653	0.6066
F1 score	0.3432	0.3325	0.3527	0.3433
	2-year forecast period			
Sensitivity	0.6232	0.5580	0.5754	0.6130
Specificity	0.6016	0.6612	0.6647	0.6443
Accuracy	0.6078	0.6316	0.6391	0.6353
F1 score	0.4772	0.4653	0.4780	0.4913

LR: Logistic regression; DT: Decision tree; RF: Random forest; XGBoost: Extreme gradient boosting.

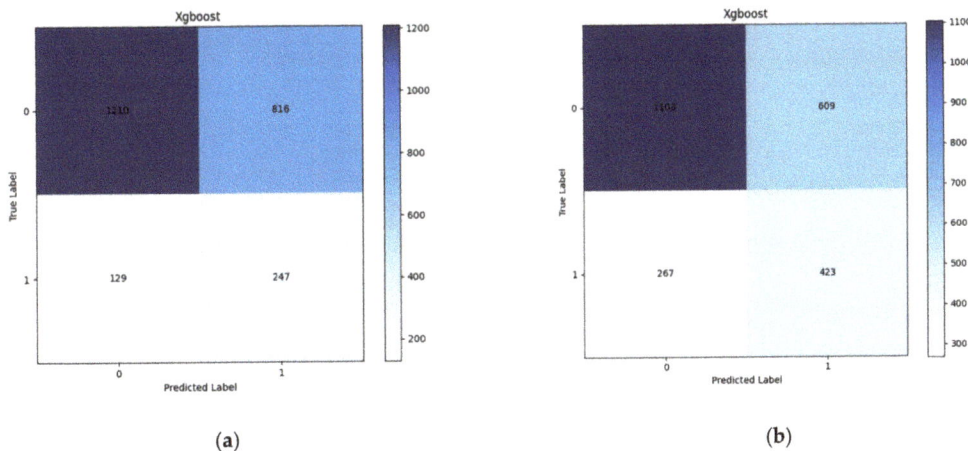

(a) (b)

Figure 3. Confusion matrices derived for prediction horizons of 1 and 2 years based on the extreme gradient boosting (XGBoost): (**a**) 1-year forecast period; (**b**) 2-year forecast period.

3.2.2. 2-Year Forecast Period

The number of incident diabetes reached 3414 (28.43%) during the 2-year follow-up. The performance of the four machine learning models is presented in Figure 2b and Table 2. The ROC value of all models for the 2-year forecast period was lower than for the 1-year forecast period. The XGBoost model still performed relatively efficiently, with a comparatively higher ROC value of 0.6707. The threshold was adjusted again because of an increased number of positive cases. The imbalance ratio decreased to 2.52, and the model for predicting 2-year risk changed accordingly. The optimal threshold was inferred by the ROC curve and increased from 0.14 (1-year forecast period) to 0.30 (2-year forecast period). Compared to the 1-year forecast period, the sensitivity of the XGBoost model decreased, and the specificity and accuracy of XGBoost increased. The F1 score rose to first. The confusion metrix of XGBoost was presented in Figure 3b.

3.3. Analysis of Feature Importance

Taking the XGBoost model with a little higher ROC value (in both forecast periods) and F1 score (in 2-year period) into account, we decided to explain the results of our work based on this machine learning model. To interpret the importance of each feature in the XGBoost model, the ranking of the input features' importance is shown in Figure 4, and the SHAP summary plot is presented in Figure 5. For two different prediction horizons, FPG, TG, and WC ranked consistently among the top three (Figure 4). The SHAP values of most features decreased to some extent during the 2-year forecast period. In view of the fact that Figure 4 can only show the correlation but not the direction of features, Figure 5 could be a good supplement. The red dots in the SHAP summary plot indicated higher feature values, and the blue dots indicated lower feature values. When the SHAP value of features was greater than zero, such as FPG, TG, WC, BMI, and ALT, that suggested that they were risk factors for diabetes onset.

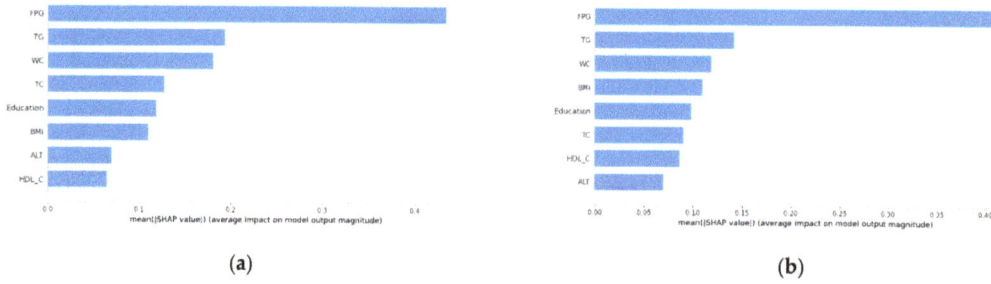

Figure 4. Feature importance in predicting incident diabetes according to the XGBoost model. The Shapley additive explanation (SHAP) algorithm is used to calculate the SHAP value which approximates how much each feature contributes to the average prediction for the dataset. (a) 1-year forecast period. (b) 2-year forecast period.

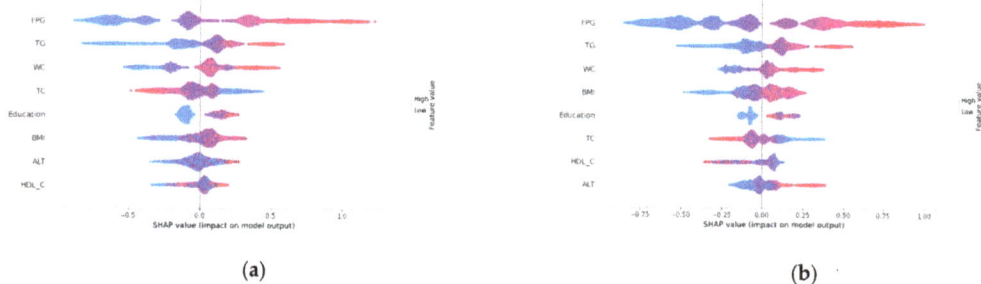

Figure 5. SHAP summary plot of the XGBoost model. (a) 1-year forecast period. (b) 2-year forecast period.

4. Discussion

In this retrospective cohort study, we established and evaluated prediction models for identifying individuals at high risk of progression from prediabetes to diabetes within 1–2 years. The XGBoost model incorporated education, BMI, WC, FPG, TC, TG, HDL-C, and ALT and provided a relatively good classification of risk among all the models overall. However, the discriminatory ability of all models decreased as the forecast period increased. In addition, it was found that there was not much difference in performance among the four models.

In both forecast periods, the XGBoost model performed relatively well. This was not unexpected; the predictive ability of XGBoost has manifested in previous studies of diabetes onset [17] and complications [18]. As an ensemble machine learning algorithm, XGBoost was not affected by the correlation of independent variables, which was exactly the problem that the LR model needed to solve. So, it might be a good choice to use the XGBoost algorithm for modeling in future studies.

Unsurprisingly, consistent with other studies [19–21], FPG was the strongest contributor to the models. We also found that the contribution of WC was higher than that of BMI in both forecast periods, which modestly supports the view that the reliability of BMI for determining obesity, a well-known major risk factor for diabetes, was questioned [22] because BMI did not distinguish fat mass from lean mass [23] and WC represented central obesity.

Notably, the proportion of biomarkers reached 62.5% (5/8) among the features included in the models. This confirmed the finding that risk evaluation constructed based on biomarkers was superior to that based on non-laboratory indicators [24]. The inclusion of biomarkers as input in the machine learning modeling will be a trend in the future.

We acknowledge that the performance of our models was not competitive with results presented in the literature for other relative machine learning research [25–27]. This may, in part, be attributed to the fact that all of the participants were elderly, who generally had several comorbid diseases. The well-known risk factors and biomarkers in elderly individuals were less sensitive to diabetes onset than in younger adults.

The insufficiency of features might also be one of the reasons why our XGBoost model did not perform as well as in other research [28], whose model included 300 features. After all, in addition to demographic and lifestyle, nutrition intake has also been found to be an important predictor of incident diabetes [29]. However, high-dimensional features generally bring about information redundancy and overfitting problem. Considering that our model included only eight features, we thought this level of performance was acceptable.

Even so, to the best of our knowledge, this was the first study to establish models designed for the prediabetes population in mainland China. The majority of previous studies [30–32] focused on the diabetes onset of the general population, ignoring the transitional and high-risk state for the development of diabetes. Given that the proportion of regression to normal glucose levels was much higher than progression towards diabetes among prediabetes [33], changing the screening objects to prediabetes seemed to be more conducive to allocating health resources.

China faces significant disease and economic burdens due to diabetes and its complications [34]. Identifying high-risk groups among prediabetic patients using the predictive machine learning model we proposed could reduce the economic burden of diabetes through the implementation of targeted lifestyle and pharmacological interventions, even more so given the fact that our model was applicable to China's national conditions. Aiming to provide free charge essential health services for all citizens, the central government launched the National Basic Public Health Service Program (BPHS), containing 14 items, of which a vital part was geriatric health services [35]. This implied that under the current health policy, no additional data collection would be needed.

Nevertheless, the present study has some limitations worth noting. The major limitation of the present study is the models' limited performance, which might be related to suboptimal sample sizes and the fewer features. Considering the particularity of our target population, further research should be undertaken to expand the sample size and explore features that are more sensitive to the geriatric population. Second, the number of incident diabetes might be underestimated, for OGTT was not included in the definition of diabetes. However, it is infeasible to use OGTT during a mass free health screening project due to its relatively expensive cost. Moreover, the data used in the study lacked the features known to be diabetes risk factors such as glycosylated hemoglobin and family history of diabetes. In addition, only participants who can be followed up were included in our study. Meanwhile, because developing models could only be based on the participants who reached the follow-up endpoint, we cannot rule out that death could have led to some selection bias. Therefore, the generalization of the research to the whole geriatric population should be cautious. Furthermore, the lack of information on lifestyle changes during follow-up might confound the predictive ability of baseline features. Finally, all the participants included in our study were Chinese, so the predictive model may not be generalizable to other ethnicities.

5. Conclusions

In conclusion, we evaluated the performance of several prediction models using four machine learning algorithms based on the demographic, anthropometric indices, and laboratory results. The XGBoost model might be an effective prediction model, which might perform well in future exploration in this field.

Author Contributions: Conceptualization, Y.G. and Y.Y.; methodology, Y.G. and Y.Y.; software, Y.H. and J.Z.; validation, Q.L., and Q.Z.; formal analysis, Q.Z.; investigation, Y.G and Y.Y.; resources, Y.G. and Y.Y.; data curation, Y.G. and Y.Y.; writing—original draft preparation, Q.Z.; writing—review and editing, Q.L.; visualization, Y.H and Q.Z.; supervision, Y.G. and Y.Y.; project administration, Y.G. and

Y.Y.; funding acquisition, Y.G. and Y.Y. All authors have read and agreed to the published version of the manuscript.

Funding: This research was funded by the Wuhan Center for Disease Control and Prevention, grant number K20-1602-011, and the Health Commission of Hubei Province, grant number WJ2021M137.

Institutional Review Board Statement: The study was conducted in accordance with the Declaration of Helsinki and approved by the Ethics Committee of Wuhan Center for Disease Control and Prevention (protocol code WHCDCIRB-K-2018023).

Informed Consent Statement: Informed consent was obtained from all subjects involved in the study.

Data Availability Statement: The authors confirm that all data underlying the findings are fully available and can be obtained after submitting a request to the corresponding author.

Acknowledgments: We thank all authors who were involved in this study. We are also thankful to Wuhan Center for Disease Control and Prevention for providing the data for analysis.

Conflicts of Interest: The authors declare no conflict of interest.

References

1. International Diabetes Federation. *IDF Diabetes Atlas, 10th ed*; International Diabetes Federation: Brussels, Belgium, 2021.
2. Caspersen, C.J.; Thomas, G.D.; Boseman, L.A.; Beckles, G.L.A.; Albright, A.L. Aging, Diabetes, and the Public Health System in the United States. *Am. J. Public Health* **2012**, *102*, 1482–1497. [CrossRef]
3. Shang, Y.; Marseglia, A.; Fratiglioni, L.; Welmer, A.-K.; Wang, R.; Wang, H.-X.; Xu, W. Natural History of Prediabetes in Older Adults from a Population-based Longitudinal Study. *J. Intern. Med.* **2019**, *286*, 326–340. [CrossRef]
4. Knowler, W.C.; Barrett-Connor, E.; Fowler, S.E.; Hamman, R.F.; Lachin, J.M.; Walker, E.A.; Nathan, D.M. Reduction in the Incidence of Type 2 Diabetes with Lifestyle Intervention or Metformin. *N. Engl. J. Med.* **2002**, *346*, 393–403. [CrossRef] [PubMed]
5. Obermeyer, Z.; Emanuel, E.J. Predicting the Future—Big Data, Machine Learning, and Clinical Medicine. *N. Engl. J. Med.* **2016**, *375*, 1216–1219. [CrossRef] [PubMed]
6. Neves, A.L.; Pereira Rodrigues, P.; Mulla, A.; Glampson, B.; Willis, T.; Darzi, A.; Mayer, E. Using Electronic Health Records to Develop and Validate a Machine-Learning Tool to Predict Type 2 Diabetes Outcomes: A Study Protocol. *BMJ Open* **2021**, *11*, e046716. [CrossRef] [PubMed]
7. Lama, L.; Wilhelmsson, O.; Norlander, E.; Gustafsson, L.; Lager, A.; Tynelius, P.; Wärvik, L.; Östenson, C.-G. Machine Learning for Prediction of Diabetes Risk in Middle-Aged Swedish People. *Heliyon* **2021**, *7*, e07419. [CrossRef]
8. Meng, X.-H.; Huang, Y.-X.; Rao, D.-P.; Zhang, Q.; Liu, Q. Comparison of Three Data Mining Models for Predicting Diabetes or Prediabetes by Risk Factors. *Kaohsiung J. Med. Sci.* **2013**, *29*, 93–99. [CrossRef]
9. Lutsey, P.L.; Pereira, M.A.; Bertoni, A.G.; Kandula, N.R.; Jacobs, D.R. Interactions Between Race/Ethnicity and Anthropometry in Risk of Incident Diabetes: The Multi-Ethnic Study of Atherosclerosis. *Am. J. Epidemiol.* **2010**, *172*, 197–204. [CrossRef]
10. World Health Organization. *International Diabetes Federation Definition and Diagnosis of Diabetes Mellitus and Intermediate Hyperglycaemia*; Report of a WHO/IDF Consultation; World Health Organization: Geneva, Switzerland, 2006.
11. American Diabetes Association Professional Practice Committee 2. Classification and Diagnosis of Diabetes: Standards of Medical Care in Diabetes—2022. *Diabetes Care* **2021**, *45*, S17–S38. [CrossRef]
12. Dreiseitl, S.; Ohno-Machado, L. Logistic Regression and Artificial Neural Network Classification Models: A Methodology Review. *J. Biomed. Inform.* **2002**, *35*, 352–359. [CrossRef]
13. Podgorelec, V.; Kokol, P.; Stiglic, B.; Rozman, I. Decision Trees: An Overview and Their Use in Medicine. *J. Med. Syst.* **2002**, *26*, 445–463. [CrossRef]
14. Breiman, L. Random Forests. *Mach. Learn.* **2001**, *45*, 5–32. [CrossRef]
15. Chen, T.; Guestrin, C. XGBoost: A Scalable Tree Boosting System. In Proceedings of the 22nd ACM SIGKDD International Conference on Knowledge Discovery and Data Mining, San Francisco, CA, USA, 13 August 2016; pp. 785–794.
16. Friedman, J.H. Greedy Function Approximation: A Gradient Boosting Machine. *Ann. Statist.* **2001**, *29*, 1189–1232. [CrossRef]
17. Xue, M.; Su, Y.; Li, C.; Wang, S.; Yao, H. Identification of Potential Type II Diabetes in a Large-Scale Chinese Population Using a Systematic Machine Learning Framework. *J. Diabetes Res.* **2020**, *2020*, 6873891. [CrossRef]
18. Li, W.; Song, Y.; Chen, K.; Ying, J.; Zheng, Z.; Qiao, S.; Yang, M.; Zhang, M.; Zhang, Y. Predictive Model and Risk Analysis for Diabetic Retinopathy Using Machine Learning: A Retrospective Cohort Study in China. *BMJ Open* **2021**, *11*, e050989. [CrossRef]
19. Lai, H.; Huang, H.; Keshavjee, K.; Guergachi, A.; Gao, X. Predictive Models for Diabetes Mellitus Using Machine Learning Techniques. *BMC Endocr. Disord.* **2019**, *19*, 101. [CrossRef]
20. Wu, Y.; Hu, H.; Cai, J.; Chen, R.; Zuo, X.; Cheng, H.; Yan, D. Machine Learning for Predicting the 3-Year Risk of Incident Diabetes in Chinese Adults. *Front. Public Health* **2021**, *9*, 626331. [CrossRef]
21. Cahn, A.; Shoshan, A.; Sagiv, T.; Yesharim, R.; Goshen, R.; Shalev, V.; Raz, I. Prediction of Progression from Pre-diabetes to Diabetes: Development and Validation of a Machine Learning Model. *Diabetes/Metab. Res. Rev.* **2020**, *36*, e3252. [CrossRef]

22. Liu, Y.; Liu, X.; Zhang, S.; Zhu, Q.; Fu, X.; Chen, H.; Guan, H.; Xia, Y.; He, Q.; Kuang, J. Association of Anthropometric Indices With the Development of Diabetes Among Hypertensive Patients in China: A Cohort Study. *Front. Endocrinol.* **2021**, *12*, 736077. [CrossRef]
23. Kopelman, P.G. Obesity as a Medical Problem. *Nature* **2000**, *404*, 635–643. [CrossRef]
24. Ahn, C.H.; Yoon, J.W.; Hahn, S.; Moon, M.K.; Park, K.S.; Cho, Y.M. Evaluation of Non-Laboratory and Laboratory Prediction Models for Current and Future Diabetes Mellitus: A Cross-Sectional and Retrospective Cohort Study. *PLoS ONE* **2016**, *11*, e0156155. [CrossRef]
25. Wang, X.; Zhai, M.; Ren, Z.; Ren, H.; Li, M.; Quan, D.; Chen, L.; Qiu, L. Exploratory Study on Classification of Diabetes Mellitus through a Combined Random Forest Classifier. *BMC Med. Inform. Decis. Mak.* **2021**, *21*, 105. [CrossRef]
26. Deberneh, H.M.; Kim, I. Prediction of Type 2 Diabetes Based on Machine Learning Algorithm. *Int. J. Environ. Res. Public Health* **2021**, *18*, 3317. [CrossRef]
27. Alghamdi, M.; Al-Mallah, M.; Keteyian, S.; Brawner, C.; Ehrman, J.; Sakr, S. Predicting Diabetes Mellitus Using SMOTE and Ensemble Machine Learning Approach: The Henry Ford ExercIse Testing (FIT) Project. *PLoS ONE* **2017**, *12*, e0179805. [CrossRef]
28. Ravaut, M.; Harish, V.; Sadeghi, H.; Leung, K.K.; Volkovs, M.; Kornas, K.; Watson, T.; Poutanen, T.; Rosella, L.C. Development and Validation of a Machine Learning Model Using Administrative Health Data to Predict Onset of Type 2 Diabetes. *JAMA Netw. Open* **2021**, *4*, e2111315. [CrossRef] [PubMed]
29. De Silva, K.; Lim, S.; Mousa, A.; Teede, H.; Forbes, A.; Demmer, R.T.; Jönsson, D.; Enticott, J. Nutritional Markers of Undiagnosed Type 2 Diabetes in Adults: Findings of a Machine Learning Analysis with External Validation and Benchmarking. *PLoS ONE* **2021**, *16*, e0250832. [CrossRef]
30. Zhang, L.; Wang, Y.; Niu, M.; Wang, C.; Wang, Z. Machine Learning for Characterizing Risk of Type 2 Diabetes Mellitus in a Rural Chinese Population: The Henan Rural Cohort Study. *Sci. Rep.* **2020**, *10*, 4406. [CrossRef]
31. Zou, Q.; Qu, K.; Luo, Y.; Yin, D.; Ju, Y.; Tang, H. Predicting Diabetes Mellitus With Machine Learning Techniques. *Front. Genet.* **2018**, *9*, 515. [CrossRef]
32. Xiong, X.; Zhang, R.; Bi, Y.; Zhou, W.; Yu, Y.; Zhu, D. Machine Learning Models in Type 2 Diabetes Risk Prediction: Results from a Cross-Sectional Retrospective Study in Chinese Adults. *Curr. Med. Sci.* **2019**, *39*, 582–588. [CrossRef]
33. Lazo-Porras, M.; Bernabe-Ortiz, A.; Ruiz-Alejos, A.; Smeeth, L.; Gilman, R.H.; Checkley, W.; Málaga, G.; Miranda, J.J. Regression from Prediabetes to Normal Glucose Levels Is More Frequent than Progression towards Diabetes: The CRONICAS Cohort Study. *Diabetes Res. Clin. Pract.* **2020**, *163*, 107829. [CrossRef]
34. Mao, W.; Yip, C.-M.W.; Chen, W. Complications of Diabetes in China: Health System and Economic Implications. *BMC Public Health* **2019**, *19*, 269. [CrossRef] [PubMed]
35. Tang, D.; Wang, J. Basic Public Health Service Utilization by Internal Older Adult Migrants in China. *Int. J. Environ. Res. Public Health* **2021**, *18*, 270. [CrossRef] [PubMed]

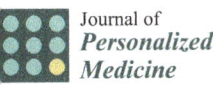

Article

Predicting the Risk of Incident Type 2 Diabetes Mellitus in Chinese Elderly Using Machine Learning Techniques

Qing Liu [1,†], Miao Zhang [1,†], Yifeng He [2], Lei Zhang [3], Jingui Zou [2], Yaqiong Yan [4] and Yan Guo [4,*]

1. Department of Epidemiology, School of Public Health, Wuhan University, Wuhan 430071, China; liuqing@whu.edu.cn (Q.L.); zhangmiao@whu.edu.cn (M.Z.)
2. School of Geodesy and Geomatics, Wuhan University, Wuhan 430079, China; heyifeng@whu.edu.cn (Y.H.); jgzou@sgg.whu.edu.cn (J.Z.)
3. School of Mathematics and Statistics, Wuhan University, Wuhan 430070, China; chris_lei@whu.edu.cn
4. Wuhan Center for Disease Control and Prevention, Wuhan 430015, China; yanyyq@whcdc.org
* Correspondence: swallow315@whcdc.org
† These authors contributed equally to this work.

Abstract: Early identification of individuals at high risk of diabetes is crucial for implementing early intervention strategies. However, algorithms specific to elderly Chinese adults are lacking. The aim of this study is to build effective prediction models based on machine learning (ML) for the risk of type 2 diabetes mellitus (T2DM) in Chinese elderly. A retrospective cohort study was conducted using the health screening data of adults older than 65 years in Wuhan, China from 2018 to 2020. With a strict data filtration, 127,031 records from the eligible participants were utilized. Overall, 8298 participants were diagnosed with incident T2DM during the 2-year follow-up (2019–2020). The dataset was randomly split into training set ($n = 101,625$) and test set ($n = 25,406$). We developed prediction models based on four ML algorithms: logistic regression (LR), decision tree (DT), random forest (RF), and extreme gradient boosting (XGBoost). Using LASSO regression, 21 prediction features were selected. The Random under-sampling (RUS) was applied to address the class imbalance, and the Shapley Additive Explanations (SHAP) was used to calculate and visualize feature importance. Model performance was evaluated by the area under the receiver operating characteristic curve (AUC), sensitivity, specificity, and accuracy. The XGBoost model achieved the best performance (AUC = 0.7805, sensitivity = 0.6452, specificity = 0.7577, accuracy = 0.7503). Fasting plasma glucose (FPG), education, exercise, gender, and waist circumference (WC) were the top five important predictors. This study showed that XGBoost model can be applied to screen individuals at high risk of T2DM in the early phrase, which has the strong potential for intelligent prevention and control of diabetes. The key features could also be useful for developing targeted diabetes prevention interventions.

Keywords: type 2 diabetes mellitus (T2DM); machine learning; prediction model; Chinese elderly

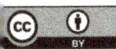

1. Introduction

Diabetes mellitus (DM) is a chronic metabolic disease characterized by hyperglycemia, which can lead to serious complications such as chronic kidney disease, acute kidney injury, cardiovascular disease, ischemic heart disease, stroke, or even death [1]. Type 2 diabetes mellitus (T2DM) is the most common type of diabetes, accounting for around 90% of all diabetes cases. According to the report of the International Diabetes Federation (IDF) in 2021, about 537 million people worldwide are suffering from diabetes and the figure is projected to rise to 643 million by 2030 and 783 million by 2045 [2]. In China, it was estimated that there were 140.9 million adults living with diabetes, accounting for 25% of patients with diabetes worldwide [3]. The rising incidence of diabetes imposes a heavy burden on individual, health system, and the whole society [4,5].

T2DM is an irreversible but preventable disease [6]. Early diagnosis and effective screening of high-risk populations can prevent or delay the occurrence or development of

T2DM and related complications [7]. Therefore, it is critical to establish an effective prediction model to assess individuals' risk of T2DM, which would help the early identification of individuals at high risk of T2DM.

Machine learning (ML) is a subfield of artificial intelligence (AI) in computer science, which uses data-driven techniques to reveal patterns and predict behavior [8,9]. In recent years, machine learning techniques have been widely applied in the medical and health field, which have proven to be accurate and efficient in disease diagnosis, treatment, and prognosis [10,11]. There are many barriers to predict the risk of diabetes, because most of the medical data are nonlinear, nonnormal, correlation structured, and complex in nature [12]. Compared with traditional statistical methods, machine learning algorithms could learn the complex non-linear interactions between risk factors by minimizing errors between predicted and observed outcomes [13]. Predictive models based on machine learning algorithms can be useful in the identification of patients with diabetes and help discover hidden patterns in risk factors of diabetes that might be missed [14]. Numerous machine learning algorithms have been utilized for the prediction of T2DM, such as logistic regression (LR) [15], support vector machines (SVM) [16], artificial neural network (ANN) [17], k-nearest neighbors (KNN) [18], decision tree (DT) [19], random forest (RF) [20], and extreme gradient boosting (XGBoost) [21]. A recent meta-analysis confirmed the good discrimination ability of machine learning models to predict T2DM in community settings, suggesting that artificial neural network performed best, followed by logistic regression, decision trees, and random forests [22]. Xie et al. constructed several machine learning models for T2DM prediction using cross-sectional data of 138,146 participants in the United States, and the experimental results showed the neural network model gave the best model performance with the highest area under the receiver operating characteristic (AUC) value of 0.7949 [23]. The study of Katarya et al. based on Pima Indian diabetes dataset found that random forest performed the best with 0.84 accuracy and 0.83 AUC [24]. Adua et al. developed four machine learning classification algorithms (Naïve-Bayes (NB), KNN, SVM, and DT) to screen for T2DM in an African population, in Ghana, and concluded that NB algorithm performed best with the AUC of 0.87 [25]. A study in Luzhou, China utilized four ML algorithms to build prediction models of diabetes mellitus by using hospital physical examination data, and it revealed that random forest was the best performing model with the highest accuracy of 0.8084 [26]. A cross-sectional study in Urumqi, China based on the national physical examination data reported that XGBoost was the best classifier with AUC of 0.9680 [27]. Obviously, prior studies demonstrated different results in T2DM prediction even using the same machine learning algorithms [28]. Despite the extensive research on T2DM prediction, there were existing obstacles to applying prior prediction models, due to the disparity of study population, the difference of data sources, as well as the unsatisfactory power of those predictive models [29]. Thus, further studies including larger samples and elderly adults are still required to facilitate the research in this area.

This study aimed to build effective prediction models for the risk of incident T2DM among Chinese elderly adults based on four machine learning algorithms: logistic regression (LR), decision tree (DT), random forest (RF), and extreme gradient boosting (XGBoost). The purpose of this study was to provide evidence supporting the prevention and control of diabetes.

2. Materials and Methods

2.1. Study Design and Participants

A retrospective cohort study was conducted using the health screening data of adults older than 65 years from 17 districts in Wuhan, China. The Wuhan Municipal Government would provide free physical examinations for the elderly aged 65 and above, which was regarded as a normalized and standardized project to benefit people. A total of 388,420 elderly people participated in the health screening in 2018. The protocol was approved by the Ethics Committee of Wuhan Center for Disease Control and Prevention (protocol code WHCDCIRB-K-2018023), and written informed consent was obtained from each participant. Baseline data were collected in 2018, and follow-up data were collected in 2019 and 2020. For longitudinal analysis of incident T2DM, excluding criteria of participants were: (1) Participants with prevalent T2DM at baseline (participants diagnosed by a fasting plasma glucose ≥7.0 mmol/L or with a self-reported previous diagnosis by health care professionals at baseline); (2) those who lost to follow-up; (3) those with duplicate data; (4) those with missing laboratory values; (5) those with outliers. After applying the exclusion criteria, a total of 127,031 participants were included in this study. The study flow chart is depicted in Figure 1.

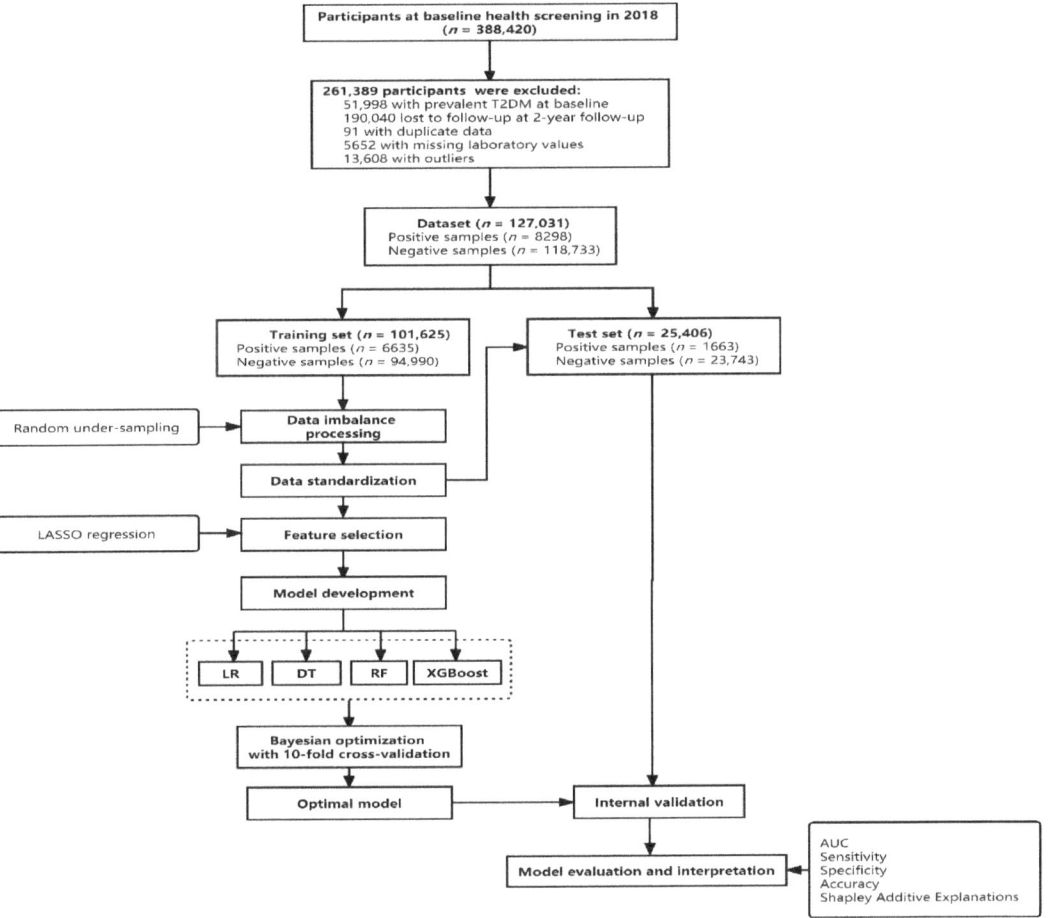

Figure 1. The study flow chart. LR, logistic regression; DT, decision tree; RF, random forest; XGBoost, extreme gradient boosting; LASSO, least absolute shrinkage and selection operator.

2.2. Candidate Predictors

The health screening data were collected and recorded at the local community health service centers in Wuhan by well-trained research staff. It included three parts: a health status questionnaire, anthropometric measures, and laboratory measures. The questionnaire included age, gender, education, marital status, medical history (hypertension, myocardial infarction, coronary heart disease, angina pectoris, fatty liver), exercise, current smoking, current drinking. Anthropometric measures were conducted by trained medical staff using standardized procedures, including weight, height, waist circumference (WC), systolic blood pressure (SBP), and diastolic blood pressure (DBP). Body mass index (BMI) was calculated as weight (kg) divided by height squared (m^2). Laboratory measures were performed at the central laboratory, including fasting plasma glucose (FPG), total cholesterol (TC), triglyceride (TG), high-density lipoprotein (HDL-C), low-density lipoprotein (LDL-C), alanine aminotransferase (ALT), aspartate transaminase (AST), total bilirubin (TBIL), serum creatinine (Scr), blood urea nitrogen (BUN), serum uric acid (SUA). The 27 candidate predictors from the health screening baseline data (Table 1) have been carefully selected based on the available variables in our dataset, clinical expertise, and prior literature evidence of their associations with T2DM [30–32].

Table 1. Baseline characteristics of the participants.

Characteristics	Total (n = 127,031)	Incident T2DM Yes (n = 8298)	Incident T2DM No (n = 118,733)	p-Value
Age, mean (SD), years	71.94 (5.10)	72.39 (5.31)	71.91 (5.08)	<0.001
Gender, n (%)				<0.001
Men	56,774 (44.69)	4114 (7.25)	52,660 (92.75)	
Women	70,257 (55.31)	4184 (5.96)	66,073 (94.04)	
Education, n (%)				<0.001
Elementary school and below	75,828 (59.69)	5597 (7.38)	70,231 (92.62)	
Junior high school	28,298 (22.28)	1522 (5.38)	26,776 (94.62)	
Technical secondary school or high school	13,742 (10.82)	695 (5.06)	13,047 (94.94)	
Junior college and above	9163 (7.21)	484 (5.28)	8679 (94.72)	
Marital status, n (%)				<0.001
Married	98,131 (77.25)	6046 (6.16)	92,085 (93.84)	
Divorced	656 (0.52)	48 (7.32)	608 (92.68)	
Widowed	27,350 (21.53)	2082 (7.61)	25,268 (92.39)	
Single	894 (0.70)	122 (13.65)	772 (86.35)	
Hypertension, n (%)				<0.001
Yes	56,847 (44.75)	4347 (7.65)	52,500 (92.35)	
No	70,184 (55.25)	3951 (5.63)	66,233 (94.37)	
Myocardial infarction, n (%)				0.621
Yes	686 (0.54)	48 (7.00)	638 (93.00)	
No	126,345 (99.46)	8250 (6.53)	118,095 (93.47)	
Coronary heart disease, n (%)				0.413
Yes	7471 (5.88)	505 (6.76)	6966 (93.24)	
No	119,560 (94.12)	7793 (6.52)	111,767 (93.48)	
Angina pectoris, n (%)				0.711
Yes	506 (0.40)	31 (6.13)	475 (93.87)	
No	126,525 (99.60)	8267 (6.53)	118,258 (93.47)	
Fatty liver, n (%)				0.020
Yes	2279 (1.79)	176 (7.72)	2103 (92.28)	
No	124,752 (98.21)	8122 (6.51)	116,630 (93.49)	
Exercise, n (%)				<0.001
Yes	74,741 (58.84)	4323 (5.78)	70,418 (94.22)	
No	52,290 (41.16)	3975 (7.60)	48,315 (92.40)	
Current smoking, n (%)				<0.001
Yes	20,498 (16.14)	1515 (7.39)	18,983 (92.61)	
No	106,533 (83.86)	6783 (6.37)	99,750 (93.63)	

Table 1. Cont.

Characteristics	Total (n = 127,031)	Incident T2DM Yes (n = 8298)	Incident T2DM No (n = 118,733)	p-Value
Current drinking, n (%)				0.908
Yes	21,429 (16.87)	1396 (6.51)	20,033 (93.49)	
No	105,602 (83.13)	6902 (6.54)	98,700 (93.46)	
BMI, mean (SD), kg/m^2	23.70 (3.26)	24.47 (3.51)	23.65 (3.24)	<0.001
WC, mean (SD), cm	84.12 (9.16)	86.30 (9.62)	83.97 (9.10)	<0.001
SBP, mean (SD), mm Hg	137.12 (20.00)	140.63 (20.38)	136.87 (19.95)	<0.001
DBP, mean (SD), mm Hg	80.09 (11.20)	81.63 (11.42)	79.99 (11.18)	<0.001
FPG, mean (SD), mmol/L	5.12 (0.69)	5.71 (0.79)	5.08 (0.66)	<0.001
TC, median (IQR), mmol/L	4.81 (4.20–5.45)	4.84 (4.20–5.49)	4.81 (4.20–5.44)	0.034
TG, median (IQR), mmol/L	1.17 (0.85–1.63)	1.28 (0.90–1.79)	1.16 (0.85–1.62)	<0.001
HDL-C, median (IQR), mmol/L	1.36 (1.15–1.62)	1.32 (1.11–1.58)	1.37 (1.15–1.62)	<0.001
LDL-C, median (IQR), mmol/L	2.60 (2.08–3.17)	2.64 (2.11–3.24)	2.60 (2.07–3.16)	<0.001
ALT, median (IQR), U/L	16.00 (12.00–21.00)	17.00 (13.00–23.00)	16.00 (12.00–20.90)	<0.001
AST, median (IQR), U/L	21.50 (18.00–26.00)	22.00 (18.00–26.00)	21.50 (18.00–26.00)	0.004
TBIL, median (IQR), μmol/L	11.90 (9.17–15.30)	12.40 (9.50–15.90)	11.90 (9.10–15.30)	<0.001
Scr, mean (SD), μmol/L	76.82 (19.93)	79.21 (20.94)	76.66 (19.85)	<0.001
BUN, median (IQR), mmol/L	5.71 (4.76–6.82)	5.67 (4.70–6.80)	5.71 (4.77–6.83)	0.037
SUA, mean (SD), μmol/L	323.80 (91.90)	333.01 (94.31)	323.15 (91.70)	<0.001

SD, standard deviation; IQR: Q1–Q3 values; T2DM, type 2 diabetes mellitus; BMI, body mass index; WC, waist circumference; SBP, systolic blood pressure; DBP, diastolic blood pressure; FBG, fasting plasma glucose; TC, total cholesterol; TG, triglycerides; HDL-C, high-density lipoprotein cholesterol; LDL-C, low-density lipoprotein cholesterol; ALT, alanine aminotransferase; AST, aspartate transaminase; TBIL, total bilirubin; Scr, serum creatinine; BUN, blood urea nitrogen; SUA, serum uric acid.

2.3. Outcome

Incident type 2 diabetes mellitus (T2DM) was diagnosed if at least one of the following two criteria were satisfied according to the American Diabetes Association (ADA): (1) a self-reported diagnosis that was determined previously by a health care professional, or (2) fasting plasma glucose (FPG) ≥ 126 mg/dL (7.0 mmol/L) [33]. In this study, self-reported T2DM was defined by asking participants whether a health care professional had ever told that he/she was diagnosed with diabetes. Fasting blood samples were collected after at least 8 h of overnight fasting and were analyzed by trained research staff at the central laboratory. Fasting plasma glucose (FPG) levels were measured using the glucose oxidase procedure.

2.4. Machine Learning Algorithms

2.4.1. Logistic Regression (LR)

LR is a classic classification algorithm that measures the relationship between a categorical dependent variable and one or more independent variables based on the sigmoid function [34]. This algorithm is a simple method for prediction which provides baseline accuracy scores to compare with other non-parametric machine learning models [14,35].

2.4.2. Decision Tree (DT)

DT is a supervised learning technique used for a classification task. A decision tree is a class discrimination tree structure, with each internal node representing an attribute (or independent variable), each branch reflecting an outcome of the test, and each leaf node corresponding to a class label (or dependent variable) [11]. The purpose of DT is to generate a decision tree with strong generalization capability [36].

2.4.3. Random Forest (RF)

RF is a typical ensemble learning algorithm that consists of multiple decision trees [37]. It can be applied to deal with regression and classification tasks. The algorithm is based on the idea of incorporating multiple decision tree classifiers to obtain the final classification result by majority voting and make accurate predictions [38]. RF can analyze complex interactions between characteristics, and is extremely adept at handling noisy and missing data [29].

2.4.4. Extreme Gradient Boosting (XGBoost)

XGBoost is an advanced ensemble algorithm, which was proposed by Chen and Guestrin in 2016 [39]. It is a scalable machine learning technique for tree boosting that can combine a series of weak classifiers to construct a stronger classifier. This classifier is an optimized implementation of the gradient boosting decision tree (GBDT) and has the advantages of high training speed, excellent performance, and can deal with large-scale data.

2.5. Model Development

The dataset was randomly split into two parts: the training set accounted for 80% ($n = 101,625$) and the test set accounted for 20% ($n = 25,406$). Since the categories of the incident T2DM in the dataset were imbalanced, the Random under-sampling (RUS) was applied to the training set to resolve the effect of class imbalance. In order to standardize the input features, the data were normalized using the Python Sklearn library [40]. The training set was standardized to mean 0 and variance 1 using the StandardScaler function from the Sklearn preprocessing library in Python, and the test set was standardized using the mean and standard deviation of the training dataset. Least Absolute Shrinkage and Selection Operator (LASSO) regression was used for feature selection in the training set to construct the prediction models. LASSO is a regression model that penalizes the absolute sizes of the coefficients, resulting in the disappearance of some regression coefficients [41]. The candidates with non-zero coefficients are selected during the feature selection. We used LASSO regression with all candidate variables to screen the final input features for the prediction models.

We trained the logistic regression (LR), decision tree (DT), and random forest (RF) models implemented using the Python Sklearn package [42]. The extreme gradient boosting (XGBoost) was implemented using the Xgboost package [39]. The input variables were the 21 features selected by LASSO regression (Table 2). For the DT, RF, and XGBoost algorithms, Bayesian optimization with 10-fold cross-validation was performed on the training set to tune the hyperparameters. Bayesian optimization was proposed by Snoek et al. [43], which has demonstrated to outperform most global optimization algorithms on benchmark functions. It has become extremely popular for tuning hyperparameters in machine learning algorithms [44]. Bayesian optimization keeps track of the previous evaluation results of the objective function and uses them to create a surrogate model such as Gaussian process which was used to find out the most optimal hyperparameters [45]. After sufficient evaluations of the objective function until reaching maximum iterations, the surrogate function becomes an accurate model for the actual objective function and the set of hyperparameters selected is optimal [46]. After 500 iterations, we find the final optimal hyperparameters of DT, RF, and XGBoost. The best hyperparameters for DT were as followed: max_depth = 19, max_features = 7, min_samples_leaf = 55, min_samples_split = 10, min_weight_fraction_ leaf = 0.031159281996108103. The best hyperparameters for RF were as followed: max_depth = 68, max_features = 8, n_estimators = 80, min_samples_leaf = 5, min_samples_split = 69, min_weight_ fraction_ leaf = 0.0009215045821160297. The best hyperparameters for XGBoost were as followed: colsample_bytree = 0.6907621204231386, gamma = 0.6991315172625473, learning_rate = 0.093311071904797607, max_depth = 3, min_child_weight = 30, reg_alpha = 0.9430563747862351, reg_lambda = 0.7001632991135449, subsample = 0.5957497121054272.

Table 2. Least Absolute Shrinkage and Selection Operator (LASSO) regression coefficients.

Predictors	Coefficient
Age	0.012
Gender	−0.026
Education	−0.027
Marital status	0.023
Hypertension	0.010
Exercise	−0.035
Current smoking	0.017
Current drinking	−0.010
WC	0.033
SBP	0.014
FPG	0.219
TC	−0.022
TG	0.020
HDL-C	0.006
LDL-C	0.009
ALT	0.037
AST	−0.026
TBIL	0.006
Scr	0.004
BUN	−0.017
SUA	−0.002

2.6. Model Evaluation

The performances of the prediction models were evaluated on the test set using tuned hyperparameters. The area under receiver operating characteristic (AUC), sensitivity, specificity, and accuracy were used to evaluate the classification performance. Sensitivity indicates the proportion of positive sets being predicted correctly, and the specificity represents the proportion of negative sets being predicted correctly. Accuracy illustrates the correct prediction of both positive and negative sets. A receiver operating characteristic (ROC) curve was drawn with the true positive rate (sensitivity) as the ordinate and the false positive rate (1-specificity) as the abscissa, which indicates the overall performance of a binary classifier system. AUC was calculated from the ROC curve. The performance metrics were calculated as follows:

$$\text{Sensitivity} = TP/(TP + FN) \tag{1}$$

$$\text{Specificity} = TN/(FP + TN) \tag{2}$$

$$\text{Accuracy} = (TP + TN)/(TP + FP + TN + FN) \tag{3}$$

Here, TP, FN, FP, and TN represent true positive, false negative, false positive, and true negative, respectively.

2.7. Model Interpretation

For further model interpretation, the Shapley Additive Explanations (SHAP) was used. SHAP is a method proposed by Lundberg and Lee in 2017, which is widely used in the interpretation of various classification and regression models [47]. In this method, the features are ranked by their contribution to the model, and the relationship between features and the outcome can be visualized. The model would produce a predicted value for each sample, and the SHAP value represented the value allocated to each feature in the sample. Its absolute value reflects the influence of the feature, and its positive or negative reflects its positive or negative effect on the predicted risk of incident T2DM. When the SHAP value > 0, it indicated that the feature contributed to a higher risk of incident T2DM; On the contrary, when the SHAP value < 0, it indicated that the feature contributed to a lower risk of incident T2DM [48].

2.8. Statistical Analysis

Data analyses were performed using SAS version 9.4 and Python version 3.10. Baseline characteristics were summarized as means ± SD (standard deviation) for normally distributed continuous variables, as median and interquartile range (IQR) for non-normally distributed continuous variables, and as numbers and percentage for categorical variables. Students' t test and Wilcoxon test were used to compare normal and non-normal continuous variables respectively and Chi-square tests or Fisher's exact test were used to compare categorical variables between subgroups. The statistical significance level was set at p-value < 0.05 (two-sided). To implement the ML algorithms, we used the Python sklearn package [42] and the Xgboost package [39].

3. Results

3.1. Baseline Characteristics

Table 1 demonstrated the participants' baseline characteristics. A total of 127,031 eligible participants were included in this study, which consisted of 8298 incident T2DM and 118,733 non-T2DM. The mean age of study participants was 71.94 ± 5.10 years old. The results showed that age, gender, education, marital status, hypertension, fatty liver, exercise, current smoking, BMI, WC, SBP, DBP, FPG, TC, TG, HDL-C, LDL-C, ALT, AST, TBIL, Scr, BUN, and SUA were all significantly associated with incident T2DM ($p < 0.05$).

3.2. Features Selected by LASSO Regression

Table 2 presented the results of the LASSO regression. Finally, 21 features were significantly associated with incident T2DM, including age, gender, education, marital status, hypertension, exercise, current smoking, current drinking, WC, SBP, FPG, TC, TG, HDL-C, LDL-C, ALT, AST, TBIL, Scr, BUN, and SUA.

3.3. Comparison of the Model Performance

Table 3 presented the results of performance of four machine learning models. The ROC curves on the training set and test set are shown in Figure 2. Overall, the XGBoost model performed best with the highest AUC value of 0.7805 on the test set, and the sensitivity, specificity, and accuracy were 0.6452, 0.7577, and 0.7503, respectively. The confusion matrix of the four machine learning models is presented in Figure 3.

Table 3. Comparison of performance of the four machine learning models.

Model	AUC	Sensitivity	Specificity	Accuracy
LR	0.7601	0.6320	0.7636	0.7550
DT	0.7280	0.5821	0.7633	0.7514
RF	0.7772	0.6428	0.7524	0.7453
XGBoost	0.7805	0.6452	0.7577	0.7503

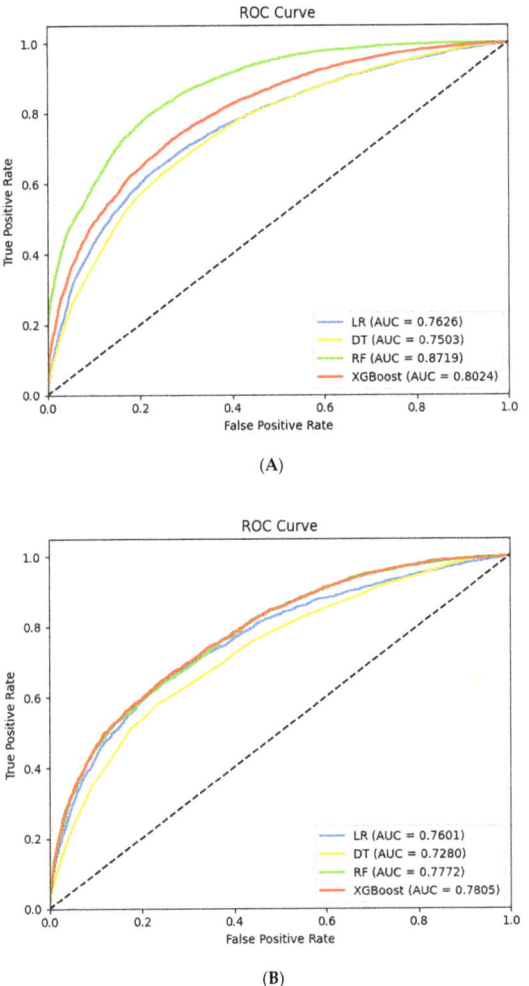

Figure 2. The receiver operating characteristics (ROC) curves of the four machine learning models on the training set (**A**) and test set (**B**).

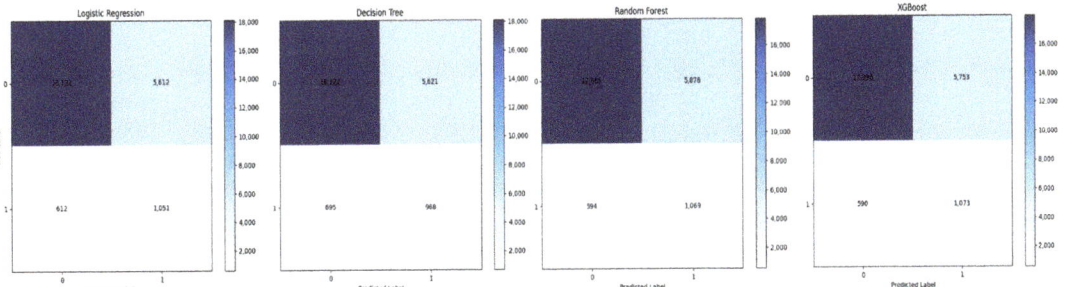

Figure 3. The confusion matrix of the four machine learning models.

3.4. Feature Importance

In this study, XGBoost performed the best out of the four models. Figure 4 presented the contributions of the 21 features on the XGBoost model output ranked by the average absolute SHAP value. FPG, education, exercise, gender, and WC were the top five important features. The SHAP values of FPG, WC, ALT, marital status, SBP, TG, hypertension, TBIL, age, smoking, Scr, and LDL-C were greater than 0, which suggested that these features were significant risk factors for incident T2DM.

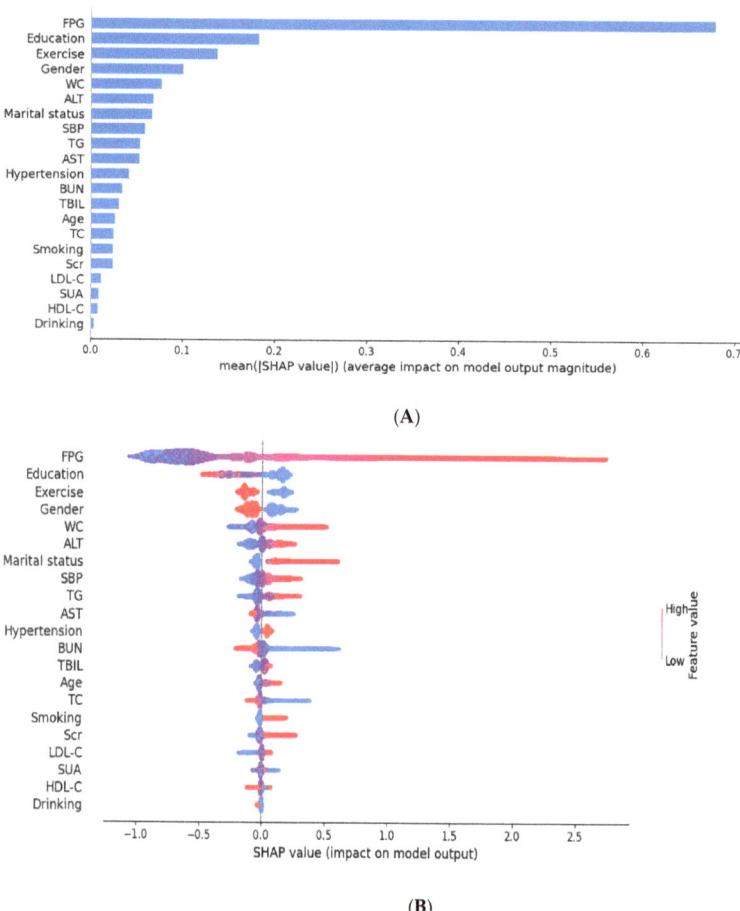

Figure 4. The interpretations for the XGBoost model. (**A**): The feature importance ranking by the SHAP value; (**B**): SHAP summary plot of the XGBoost model. Each dot represents a sample, with blue indicating a low feature value and red indicating a high feature value. The higher the SHAP value of a feature, the higher the risk of incident T2DM. Smoking was defined as current smoking; drinking was defined as current drinking.

4. Discussion

In this retrospective study, we applied four machine learning algorithms to build prediction models for the risk of incident T2DM among Chinese elderly. It is found that the XGBoost model with 21 features demonstrated the best performance for predicting T2DM. This suggested that the prediction model derived in the present study could be applied to screen out individuals at high risk of T2DM, which could benefit the prevention and control of diabetes.

To date, the research of diabetes prediction models tended to focus on white populations [49–52], and Asian populations especially for the elderly have received relatively little attention. This study utilized a large longitudinal dataset obtained from Chinese elderly to establish prediction models for T2DM. The prediction results confirmed that the XGBoost model performed best with the highest AUC value of 0.7805 in predicting the probability that an individual develops T2DM. It was a good example of success for the XGBoost's application in the research of diabetes risk prediction. This finding was consistent with earlier studies [14,21,27,53], which identified the good prediction power of the XGBoost model, with AUC values ranging from 0.8300 to 0.9680. Different from this study, a previous Korean population-based cohort study demonstrated that the ensemble models (e.g., stacking classifier) had better performance than the single models including XGBoost [54]. A rural cohort study in Henan province of China showed good predictive efficiency for the prediction models of T2DM, with AUC values ranging from 0.811 to 0.872 using laboratory data [55]. Compared with previous research, the AUC value in this study was relatively not satisfactory enough. A potential reason could be due to the differences of the study population and input features in the models, which could impact the predictive performance to some extent. Different from our study, the study population of prior studies [14,21,27,53] were middle-aged adults and fewer predictors were applied in the prediction of diabetes. To our knowledge, this was the first study that targeted the elderly population ($\geq$65 years) in China to build predictive models for diabetes using machine learning techniques, which would have great implications for designing diabetes prevention focusing on the elderly. With the development of artificial intelligence, machine learning techniques have been widely applied in the medical field, especially for prediction models for diabetes [49,51,53,56–58]. It is worth noting that the advantages of machine learning models are well-documented empirically compared with traditional statistical methods, but its disadvantage is the lack of model interpretability [13]. XGBoost was often considered as a black box model, because it tends to have better accuracy for predictions compared with linear models while it loses the model interpretability at the same time [39]. Thus, we applied the Shapley Additive Explanations (SHAP) method developed by Lundberg and Lee [47] to better explain the contribution of each feature to the model. This is crucial for healthcare workers to get over the model interpretability barrier to apply predictive models in clinical practice.

Notably, the results of the feature importance analysis indicated the contribution of different feature to the model. These features such as FPG, education, exercise, gender, WC, etc., made substantial contributions to the prediction model. This was in accordance with the results observed in prior similar research [14,53,59]. Early identification of key risk factors had important implications for the risk assessment and prevention of diabetes. Our model results identified that FPG was the most significant predictor of T2DM. Individuals with higher blood glucose would have a greater likelihood of developing diabetes. An explanation for this was that hyperglycemia was correlated with insulin resistance [60]. As mentioned in the literature review, blood glucose was the main traditionally diabetes predictor and also widely used for diagnosis of diabetes [61]. This indicated that blood glucose control plays a key role in the prevention of T2DM, especially for the elderly.

As is shown in the present study, education and exercise showed negative associations with the risk of incident T2DM. Several studies have suggested that diabetes is associated with a low level of education [62–66]. A cohort study among American adults has confirmed that educational level was linked to the onset of diabetes [66]. Individuals with less than a high school educational level (hazard rate [HR] 1.58; 95% CI, 1.26–1.97) were more likely to develop diabetes. It is possible that people with higher education would have better health literacy, so they paid more attention to health management to prevent diabetes [65]. Prior studies have also noted the key role of exercise [67,68] and found that exercise intervention could decrease the risk of developing diabetes by 46% [68]. The China Da Qing Diabetes

Prevention Study has identified the long-term effects of exercise interventions in reducing the incidence of T2DM [67]. It was shown that exercise intervention groups had a 49% decreased incidence of T2DM (hazard rate ratio [HRR], 0.51; 95% CI, 0.31–0.83) over the past two decades. There is need for implementing diabetes prevention programs, emphasizing the importance of regular exercise, and focusing particularly on lower educated populations. In our study, another interesting finding was that men were more likely to develop T2DM compared to women, which agreed with results from earlier studies [69,70]. Previous meta-analysis also demonstrated that gender was a dependent risk factor of T2DM in mainland China [71]. It found that the female gender (odds ratio [OR], 0.87, 95% CI, 0.78–0.97) was significantly negatively associated with the risk of T2DM. This could be explained by the fact that most risk factors (e.g., smoking and alcohol consumption, and physical inactivity) were more prevalent in men than women [72]. Therefore, more attention should be paid to men. As a measure of central/abdominal obesity, WC was also proved to be a strong predictor of T2DM. The significance of WC has been illustrated in other studies [17,73]. A 13-year prospective cohort study reported that a higher WC was linked to an increased risk of diabetes and the age-adjusted relative risks (RRs) across quintiles of WC were 1.0, 2.0, 2.7, 5.0, and 12.0, respectively [74]. Our findings further supported that the routine measurement of waist circumference would help clinical workers make preventive recommendations for individuals at high risk of diabetes.

Diabetes has become a major human health challenge and a global health burden because of its high morbidity and mortality rates [75,76]. The XGBoost prediction model established in this study showed promising performance. It had important public health implications, which could help clinicians screen out populations with a high risk of diabetes. The key features identified in this study not only captured each person's socio-demographic variables, but also medical history, anthropometric and clinical laboratory variables, which could be effective for formulating and implementing targeted diabetes prevention strategies to reduce the disease burden.

Despite of the above encouraging findings, the current study has several limitations. First, only the participants who attended both the baseline survey and 2-year follow-up were included in this study, which might potentially introduce a selection bias and limit the generalizability of the results. Second, some important risk factors of T2DM such as HbA1c, and insulin were not accounted for in the prediction models due to lack of relevant data. Third, some diabetes cases would be misclassified as non-T2DM because the oral glucose tolerance test (OGTT) was not included for the diagnosis of T2DM. However, the high cost and large sample size make it infeasible and difficult to perform oral glucose tolerance tests for all participants. Fourth, we only performed internal validation, and these prediction models need to be further validated in an external validation set in future work. Moreover, further work is warranted to consider auto encoder, to extract the type 2 diabetes mellitus (T2DM) features automatically, which can improve the classification efficiency of T2DM to some extent.

5. Conclusions

The current study developed four predictive models based on ML algorithms for the risk of incident T2DM in Chinese elderly. Our findings demonstrated that the XGBoost model achieved the best predictive performance for T2DM. Additionally, FPG, education, exercise, gender, and WC were the strongest predictors in the prediction model, which would benefit clinical practice in developing targeted diabetes prevention and control interventions.

Author Contributions: Conceptualization, Y.G. and Y.Y.; methodology, Y.G. and Y.Y.; software, Y.H., L.Z. and J.Z.; validation, Q.L. and M.Z.; formal analysis, M.Z.; investigation, Y.G. and Y.Y.; resources, Y.G. and Y.Y.; data curation, Y.G. and Y.Y.; writing—original draft preparation, M.Z.; writing—review and editing, Q.L.; visualization, Y.H., L.Z. and M.Z.; supervision, Y.G. and Y.Y.; project administration, Y.G. and Y.Y.; funding acquisition, Y.G. and Y.Y. All authors have read and agreed to the published version of the manuscript.

Funding: This research was funded by Wuhan Center for Disease Control and Prevention, grant number K20-1602-011 and Health Commission of Hubei Province, grant number WJ2021M137.

Institutional Review Board Statement: The study was conducted in accordance with the Declaration of Helsinki, and approved by the Ethics Committee of Wuhan Center for Disease Control and Prevention (protocol code WHCDCIRB-K-2018023).

Informed Consent Statement: Informed consent was obtained from all subjects involved in the study. Written informed consent has been obtained from the patient(s) to publish this paper.

Data Availability Statement: The data presented in this study are available from the corresponding author upon reasonable request.

Acknowledgments: Thanks to the participants for taking part in the study. The authors are also grateful for the financial support from Wuhan Center for Disease Control and Prevention.

Conflicts of Interest: The authors declare no conflict of interest.

References

1. World Health Organization. Diabetes. Available online: https://www.who.int/health-topics/diabetes#tab=tab_1 (accessed on 11 January 2022).
2. International Diabetes Federation. Diabetes around the World in 2021. Available online: https://diabetesatlas.org/ (accessed on 11 January 2022).
3. International Diabetes Federation. IDF Atlas 10th Edition. Available online: https://diabetesatlas.org/atlas/tenth-edition/ (accessed on 11 January 2022).
4. Ma, R.C.W.; Tsoi, K.Y.; Tam, W.H.; Wong, C.K.C. Developmental origins of type 2 diabetes: A perspective from China. *Eur. J. Clin. Nutr.* **2017**, *71*, 870–880. [CrossRef] [PubMed]
5. Huang, Y.; Vemer, P.; Zhu, J.; Postma, M.J.; Chen, W. Economic burden in Chinese patients with diabetes mellitus using electronic insurance claims data. *PLoS ONE* **2016**, *11*, e0159297. [CrossRef] [PubMed]
6. Li, Y.; Wang, D.D.; Ley, S.H.; Vasanti, M.; Howard, A.G.; He, Y.; Hu, F.B. Time trends of dietary and lifestyle factors and their potential impact on diabetes burden in China. *Diabetes Care* **2017**, *40*, 1685–1694. [CrossRef]
7. Peer, N.; Balakrishna, Y.; Durao, S. Screening for type 2 diabetes mellitus. *Cochrane Database Syst. Rev.* **2020**, *5*, 1465–1858.
8. Topol, E.J. High-performance medicine: The convergence of human and artificial intelligence. *Nat. Med.* **2019**, *25*, 44–56. [CrossRef]
9. Nelson, C.A.; Pérez-Chada, L.M.; Creadore, A.; Li, S.J.; Lo, K.; Manjaly, P.; Pournamdari, A.B.; Tkachenko, E.; Barbieri, J.S.; Ko, J.M.; et al. Patient perspectives on the use of artificial intelligence for skin cancer screening: A qualitative study. *JAMA Derm.* **2020**, *156*, 501–512. [CrossRef] [PubMed]
10. Anwar, F.; Qurat Ul, A.; Ejaz, M.Y.; Mosavi, A. A comparative analysis on diagnosis of diabetes mellitus using different approaches—A survey. *Inf. Med Unlocked* **2020**, *21*, 100482. [CrossRef]
11. Rigla, M.; García-Sáez, G.; Pons, B.; Hernando, M.E. Artificial intelligence methodologies and their application to diabetes. *J. Diabetes Sci. Technol.* **2018**, *12*, 303–310. [CrossRef]
12. Maniruzzaman, M.; Kumar, N.; Menhazul Abedin, M.; Shaykhul Islam, M.; Suri, H.S.; El-Baz, A.S.; Suri, J.S. Comparative approaches for classification of diabetes mellitus data: Machine learning paradigm. *Comput. Methods Programs Biomed.* **2017**, *152*, 23–34. [CrossRef]
13. Dreiseitl, S.; Ohno-Machado, L. Logistic regression and artificial neural network classification models: A methodology review. *J. Biomed. Inform.* **2002**, *35*, 352–359. [CrossRef]
14. Dinh, A.; Miertschin, S.; Young, A.; Mohanty, S.D. A data-driven approach to predicting diabetes and cardiovascular disease with machine learning. *BMC Med. Inf. Decis. Mak.* **2019**, *19*, 211. [CrossRef] [PubMed]
15. Moon, S.; Jang, J.Y.; Kim, Y.; Oh, C.M. Development and validation of a new diabetes index for the risk classification of present and new-onset diabetes: Multicohort study. *Sci. Rep.* **2021**, *11*, 15748. [CrossRef] [PubMed]
16. Yu, W.; Liu, T.; Valdez, R.; Gwinn, M.; Khoury, M.J. Application of support vector machine modeling for prediction of common diseases: The case of diabetes and pre-diabetes. *BMC Med. Inf. Decis. Mak.* **2010**, *10*, 16. [CrossRef] [PubMed]
17. Borzouei, S.; Soltanian, A.R. Application of an artificial neural network model for diagnosing type 2 diabetes mellitus and determining the relative importance of risk factors. *Epidemiol. Health* **2018**, *40*, e2018007. [CrossRef] [PubMed]
18. Garcia-Carretero, R.; Vigil-Medina, L.; Mora-Jimenez, I.; Soguero-Ruiz, C.; Barquero-Perez, O.; Ramos-Lopez, J. Use of a K-nearest neighbors model to predict the development of type 2 diabetes within 2 years in an obese, hypertensive population. *Med. Biol. Eng. Comput.* **2020**, *58*, 991–1002. [CrossRef] [PubMed]
19. Pei, D.; Yang, T.; Zhang, C. Estimation of diabetes in a high-risk adult Chinese population using J48 Decision Tree model. *Diabetes Metab. Syndr. Obes.* **2020**, *13*, 4621–4630. [CrossRef]

20. Ooka, T.; Johno, H.; Nakamoto, K.; Yoda, Y.; Yokomichi, H.; Yamagata, Z. Random forest approach for determining risk prediction and predictive factors of type 2 diabetes: Large-scale health check-up data in Japan. *BMJ Nutr. Prev. Health* **2021**, *4*, 140–148. [CrossRef]
21. Wang, L.; Wang, X.; Chen, A.; Jin, X.; Che, H. Prediction of type 2 diabetes risk and its effect evaluation based on the XGBoost model. *Healthcare* **2020**, *8*, 247. [CrossRef]
22. Silva, K.; Lee, W.K.; Forbes, A.; Demmer, R.T.; Barton, C.; Enticott, J. Use and performance of machine learning models for type 2 diabetes prediction in community settings: A systematic review and meta-analysis. *Int. J. Med. Inf.* **2020**, *143*, 104268. [CrossRef]
23. Xie, Z.; Nikolayeva, O.; Luo, J.; Li, D. Building risk prediction models for type 2 diabetes using machine learning techniques. *Prev. Chronic Dis.* **2019**, *16*, E130. [CrossRef]
24. Katarya, R.; Jain, S. Comparison of different machine learning models for diabetes detection. In Proceedings of the 2020 IEEE International Conference on Advances and Developments in Electrical and Electronics Engineering (ICADEE), Coimbatore, India, 10–11 December 2020; IEEE: Piscataway, NJ, USA, 2020; pp. 117–121.
25. Adua, E.; Kolog, E.A.; Afrifa-Yamoah, E.; Amankwah, B.; Obirikorang, C.; Anto, E.O.; Acheampong, E.; Wang, W.; Tetteh, A.Y. Predictive model and feature importance for early detection of type II diabetes mellitus. *Transl. Med. Commun.* **2021**, *6*, 17. [CrossRef]
26. Zou, Q.; Qu, K.; Luo, Y.; Yin, D.; Ju, Y.; Tang, H. Predicting diabetes mellitus with machine learning techniques. *Front. Genet.* **2018**, *9*, 515. [CrossRef] [PubMed]
27. Xue, M.; Su, Y.; Li, C.; Wang, S.; Yao, H. Identification of potential type II diabetes in a large-scale Chinese population using a systematic machine learning framework. *J. Diabetes Res.* **2020**, *2020*, 6873891. [CrossRef] [PubMed]
28. Kuo, K.M.; Talley, P.; Kao, Y.; Huang, C.H. A multi-class classification model for supporting the diagnosis of type II diabetes mellitus. *PeerJ* **2020**, *8*, e9920. [CrossRef]
29. Zhao, H.; Zhang, X.; Xu, Y.; Gao, L.; Ma, Z.; Sun, Y.; Wang, W. Predicting the risk of hypertension based on several easy-to-collect risk factors: A machine learning method. *Front. Public Health* **2021**, *9*, 619429. [CrossRef]
30. Agardh, E.; Allebeck, P.; Hallqvist, J.; Moradi, T.; Sidorchuk, A. Type 2 diabetes incidence and socio-economic position: A systematic review and meta-analysis. *Int. J. Epidemiol.* **2011**, *40*, 804–818. [CrossRef]
31. Smith, A.D.; Crippa, A.; Woodcock, J.; Brage, S. Physical activity and incident type 2 diabetes mellitus: A systematic review and dose-response meta-analysis of prospective cohort studies. *Diabetologia* **2016**, *59*, 2527–2545. [CrossRef]
32. Lu, J.; Li, M.; Peng, K.; Xu, M.; Xu, Y.; Chen, Y.; Wang, T.; Zhao, Z.; Dai, M.; Zhang, D.; et al. Predictive value of fasting glucose, postload glucose, and hemoglobin A1c on risk of diabetes and complications in Chinese adults. *Diabetes Care* **2019**, *42*, 1539–1548. [CrossRef]
33. American Diabetes Association. 2. Classification and diagnosis of diabetes: Standards of medical care in diabetes—2021. *Diabetes Care* **2021**, *44*, S15–S33. [CrossRef]
34. Choi, R.Y.; Coyner, A.S.; Kalpathy-Cramer, J.; Chiang, M.F.; Campbell, J.P. Introduction to machine learning, neural networks, and deep learning. *Transl. Vis. Sci. Technol.* **2020**, *9*, 14.
35. Cox, D.R. The regression analysis of binary sequences. *J. R. Stat. Soc. Ser. B Stat. Methodol.* **1958**, *20*, 215–242. [CrossRef]
36. Quinlan, J.R. Induction of decision trees. *Mach. Learn.* **1986**, *1*, 81–106. [CrossRef]
37. Breiman, L. Random Forests. *Mach. Learn.* **2001**, *45*, 5–32. [CrossRef]
38. Muhammad, L.J.; Algehyne, E.A.; Usman, S.S. Predictive supervised machine learning models for diabetes mellitus. *SN Comput. Sci.* **2020**, *1*, 240. [CrossRef]
39. Chen, T.; Guestrin, C. XGBoost: A scalable tree boosting system. In Proceedings of the 22nd ACM SIGKDD International Conference on Knowledge Discovery and Data Mining, San Francisco, CA, USA, 13–17 August 2016; Association for Computing Machinery: New York, NY, USA, 2016; pp. 785–794.
40. Taye, G.T.; Shim, E.B.; Hwang, H.-J.; Lim, K.M. Machine learning approach to predict ventricular fibrillation based on QRS complex shape. *Front. Physiol.* **2019**, *10*, 1193. [CrossRef]
41. Tibshirani, R. Regression shrinkage and selection via the Lasso. *J. R. Stat. Soc. Ser. B Stat. Methodol.* **1996**, *58*, 267–288. [CrossRef]
42. Pedregosa, F.; Varoquaux, G.; Gramfort, A.; Michel, V.; Thirion, B.; Grisel, O.; Blondel, M.; Prettenhofer, P.; Weiss, R.; Dubourg, V.; et al. Scikit-learn: Machine learning in Python. *J. Mach. Learn. Res.* **2011**, *12*, 2825–2830.
43. Snoek, J.; Larochelle, H.; Adams, R.P. Practical Bayesian optimization of machine learning algorithms. In Proceedings of the Advances in Neural Information Processing Systems 25 (NIPS 2012), Lake Tahoe, NV, USA, 3–6 December 2012; Neural Information Processing Systems Foundation, Inc. (NIPS): La Jolla, CA, USA, 2013; pp. 2951–2959.
44. Frazier, P.I. A tutorial on Bayesian optimization. *arXiv* **2018**, arXiv:1807.02811.
45. Data, M.I.T.C.; Dernoncourt, F.; Nemati, S.; Kassis, E.B.; Ghassemi, M.M. Hyperparameter Selection. In *Secondary Analysis of Electronic Health Records*; Springer: Cham, Switzerland, 2016; pp. 419–427.
46. Koul, N.; Manvi, S.S. Framework for classification of cancer gene expression data using Bayesian hyper-parameter optimization. *Med. Biol. Eng. Comput.* **2021**, *59*, 2353–2371. [CrossRef]
47. Lundberg, S.M.; Lee, S.I. A unified approach to interpreting model predictions. In Proceedings of the Advances in Neural Information Processing Systems 30 (NIPS 2017), Long Beach, CA, USA, 4–9 December 2017; Curran Associates Inc.: Red Hook, NY, USA, 2017; pp. 4766–4775.

48. Xue, B.; Li, D.; Lu, C.; King, C.R.; Wildes, T.; Avidan, M.S.; Kannampallil, T.; Abraham, J. Use of machine learning to develop and evaluate models using preoperative and intraoperative data to identify risks of postoperative complications. *JAMA Netw. Open* **2021**, *4*, e212240. [CrossRef]
49. Ravaut, M.; Harish, V.; Sadeghi, H.; Leung, K.K.; Volkovs, M.; Kornas, K.; Watson, T.; Poutanen, T.; Rosella, L.C. Development and validation of a machine learning model using administrative health data to predict onset of type 2 diabetes. *JAMA Netw. Open* **2021**, *4*, e2111315. [CrossRef] [PubMed]
50. Lai, H.; Huang, H.; Keshavjee, K.; Guergachi, A.; Gao, X. Predictive models for diabetes mellitus using machine learning techniques. *BMC Endocr. Disord.* **2019**, *19*, 101. [CrossRef] [PubMed]
51. Wei, H.; Sun, J.; Shan, W.; Xiao, W.; Wang, B.; Ma, X.; Hu, W.; Wang, X.; Xia, Y. Environmental chemical exposure dynamics and machine learning-based prediction of diabetes mellitus. *Sci. Total Env.* **2022**, *806*, 150674. [CrossRef] [PubMed]
52. Sadeghi, S.; Khalili, D.; Ramezankhani, A.; Mansournia, M.A.; Parsaeian, M. Diabetes mellitus risk prediction in the presence of class imbalance using flexible machine learning methods. *BMC Med. Inf. Decis. Mak.* **2022**, *22*, 36. [CrossRef]
53. Wu, Y.; Hu, H.; Cai, J.; Chen, R.; Zuo, X.; Cheng, H.; Yan, D. Machine learning for predicting the 3-year risk of incident diabetes in Chinese adults. *Front. Public Health* **2021**, *9*, 626331. [CrossRef]
54. Deberneh, H.M.; Kim, I. Prediction of type 2 diabetes based on machine learning algorithm. *Int. J. Environ. Res. Public Health* **2021**, *18*, 3317. [CrossRef]
55. Zhang, L.; Wang, Y.; Niu, M.; Wang, C.; Wang, Z. Machine learning for characterizing risk of type 2 diabetes mellitus in a rural Chinese population: The Henan Rural Cohort Study. *Sci. Rep.* **2020**, *10*, 4406. [CrossRef]
56. Rufo, D.D.; Debelee, T.G.; Ibenthal, A.; Negera, W.G. Diagnosis of diabetes mellitus using gradient boosting machine (LightGBM). *Diagnostics* **2021**, *11*, 1714. [CrossRef]
57. Farran, B.; AlWotayan, R.; Alkandari, H.; Al-Abdulrazzaq, D.; Channanath, A.; Thanaraj, T.A. Use of non-invasive parameters and machine-learning algorithms for predicting future risk of type 2 diabetes: A retrospective cohort study of health data from Kuwait. *Front. Endocrinol.* **2019**, *10*, 624. [CrossRef]
58. Yang, T.; Zhang, L.; Yi, L.; Feng, H.; Li, S.; Chen, H.; Zhu, J.; Zhao, J.; Zeng, Y.; Liu, H. Ensemble learning models based on noninvasive features for type 2 diabetes screening: Model development and validation. *JMIR Med. Inf.* **2020**, *8*, e15431. [CrossRef]
59. Maniruzzaman, M.; Rahman, M.J.; Ahammed, B.; Abedin, M.M. Classification and prediction of diabetes disease using machine learning paradigm. *Health Inf. Sci. Syst.* **2020**, *8*, 7. [CrossRef] [PubMed]
60. Lorenzo, C.; Wagenknecht, L.E.; Hanley, A.J.G.; Rewers, M.J.; Karter, A.J.; Haffner, S.M. A1C between 5.7 and 6.4% as a marker for identifying pre-diabetes, insulin sensitivity and secretion, and cardiovascular risk factors: The Insulin Resistance Atherosclerosis Study (IRAS). *Diabetes Care* **2010**, *33*, 2104–2109. [CrossRef] [PubMed]
61. Abbasi, A.; Sahlqvist, A.-S.; Lotta, L.; Brosnan, J.M.; Vollenweider, P.; Giabbanelli, P.; Nunez, D.J.; Waterworth, D.; Scott, R.A.; Langenberg, C.; et al. A systematic review of biomarkers and risk of incident type 2 diabetes: An overview of epidemiological, prediction and aetiological research literature. *PLoS ONE* **2016**, *11*, e0163721. [CrossRef] [PubMed]
62. Meng, X.-H.; Huang, Y.-X.; Rao, D.-P.; Zhang, Q.; Liu, Q. Comparison of three data mining models for predicting diabetes or prediabetes by risk factors. *Kaohsiung J. Med. Sci.* **2013**, *29*, 93–99. [CrossRef] [PubMed]
63. Cao, G.; Cui, Z.; Ma, Q.; Wang, C.; Xu, Y.; Sun, H.; Ma, Y. Changes in health inequalities for patients with diabetes among middle-aged and elderly in China from 2011 to 2015. *BMC Health Serv. Res.* **2020**, *20*, 719. [CrossRef] [PubMed]
64. Espelt, A.; Kunst, A.E.; Palència, L.; Gnavi, R.; Borrell, C. Twenty years of socio-economic inequalities in type 2 diabetes mellitus prevalence in Spain, 1987–2006. *Eur. J. Public Health* **2012**, *22*, 765–771. [CrossRef]
65. Asadi-Lari, M.; Khosravi, A.; Nedjat, S.; Mansournia, M.A.; Majdzadeh, R.; Mohammad, K.; Vaez-Mahdavi, M.R.; Faghihzadeh, S.; Haeri Mehrizi, A.A.; Cheraghian, B. Socioeconomic status and prevalence of self-reported diabetes among adults in Tehran: Results from a large population-based cross-sectional study (Urban HEART-2). *J. Endocrinol. Investig.* **2016**, *39*, 515–522. [CrossRef]
66. Pantell, M.S.; Prather, A.A.; Downing, J.M.; Gordon, N.P.; Adler, N.E. Association of social and behavioral risk factors with earlier onset of adult hypertension and diabetes. *JAMA Netw. Open* **2019**, *2*, e193933. [CrossRef]
67. Li, G.; Zhang, P.; Wang, J.; Gregg, E.W.; Yang, W.; Gong, Q.; Li, H.; Li, H.; Jiang, Y.; An, Y.; et al. The long-term effect of lifestyle interventions to prevent diabetes in the China Da Qing Diabetes Prevention Study: A 20-year follow-up study. *Lancet* **2008**, *371*, 1783–1789. [CrossRef]
68. Pan, X.-R.; Li, G.-W.; Hu, Y.-H.; Wang, J.-X.; Yang, W.-Y.; An, Z.-X.; Hu, Z.-X.; Lin, J.; Xiao, J.-Z.; Cao, H.-B.; et al. Effects of diet and exercise in preventing NIDDM in people with impaired glucose tolerance: The Da Qing IGT and Diabetes Study. *Diabetes Care* **1997**, *20*, 537–544. [CrossRef]
69. Anjana, R.M.; Deepa, M.; Pradeepa, R.; Mahanta, J.; Narain, K.; Das, H.K.; Adhikari, P.; Rao, P.V.; Saboo, B.; Kumar, A.; et al. Prevalence of diabetes and prediabetes in 15 states of India: Results from the ICMR-INDIAB population-based cross-sectional study. *Lancet Diabetes Endocrinol.* **2017**, *5*, 585–596. [CrossRef]
70. Subramani, S.K.; Yadav, D.; Mishra, M.; Pakkirisamy, U.; Mathiyalagen, P.; Prasad, G. Prevalence of type 2 diabetes and prediabetes in the Gwalior-Chambal region of central India. *Int. J. Environ. Res. Public Health* **2019**, *16*, 4708. [CrossRef] [PubMed]
71. Zhou, T.; Liu, X.; Liu, Y.; Li, X. Spatio-temporal patterns of the associations between type 2 diabetes and its risk factors in mainland China: A systematic review and meta-analysis. *Lancet* **2018**, *392*, S32. [CrossRef]

72. Aryal, K.K.; Mehata, S.; Neupane, S.; Vaidya, A.; Dhimal, M.; Dhakal, P.; Rana, S.; Bhusal, C.L.; Lohani, G.R.; Paulin, F.H.; et al. The burden and determinants of non communicable diseases risk factors in Nepal: Findings from a nationwide STEPS survey. *PLoS ONE* **2015**, *10*, e0134834. [CrossRef] [PubMed]
73. Xu, Z.; Qi, X.; Dahl, A.K.; Xu, W. Waist-to-height ratio is the best indicator for undiagnosed type 2 diabetes. *Diabet. Med.* **2013**, *30*, e201–e207. [CrossRef]
74. Wang, Y.; Rimm, E.B.; Stampfer, M.J.; Willett, W.C.; Hu, F.B. Comparison of abdominal adiposity and overall obesity in predicting risk of type 2 diabetes among men. *Am. J. Clin. Nutr.* **2005**, *81*, 555–563. [CrossRef]
75. Bommer, C.; Heesemann, E.; Sagalova, V.; Manne-Goehler, J.; Atun, R.; Bärnighausen, T.; Vollmer, S. The global economic burden of diabetes in adults aged 20–79 years: A cost-of-illness study. *Lancet Diabetes Endocrinol.* **2017**, *5*, 423–430. [CrossRef]
76. Rowley, W.R.; Bezold, C.; Arikan, Y.; Byrne, E.; Krohe, S. Diabetes 2030: Insights from yesterday, today, and future trends. *Popul. Health Manag* **2017**, *20*, 6–12. [CrossRef]

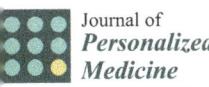

Article

Predicting the Need for Therapeutic Intervention and Mortality in Acute Pancreatitis: A Two-Center International Study Using Machine Learning

Na Shi [1,†], Lan Lan [2,*,†], Jiawei Luo [3], Ping Zhu [1], Thomas R. W. Ward [4], Peter Szatmary [4], Robert Sutton [4], Wei Huang [1,4], John A. Windsor [5], Xiaobo Zhou [6] and Qing Xia [1,*]

1. Department of Integrated Traditional Chinese and Western Medicine, Sichuan Provincial Pancreatitis Centre and West China-Liverpool Biomedical Research Centre, West China Hospital, Sichuan University, Chengdu 610044, China; nashi@scu.edu.cn (N.S.); zhuping@wchscu.cn (P.Z.); dr_wei_huang@scu.edu.cn (W.H.)
2. IT Center, Beijing Tiantan Hospital, Capital Medical University, Beijing 100070, China
3. West China Biomedical Big Data Centre, West China Hospital, Sichuan University, Chengdu 610041, China; luojiawei@wchscu.cn
4. Liverpool Pancreatitis Study Group, Royal Liverpool University Hospital, Institute of Translational Medicine, University of Liverpool, Liverpool L6 93BX, UK; thomasrwward@doctors.org.uk (T.R.W.W.); pszatmary@me.com (P.S.); r.sutton@liverpool.ac.uk (R.S.)
5. Surgical and Translational Research Centre, Faculty of Medical and Health Sciences, University of Auckland, Auckland 1023, New Zealand; j.windsor@auckland.ac.nz
6. School of Biomedical Informatics, University of Texas Health Science Centre at Houston, Houston, TX 77030, USA; xiaobo.zhou@uth.tmc.edu
* Correspondence: lanlan_xxzx@bjtth.org (L.L.); xiaqing@medmail.com.cn (Q.X.)
† Theses authors contributed equally to this study.

Abstract: Background: Current approaches to predicting intervention needs and mortality have reached 65–85% accuracy, which falls below clinical decision-making requirements in patients with acute pancreatitis (AP). We aimed to accurately predict therapeutic intervention needs and mortality on admission, in AP patients, using machine learning (ML). Methods: Data were obtained from three databases of patients admitted with AP: one retrospective (Chengdu) and two prospective (Liverpool and Chengdu) databases. Intervention and mortality differences, as well as potential predictors, were investigated. Univariate analysis was conducted, followed by a random forest ML algorithm used in multivariate analysis, to identify predictors. The ML performance matrix was applied to evaluate the model's performance. Results: Three datasets of 2846 patients included 25 potential clinical predictors in the univariate analysis. The top ten identified predictors were obtained by ML models, for predicting interventions and mortality, from the training dataset. The prediction of interventions includes death in non-intervention patients, validated with high accuracy (96%/98%), the area under the receiver-operating-characteristic curve (0.90/0.98), and positive likelihood ratios (22.3/69.8), respectively. The post-test probabilities in the test set were 55.4% and 71.6%, respectively, which were considerably superior to existing prognostic scores. The ML model, for predicting mortality in intervention patients, performed better or equally with prognostic scores. Conclusions: ML, using admission clinical predictors, can accurately predict therapeutic interventions and mortality in patients with AP.

Keywords: acute pancreatitis; machine learning; predictor; interventions; mortality

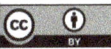

1. Introduction

Acute pancreatitis (AP) is one of the most common admission diagnoses relating to an acute gastrointestinal pathology. Approximately 25% of patients with AP develop infected pancreatic necrosis (IPN) and/or organ failure (OF), with mortality rates of 20–50% [1,2].

While the outcome of patients with AP has improved over recent decades, AP incidence and associated disability remain high [3], and specific drug therapies remain unavailable [4]. One of the challenges of therapeutic trials for AP is the inaccuracy in early severity and complication prediction, resulting in heterogeneous treatment groups. A review of current predictors of AP outcome [5] (including IPN, OF, and the need for intervention) demonstrated that the accuracy of current systems ranges from 65% to 85%, implying a misclassification error of 15–35%. This degree of inaccuracy in the prediction has clinical and research practice consequences.

Improving the accuracy of early severity prediction is of paramount importance and a matter of significant international effort. Various individual serum biomarkers have been investigated. However, they have failed to improve the clinical utility of existing simple and inexpensive scoring systems [6–10]. Combinations of markers and/or scoring systems potentially add value but lack external and/or multicenter validation [11–14]. The development and increasing accessibility of omics platforms have provided opportunities for prognostication based on genetic [15], transcriptomic [16], proteomic [17–20], metabolic profiling [21,22], and multi-platform omics analyses [23] Nevertheless, the application of these platforms in AP remains in its infancy.

The premise of machine learning (ML) in disease prognostication is to incorporate the wisdom embedded within decisions made by multiple clinicians, and the outcomes of their patients, in order to inform the individualized patient treatment [24]. ML is a broad field involving computer science and statistics, and broadly speaking, it involves a machine-led selection of iterative computational models to progressively improve the model's performance in a specific task. The ability to handle vast datasets in an inherently unbiased manner has led to the growing interest in, and use of, ML-based applications in multiple areas of medicine [25–28]. This includes the use of ML in the diagnosis, prognosis, and predicted treatment response in patients with gastrointestinal diseases, although the lack of high-quality datasets continues to present a problem [29].

In AP, ML has been used to aid in the prediction of OF [30–32] and severity [33–35]; however, thus far, no study has accurately and timeously predicted the need for therapeutic intervention [36]. The identification of high-risk patients who require specialist intervention is critical, as these patients are, not only, at considerable risk of adverse disease outcomes but timely management has considerable implications for the health-care system. This includes the possible need to provide services that may not be available throughout the day, or every day in the week, and the provision of services may mean a transfer to a different hospital in some care settings.

Although there have been attempts to standardize the language surrounding indications for intervention in AP [37], there are numerous instances (e.g., ongoing OF or other severe gastrointestinal symptoms, due to the mass effect of walled-off necrosis or disconnected pancreatic duct syndrome) [38] that warrant intervention under the care of an experienced pancreatologist. These can often be difficult to classify or use to provide general guidance on the use of traditional methods.

Therefore, this study aimed to apply an ML algorithm to preoperatively predict the need for intervention and mortality in patients admitted with AP.

2. Materials and Methods

2.1. Overview

Data on patients with AP were collected, retrospectively (single center, Chengdu) and prospectively (two centers, Liverpool and Chengdu), and analyzed following the STROBE guidelines for observational studies [39]. Confirmation that specific ethical approval was not required was provided by the Institutional Review Board of West China Hospital of Sichuan University (WCH/SCU), due to prior approval for the use of retrospective data. Informed consent was obtained from patients admitted to Royal Liverpool University Hospital (RLUH), and ethical approval was not required because anonymized data were used. Predictors and outcomes from both retrospective and prospective databases were used to develop and test predictive models for intervention and mortality.

2.2. Cohorts and Data Collection

Eligible patients were identified from the Hospital Information System by using the International Classification of Diseases, 10th edition, code K85. All patients were admitted to WCH/SCU or RLUH, within 48 h of abdominal pain onset, with a diagnosis of AP, as defined by the revised Atlanta classification [37]. Patients in the retrospective cohort were admitted between 1 October 2009 and 30 September 2013. Patients in the prospective cohorts were admitted between 1 September 2014 and 31 December 2015 (WCH/SCU) or between 1 June 2010 and 30 June 2017 (RLUH). Data collection in both centers was based on a predefined pro forma and coordinated by experienced researchers, with quality assurance and control measures in place at every step of the study process.

2.3. Potential Predictors

Demographic variables (age, sex, comorbidities, abdominal pain onset time, and etiology), available quantitative laboratory tests on admission common to all three cohorts (white blood cell [WBC], neutrophils, lymphocytes, hematocrit, urea, creatinine, albumin, and C-reactive protein [CRP]), and clinical severity scores on admission (sequential organ failure assessment [SOFA] [40], systemic inflammatory response syndrome [SIRS] [41], bedside index, for severity in acute pancreatitis [BISAP] [42], acute physiology, and chronic health examination [APACHE] II [43], as well as modified computerized tomographic severity index [MCTSI]) [44] were collected. Additional clinical variables, including pleural effusion, local complications, OF, pancreatic, and extrapancreatic infection (bacteremia and others) were also recorded (worst during hospitalization or before surgery), as were daily assessments of type, onset, and duration of OF.

2.4. Definition of Groups

The patients were divided into conservative-treatment (no intervention) and invasive-intervention (including pancreatic cyst percutaneous catheter drainage and necrosectomy) groups for further analysis.

2.5. Statistical Analysis and Model Development

The chi-squared test was used to analyze categorical data, and the Kruskal–Wallis test was used for ranked variables. The rank-sum test was used for skewed and continuous data. Random forest (RF) ML [45] multivariate analysis was used to construct the algorithms and resolve the impact of data imbalances on predictions (2714 cases in the non-intervention group, more than 20 times of the 132 cases in the intervention group). RF can process high-dimensional samples and does not require dimensionality reduction for datasets with numerous variables. It is worth noting that RF is an ensemble method that utilizes many classifiers to work together, and it has high accuracy and superiority on unbalanced datasets. The mean decrease in the Gini value of each variable, indicating the importance of the variable to the outcome, was obtained by the varImpPlot function using the R software. We comprehensively evaluated the model's performance, using the area under receiver-operating-characteristic curve (AUC) analysis, and evaluated the post-test probabilities by calculating the positive and negative likelihood ratios.

All the analytic processes were performed using R software (version 3.6.3).

2.5.1. Data Sources

Since there were three datasets in this study: (1) a retrospective cohort from WCH/SCU, (2) a prospective cohort from WCH/SCU, (3) and a prospective cohort from RLUH, the differences between various data collection times and populations might have had varying effects on outcomes. Therefore, the differences affecting the research outcomes were analyzed. First, we used the three datasets, separately, to predict intervention needs and mortality. Thereafter, we aggregated the three datasets into a single dataset for the prediction. We found that the results of modelling the three datasets separately, and those of integrating them into one dataset, were similar. In addition, this study was a retrospective analysis of data collected in a previous period. Therefore, we consolidated the three different data sources into a single dataset before analysis and modeling.

2.5.2. Univariate Analysis

The impact of each individual variable on "need for intervention" and "mortality" was examined using univariate analysis. Where the resulting p-value was <0.10, the variable was included in multivariable analysis.

2.5.3. Performance of the ML Algorithm

For multivariate analysis, an RF ML approach was used. Patients were divided into three groups for modeling: (1) intervention and conservative management, (2) mortality and survival among intervention patients, and (3) mortality and survival among conservatively managed patients. The larger the mean decrease in the Gini value, the greater the impact of the variable. We extracted the characteristics of the intervention and deceased patients, compared with those of non-intervention and surviving patients, and evaluated the model's performance using evaluation indicators (accuracy, AUC, sensitivity, specificity, and likelihood ratio). Accuracy was evaluated based on the percentage of correct predictions. To predict the performance of ML, accuracy was evaluated based on the proportion of correct predictions in the total sample. As a rule of thumb, a test with a high predictive value has a positive likelihood ratio >5, usually closer to 10, and occasionally higher [46]. In all three groups, the total dataset was divided into training, validation, and test datasets according to a specific ratio of 6:2:2. The training set was used to develop the model, the validation set was used to adjust the parameters, and the test set was used to obtain the final result, which was the average performance with 30 repetitions (Figure 1). The hyperparameters of random forest include the number of trees (ntree), the number of variables required to build a single tree (nvariable), and the minimum sample size of leaf nodes (nodesize). Through parameter sensitivity analysis (Supplementary Table S1), the final chosen hyperparameters were: ntree = 500, nvariable = 4, and nodesize = 1.

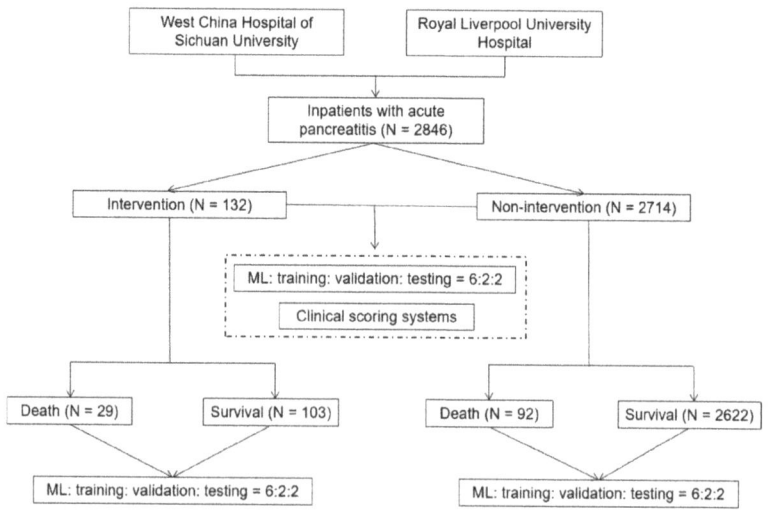

Figure 1. The flow chart of this study.

3. Results

3.1. Comparison of Characteristics between Intervention and Non-Intervention Patients with AP

A retrospective cohort of 2018 patients (WCH/SCU) and two prospective cohorts of 259 and 569 patients (WCH/SCU and RLUH, respectively) were included in the analysis. The proportions of intervention and mortality (chi-squared test; $p = 0.432$ and $p = 0.411$, respectively) were similar across all cohorts, indicating that any observed differences in the number of interventions and/or mortality were unlikely to be due to inherent differences in the source data.

The clinical characteristics of the 2846 patients are summarized in Table 1. The number of patients requiring therapeutic intervention was 132 (4.6%), while 2714 (95.4%) were managed conservatively. The most common etiologies (in order) were biliary, hypertriglyceridemia, and alcohol consumption. The median age of all participants was 46 years (interquartile range, 38–58 years), and 64.0% were men. There were no significant differences in age, sex, Charlson comorbidity index, or etiology between the two groups. The time from pain to admission was 6 h longer in the intervention group ($p < 0.05$).

WBC, neutrophil, hematocrit, urea, creatinine, and CRP in the intervention group were significantly higher than those in the non-intervention group, while albumin levels were lower (all $p < 0.05$). The admission clinical scoring systems, including SOFA, BISAP, SIRS, APACHE II, and worst MCTSI, were all higher among intervention patients, with the ratio of severe cases being three times higher than that in the non-intervention group.

Patients requiring intervention exhibited significantly worse clinical outcomes: 98/132 (74.2%) developed acute peripancreatic fluid collection, and 84/132 (63.6%) developed pancreatic and/or peripancreatic necrosis. Out of the 84 patients with necrosis, 81 were confirmed to have infectious necrosis; 99/132 (75%), 42/132 (31.8%), and 29/132 (22%) therapeutic-intervention patients developed persistent pulmonary, circulatory, and renal failure, respectively, with the duration of all three types' OF lasting longer than those in the non-intervention group. Extrapancreatic infection was also more prevalent in the intervention group, regardless of bacteremia or lung infection.

Table 1. Characteristics between intervention and non-intervention patients with AP.

Characteristic	Total (n = 2846)	Intervention (n = 132)	Non-Intervention (n = 2714)	p
Demographics				
Age, year (M[Q])	46 (38–58)	48 (39–62)	46 (38–57)	0.125
Male (%)	1822 (64.0)	88 (66.7)	1734 (63.9)	0.578
CCI (M[Q])	0 (0–1)	0 (0–1)	0 (0–1)	0.260
Modified CCI, (M[Q])	0 (0–1)	0 (0–2)	0 (0–1)	0.176
ASA (%)				0.005
I	2120 (74.5)	108 (81.8)	2012 (74.1)	
II	573 (20.1)	13 (9.8)	560 (20.6)	
III	153 (5.4)	11 (9.3)	142 (5.2)	
From onset to admission, h (M[Q])	18 (10–27)	24 (10–33)	18 (10–27)	0.001
Aetiology (%)				0.063
Biliary	1069 (37.6)	65 (49.2)	1004 (37.0)	
Hypertriglyceridemia	805 (28.3)	33 (25.0)	772 (28.4)	
Alcoholics	216 (7.6)	8 (6.1)	208 (7.7)	
ERCP	20 (0.7)	0 (0.0)	20 (0.7)	
Drug-induced	8 (0.3)	1 (0.8)	7 (0.3)	
Others	728 (25.6)	25 (18.9)	703 (25.9)	
Laboratory tests				
WBC, 10^9/L (M[Q])	12.9 (10.01–16.30)	14.3 (10.43–17.35)	12.87 (10–16.26)	0.011
Neutrophils, 10^9/L (M[Q])	11.00 (8.10–14.34)	12.66 (9.17–15.61)	10.95 (8.05–14.28)	0.001
Lymphocyte, 10^9/L (M[Q])	1.01 (0.70–1.49)	0.96 (0.62–1.53)	1.02 (0.70–1.49)	0.352
Hematocrit, % (M[Q])	43 (39–46)	45 (40–49)	43 (39.3–46)	0.003
Urea, mmol/L (M[Q])	5.00 (3.72–6.60)	6.36 (4.79–8.61)	4.92 (3.70–6.47)	<0.001 *
Creatinine, μmmol/L (M[Q])	74 (62–89)	87 (68–134)	73 (62–88)	<0.001 *
Albumin, g/L (M[Q])	42.0 (38.2–45.3)	37.3 (32.3–43.2)	42.1 (38.6–45.4)	<0.001 *
CRP, mg/L (M[Q])	28.7 (3.31–142)	158 (20–22)	26 (2.7–136)	<0.001 *

Table 1. Cont.

Characteristic	Total (n = 2846)	Intervention (n = 132)	Non-Intervention (n = 2714)	p
Clinical scoring systems				
SOFA (M[Q])	0 (0–2)	2 (0–3)	0 (0–1)	<0.001 *
BISAP (M[Q])	1 (0–2)	2 (1–2)	1 (0–2)	<0.001 *
SIRS (M[Q])	1 (1–2)	2 (1–3)	1 (1–2)	<0.001 *
APACHE II (M[Q])	4 (2–7)	7 (4–11)	4 (2–7)	<0.001 *
RAC (%)				<0.001 *
Mild	1373 (48.2)	4 (3.0)	1369 (50.4)	
Moderately severe	888 (31.2)	29 (22.0)	859 (31.7)	
Severe	585 (20.6)	99 (75.0)	486 (17.9)	
Worst MCTSI (M[Q])	2 (0–6)	8 (6–10)	2 (0–6)	<0.001 *
From admission to worst MCTSI, day (M[Q])	0 (0–2)	2 (1–9)	0 (0–1)	<0.001 *
Clinical outcomes				
Local complication				
APFC (%)	1121 (39.4)	98 (74.2)	1023 (37.7)	<0.001 *
Necrosis (%)	416 (14.6)	84 (63.6)	332 (12.2)	<0.001 *
Single organ failure				
Pulmonary failure (%)				<0.001 *
TOF	417 (14.7)	8 (6.1)	409 (15.1)	
POF	578 (20.3)	99 (75.0)	479 (17.6)	
Onset of pulmonary failure, day (M[Q])	0 (0–1)	1 (1–2)	0 (0–1)	<0.001 *
Duration of pulmonary failure, day (M[Q])	0 (0–1)	12.5 (1–24)	0 (0–1)	<0.001 *
Circulatory failure (%)				<0.001 *
TOF	42 (1.5)	9 (6.8)	33 (1.2)	
POF	111 (3.9)	42 (31.8)	69 (2.5)	
Onset of circulatory failure, day (M[Q])	0 (0–0)	0 (0–3)	0 (0–0)	<0.001 *
Duration of circulatory failure, day (M[Q])	0 (0–0)	0 (0–3)	0 (0–0)	<0.001 *
Renal failure (%)				<0.001 *
TOF	57 (2.0)	15 (11.4)	42 (1.5)	
POF	104 (3.7)	29 (22.0)	75 (2.8)	
Onset of renal failure, day (M[Q])	0 (0–0)	0 (0–1)	0 (0–0)	<0.001 *
Duration of renal failure, day (M[Q])	0 (0–0)	0 (0–1)	0 (0–0)	<0.001 *
Pleural effusion (%)	268 (9.4)	15 (11.4)	253 (9.3)	0.528
IPN (%)	85 (3.0)	81 (61.4)	4 (0.1)	<0.001 *
Extrapancreatic infection (%)				<0.001 *
Bacteremia	75 (2.6)	24 (18.2)	51 (1.9)	
Lung and others	147 (5.2)	31 (23.5)	116 (4.3)	

AP, acute pancreatitis; CCI, Charlson comorbidity index; ASA, American society of anesthesiologists; ERCP, endoscopic retrograde cholangiopancreatography; WBC, white blood cell count; CRP, C-reactive protein; SOFA, sequential organ failure assessment; BISAP, bedside index of severity in acute pancreatitis; SIRS, systemic inflammatory response syndrome; APACHE II, acute physiology and chronic health evaluation II; RAC, revised Atlanta classification; MCTSI, modified computerized tomographic severity index; APFC, acute peripancreatic fluid collection; IPN, infected pancreatic necrosis; TOF, transient organ failure; POF, persistent organ failure; M[Q], median and inter-quartile range for quantitative data; (%), number and percentage for categorical variables; * $p < 0.05$, indicates statistical significance.

The comparisons between death and survival among intervention patients, as well as among non-intervention patients, are shown in Supplementary Table S2 and Supplementary Table S3, respectively.

3.2. Important Features and Predictors for Intervention and Mortality

As shown in Table 2, important features (variables) associated with intervention and death differed. Compared with that in non-intervention patients, the duration of pulmonary failure was the most important factor in intervention patients. The remaining nine important variables for intervention patients, ranging from heavy to light, were neutrophils, albumin, lymphocytes, creatinine, age, hematocrit, onset of circulatory failure, APACHE II, and duration of circulatory failure. OF characteristics were all important variables for death among both intervention and non-intervention patients, especially for the occurrence of circulatory and renal failure. Circulatory failure, onset of circulatory failure, duration of circulatory failure, renal failure, duration of renal failure, duration of pulmonary failure, and APACHE II were all important variables for death in both intervention and non-intervention groups. The difference was that urea and CRP were important indicators of death in intervention patients, while creatine and WBC were important indicators in non-intervention patients.

Table 2. Top 10 important features for intervention or mortality among the three groups.

Intervention		Death in Intervention		Death in Non-Intervention	
Variable	Mean Decrease Gini	Variable	Mean Decrease Gini	Variable	Mean Decrease Gini
Duration of pulmonary failure	23.78	Duration of renal failure	2.54	Renal failure	10.99
Neutrophils	10.18	Duration of circulatory failure	2.52	Circulatory failure	10.00
Albumin	9.91	Onset of circulatory failure	2.35	Duration of circulatory failure	8.62
Lymphocytes	9.06	Circulatory failure	2.21	Onset of circulatory failure	7.70
Creatine	8.36	Renal failure	1.60	Duration of renal failure	6.37
Age	8.27	Creatinine	1.59	Onset of renal failure	5.46
Hematocrit	8.09	Duration of pulmonary failure	1.38	APACHE II	4.72
Onset of circulatory failure	7.95	Urea	1.19	Duration of pulmonary failure	4.45
APACHE II	6.70	APACHE II	1.19	Creatinine	4.09
Duration of circulatory failure	5.48	CRP	0.92	WBC	3.80

APACHE II, acute physiology and chronic health evaluation II; CRP, C-reactive protein; WBC, white blood cell count.

Figure 2 shows the relationship between important variables (the top five) and the outcome. The first column (a) displays the top features for intervention, the second column (b) is for death in the intervention group, and the third column (c) is for death in the non-intervention group. A scatter plot was used to show the relationship between categorical variables and the outcome, and a box plot was used to show the relationship between quantitative data and the outcome. Pulmonary failure persisted significantly longer in the intervention groups than in the non-intervention groups, along with higher neutrophil and creatinine levels and a lower albumin level, while the lymphocyte level was similar between these two groups. The top five important features of death were all about circulatory and renal failure. The difference between the intervention and non-intervention groups, among deceased patients, was that the duration of renal and circulatory failure had an impact on death in the intervention group, while the most important variables for death in the non-intervention group were the rate of renal failure and circulatory failure.

3.3. Prediction and Diagnostic Performance for Intervention and Mortality

Regarding the prediction of intervention, the accuracy of ML-based intervention prediction was 96%, thus indicating that predicting both the positive and negative categories of the model was highly accurate. The model identified 74% (sensitivity) of patients requiring intervention. Overall, the AUC was approximately 90%, and the positive likelihood ratio was 22.3. The death in the intervention patients were 86% recognized (sensitivity), the AUC reached 89%, and the positive likelihood ratio was 6.14. In terms of death in non-intervention prediction, the ML-based model performed better, the AUC could reach 98%, and the positive likelihood ratio was 69.6 (Table 3). The performance of all three ML models on the test dataset was consistent with the above-mentioned.

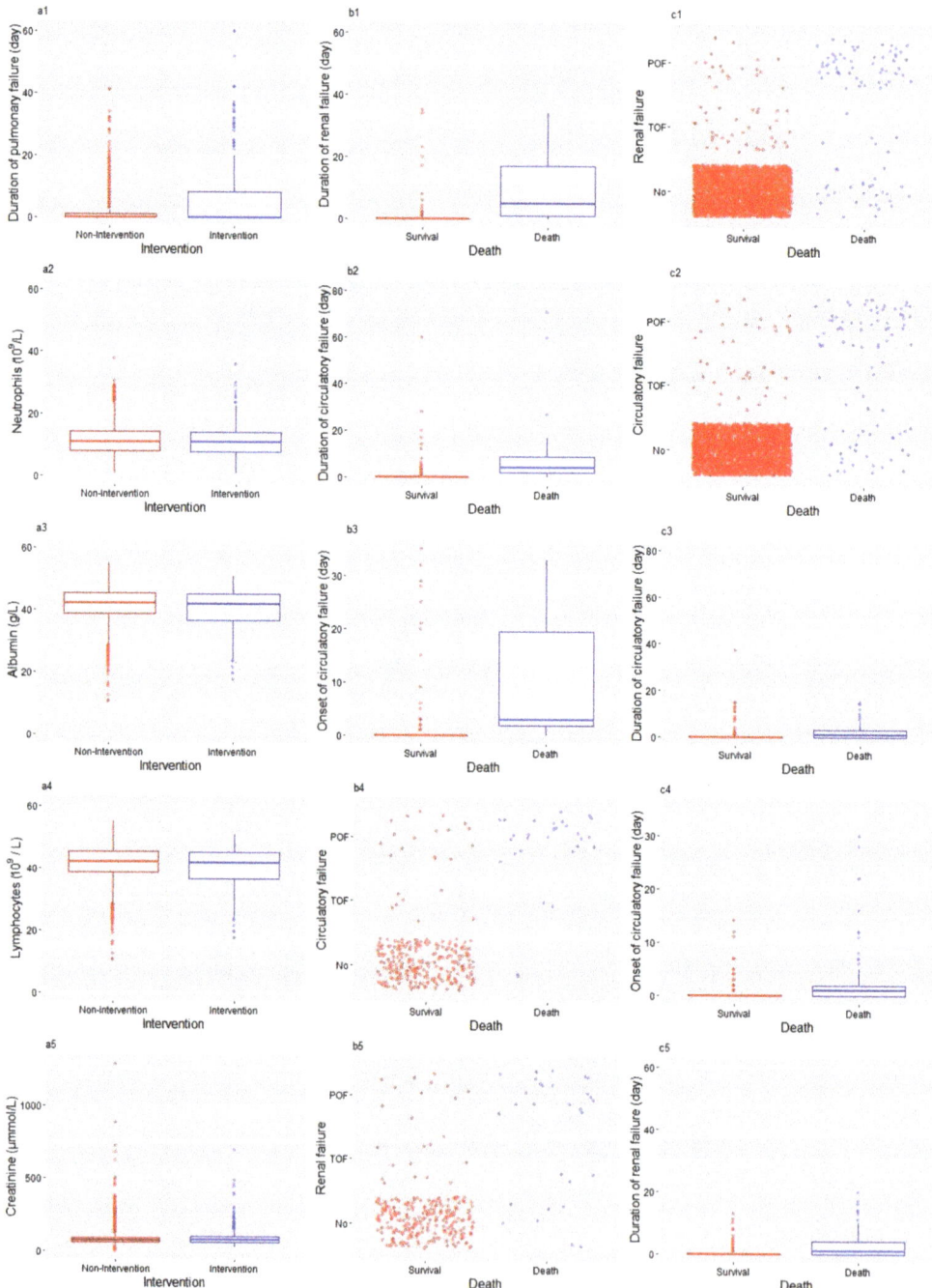

Figure 2. The relationship between important variable (the top five) and outcome. The first column (**a1–a5**) displays the top features for intervention, the second column (**b1–b5**) is for death in the intervention group, and the third column (**c1–c5**) is for death in the non-intervention group.

Table 3. Performance of prediction for the three groups.

	Accuracy	AUC	Sensitivity	Specificity	Likelihood Ratio (+)	Likelihood Ratio (−)
Predicting Intervention in AP (n = 2846)						
Validation (n = 569)	0.96	0.90	0.74	0.97	22.3	0.27
Test (n = 569)	0.97	0.91	0.76	0.97	25.5	0.35
Predicting Death in Intervention (n = 132)						
Validation (n = 26)	0.84	0.89	0.74	0.86	6.14	0.30
Test (n = 26)	0.82	0.89	0.82	0.82	4.80	0.28
Predicting Death in Non-Intervention (n = 2714)						
Validation (n = 543)	0.98	0.98	0.76	0.99	69.6	0.25
Test (n = 543)	0.98	0.99	0.77	0.99	71.9	0.31

3.4. Comparison of the Models with Prognostic Scores

Furthermore, the predictive performance for intervention and mortality, in patients with AP, from the test set was compared among ML models, SOFA, BISAP, SIRS, APACHE II, and worst MCTSI by calculating the positive likelihood ratios and post-test probabilities. In the test set, 4.64% of patients with AP required intervention. The existing prognostic scores on admission showed minimal to small changes, with an increase in the likelihood of intervention in patients with AP with extremely low sensitivities, while only the ML model moderately increased the rate, with a positive likelihood ratio of 25.5 and post-test probability of 55.4%. On predicting mortality in all intervention patients, the ML model performed better, or equally, with prognostic scores. Interestingly, the ML model significantly improved the likelihood ratio (71.9) in predicting mortality in non-intervention patients, increasing the 3.39% pre-test probability to 71.6% (post-test probability), while the worst MCTSI showed nearly no change. The details are presented in Table 4.

Table 4. Performance of prediction with ML models and clinical scoring systems in the test set.

	Sensitivity	Specificity	Likelihood Ratio (+)	Post-Test Probability (%)
Intervention (4.64% pre-test probability)				
ML model	0.76	0.97	25.5	55.4
SOFA	0.08	0.98	5.0	19.6
BISAP	0.08	0.98	4.3	17.3
SIRS	0.06	0.98	3.2	13.5
APACHE II	0.08	0.98	5.4	20.8
Worst MCTSI	0.13	0.99	12.7	38.2
Death in intervention (21.97% pre-test probability)				
ML model	0.82	0.82	4.8	57.5
SOFA	0.69	0.78	3.7	51.0
BISAP	0.52	0.96	4.4	55.3
SIRS	0.44	0.84	2.3	39.3
APACHE II	0.69	0.92	6.4	64.3
Worst MCTSI	0.48	0.69	2.0	36.0
Death in non-intervention (3.39% pre-test probability)				
ML model	0.77	0.99	71.9	71.6
SOFA	0.11	0.99	21.5	43.0
BISAP	0.14	0.99	32.5	53.3
SIRS	0.07	0.99	12.7	30.8
APACHE II	0.15	0.99	30.2	51.4
Worst MCTSI	0.03	0.96	1.0	3.4

ML, machine learning; SOFA, sequential organ failure assessment; BISAP, bedside index of severity in acute pancreatitis; SIRS, systemic inflammatory response syndrome; APACHE II, acute physiology and chronic health evaluation II; MCTSI, modified computerized tomographic severity index.

4. Discussion

To the best of our knowledge, this is the first study to use ML to quantify AP intervention indications and predictors of mortality on admission. Based on substantial international AP data from two centers, we found the duration of pulmonary failure to be an important indicator of intervention, followed by neutrophils and albumin, and OF characteristics were important predictors of death, in patients with AP, by ML. Using our models, we can predict whether patients with AP require intervention at an early stage of hospitalization, thus providing an important reference for timely consideration of whether to transfer to the intervention department or a higher-level hospital that can perform intervention. Furthermore, a pre-judgment can also be made regarding death, especially in those non-intervention patients with AP.

The use of big data to capture patient-level outcomes has increased exponentially over the past 10 years, providing a strong foundation for continuing investigations on questions more specific to surgery [47]. ML algorithms, based on big data from multiple sources, are being developed to help deliver care, inform health policy, and reduce waste, since various data sources can potentially yield a rich matched data set [48,49]. ML applications can improve the accuracy of treatment protocols and health outcomes through algorithmic processes [50]. While guidelines present evidence-based international consensus statements on AP management, mainly through the collaboration of a panel of experts, new and more instructive guidelines require more data to be implemented in this era of big data.

Clinicians worldwide seem to be following the same initial, guideline-based management protocol to the greatest extent possible; nonetheless, surgeons hold different opinions regarding multidisciplinary strategies for endoscopy, radiology, and interventions. Most guidelines and related randomized controlled trials compared intervention methods [51–56] or timing [57] of interventions but investigated indicators minimally. In addition, although IPN is the intervention recommended by most AP treatment guides for necrotizing pancreatitis [38,58–60], it is often determined when the intervention approaches in clinical practice. Clinical indicators for predicting interventions on admission, using real-world big data, can balance clinical efficacy with cost effectiveness. To identify intervention patients in the early stage of hospitalization, we intended to use the data obtained on admission, as well as the worst preoperative imaging manifestations and OF characteristics, to identify predictors of intervention.

A prediction model was ultimately established. The better the predictive performance, the higher the accuracy of predicting whether a new patient with AP will be operated on or die. There were no existing prognostic scores for intervention in patients with AP, as our results demonstrated that the existing available AP-related prognostic systems showed low predictive performance for intervention. Our results revealed that the AUC for the prediction of intervention was not low, the intervention patient-recognition rate (sensitivity) was 74%, and patients who did not require surgery had recognition rates (specificity) exceeding 90%, suggesting that the model is useful for the initial screening of interventions that do not require surgery. Patients with AP who do not require intervention are ruled out first (because of high accuracy and specificity), and the remaining patients can be further observed to determine whether intervention is warranted, thus saving medical resources. Moreover, a positive likelihood ratio >5 indicated our model's good predictive effect, while other prognostic scores at the early stage of the disease almost lacked predictive value in predicting interventions in patients with AP.

The predictive performance for mortality was better with an AUC > 95% and a positive likelihood ratio > 10. This suggests that the model can be used to predict death in both interventions, more so in non-intervention patients, and attention can be focused on advancement. Regarding the top 10 variables important for death, whether the patient is operated on or not, the important variable was organ function, differing greatly from the variables important to intervention, and the other two studies predicted hospital mortality in patients with AP (Supplementary Table S4). The Dutch Pancreatitis Study Group concluded that infection, onset, and duration of OF were not associated with death in necrotizing pancreatitis [61], findings that are inconsistent with ours [62–64]. This may be because of the single center and multicenter analyses differed in their results. Therefore, we used a two-center study to further confirm that OF was more important than infection as a predictor of death in AP, based extensive AP data.

Our study also has some limitations. Firstly, most of the data were collected on admission; however, the condition of the patients with AP changed over time. To predict surgery and death more accurately, more time-consuming variables or more frequent data collection are required for predictive research. Secondly, if invasive intervention was required, we usually performed selective percutaneous catheter drainage (pancreatic necrosis less than 30%) or a retroperitoneal pancreatic necrosectomy approach (pancreatic necrosis greater than 30%), but we did not perform percutaneous or endoscopic transgastric drainage routinely [62]. Comparison between open and minimally invasive procedures would modify the current model and require further analysis. Thirdly, the retrospective collection of data may not contain all the features needed for current or future studies, which makes it impossible to guarantee homogeneity between the local data and study data in model reproduction. Therefore, more prospective data sources in multi-regional and multi-center studies may strengthen the interpretation of model validation methods and, consequently, establish general models that can be widely promoted.

5. Conclusions

ML models are potentially useful in predicting intervention and death, in patients with AP, using clinical indicators on admission.

Supplementary Materials: The following supporting information can be downloaded at: https://www.mdpi.com/article/10.3390/jpm12040616/s1, Table S1. Parameter sensitivity analysis. Table S2. Characteristics between died and survived intervention patients with AP. Table S3. Characteristics between died and survived non-intervention patients with AP. Table S4. Characteristics of studies predicted hospital mortality in patients with AP [65,66].

Author Contributions: N.S. and L.L. contributed equally to this study. Conceptualization, X.Z. and J.A.W.; Methodology, L.L., P.Z. and T.R.W.W.; Formal Analysis, L.L. and J.L.; Data Curation, N.S. and W.H.; Writing–Original Draft Preparation, N.S. and L.L.; Writing–Review & Editing, P.S., W.H., Q.X., J.A.W. and X.Z.; Supervision, Q.X. and X.Z.; Project Administration, Q.X. and R.S.; Funding Acquisition, N.S., X.Z. and Q.X. All authors have read and agreed to the published version of the manuscript.

Funding: This work was supported by the NZ-China Strategic Research Alliance 2016 Award (China: 2016YFE0101800, Q.X. and W.H.; New Zealand: J.A.W.); This study was supported by Sichuan Provincial Department of Science and Technology (Grant No. 19ZDYF1765, 2020YFS0235). 1.3.5 project for disciplines of excellence, West China Hospital, Sichuan University (Grant No. ZYJC18010). Center of Excellence-International Collaboration Initiative Grant (Grant No. 139170052).

Institutional Review Board Statement: Ethical approval was not required was provided by the Institutional Review Board of West China Hospital of Sichuan University (WCH/SCU) due to prior approval for the use of retrospective data. Informed consent was obtained from patients admitted to Royal Liverpool University Hospital (RLUH) and ethical approval was not required because anonymized data were used.

Informed Consent Statement: Patient consent was waived due to prior approval for the use of retrospective data or anonymized data were used.

Data Availability Statement: Restrictions apply to the availability of data generated or analysed during this study to preserve patient confidentiality or because they were used under license. The corresponding author will on request detail the restrictions and any conditions under which access to some data may be provided.

Acknowledgments: These authors thank all the staff from the pancreas multidisciplinary teams at West China Hospital of Sichuan University and Royal Liverpool University Hospital for their continuous support.

Conflicts of Interest: The authors declare no conflict of interest.

References

1. Peery, A.F.; Crockett, S.D.; Murphy, C.C.; Lund, J.L.; Dellon, E.S.; Williams, J.L.; Jensen, E.T.; Shaheen, N.J.; Barritt, A.S.; Lieber, S.R.; et al. Burden and Cost of Gastrointestinal, Liver, and Pancreatic Diseases in the United States: Update 2018. *Gastroenterology* **2019**, *156*, 254–272.e11. [CrossRef] [PubMed]
2. Boxhoorn, L.; Voermans, R.P.; Bouwense, S.A.; Bruno, M.J.; Verdonk, R.C.; Boermeester, M.A.; van Santvoort, H.C.; Besselink, M.G. Acute pancreatitis. *Lancet* **2020**, *396*, 726–734. [CrossRef]
3. Xiao, A.Y.; Tan, M.L.; Wu, L.M.; Asrani, V.M.; Windsor, J.A.; Yadav, D.; Petrov, M.S. Global incidence and mortality of pancreatic diseases: A systematic review, meta-analysis, and meta-regression of population-based cohort studies. *Lancet Gastroenterol. Hepatol.* **2016**, *1*, 45–55. [CrossRef]
4. Moggia, E.; Koti, R.; Belgaumkar, A.P.; Fazio, F.; Pereira, S.P.; Davidson, B.R.; Gurusamy, K.S. Pharmacological interventions for acute pancreatitis. *Cochrane Database Syst. Rev.* **2017**, *4*, CD011384. [CrossRef]
5. Gomatos, I.P.; Xiaodong, X.; Ghaneh, P.; Halloran, C.; Raraty, M.; Lane, B.; Sutton, R.; Neoptolemos, J.P. Prognostic markers in acute pancreatitis. *Expert Rev. Mol. Diagn.* **2014**, *14*, 333–346. [CrossRef]
6. Staubli, S.M.; Oertli, D.; Nebiker, C.A. Laboratory markers predicting severity of acute pancreatitis. *Crit. Rev. Clin. Lab. Sci.* **2015**, *52*, 273–283. [CrossRef]
7. Liu, T.; Huang, W.; Szatmary, P.; Abrams, S.T.; Alhamdi, Y.; Lin, Z.; Greenhalf, W.; Wang, G.; Sutton, R.; Toh, C.H. Accuracy of circulating histones in predicting persistent organ failure and mortality in patients with acute pancreatitis. *Br. J. Surg.* **2017**, *104*, 1215–1225. [CrossRef]
8. Goswami, P.; Sonika, U.; Moka, P.; Sreenivas, V.; Saraya, A. Intestinal Fatty Acid Binding Protein and Citrulline as Markers of Gut Injury and Prognosis in Patients With Acute Pancreatitis. *Pancreas* **2017**, *46*, 1275–1280. [CrossRef]
9. De-Madaria, E.; Molero, X.; Bonjoch, L.; Casas, J.; Cardenas-Jaen, K.; Montenegro, A.; Closa, D. Oleic acid chlorohydrin, a new early biomarker for the prediction of acute pancreatitis severity in humans. *Ann. Intensive Care* **2018**, *8*, 1. [CrossRef]
10. Huang, Q.; Wu, Z.; Chi, C.; Wu, C.; Su, L.; Zhang, Y.; Zhu, J.; Liu, Y. Angiopoietin-2 Is an Early Predictor for Acute Gastrointestinal Injury and Intestinal Barrier Dysfunction in Patients with Acute Pancreatitis. *Dig. Dis. Sci.* **2021**, *66*, 114–120. [CrossRef]
11. Hong, W.; Lillemoe, K.D.; Pan, S.; Zimmer, V.; Kontopantelis, E.; Stock, S.; Zippi, M.; Wang, C.; Zhou, M. Development and validation of a risk prediction score for severe acute pancreatitis. *J. Transl. Med.* **2019**, *17*, 146. [CrossRef] [PubMed]
12. Wu, H.; Li, J.; Zhao, J.; Li, S. A new scoring system can be applied to predict the organ failure related events in acute pancreatitis accurately and rapidly. *Pancreatology* **2020**, *20*, 622–628. [CrossRef] [PubMed]
13. Tan, J.W.; Zhang, X.Q.; Geng, C.M.; Peng, L.L. Development of the National Early Warning Score-Calcium Model for Predicting Adverse Outcomes in Patients With Acute Pancreatitis. *J. Emerg. Nurs.* **2020**, *46*, 171–179. [CrossRef] [PubMed]
14. Rasch, S.; Pichlmeier, E.M.; Phillip, V.; Mayr, U.; Schmid, R.M.; Huber, W.; Lahmer, T. Prediction of Outcome in Acute Pancreatitis by the qSOFA and the New ERAP Score. *Dig. Dis. Sci.* **2022**, *67*, 1371–1378. [CrossRef]
15. Fan, L.; Hui, X.; Mao, Y.; Zhou, J. Identification of Acute Pancreatitis-Related Genes and Pathways by Integrated Bioinformatics Analysis. *Dig. Dis. Sci.* **2020**, *65*, 1720–1732. [CrossRef]
16. Blenkiron, C.; Askelund, K.J.; Shanbhag, S.T.; Chakraborty, M.; Petrov, M.S.; Delahunt, B.; Windsor, J.A.; Phillips, A.R. MicroRNAs in mesenteric lymph and plasma during acute pancreatitis. *Ann. Surg.* **2014**, *260*, 341–347. [CrossRef]
17. Waldron, R.T.; Lugea, A.; Gulla, A.; Pandol, S.J. Proteomic Identification of Novel Plasma Biomarkers and Pathobiologic Pathways in Alcoholic Acute Pancreatitis. *Front. Physiol.* **2018**, *9*, 1215. [CrossRef]
18. Garcia-Hernandez, V.; Sanchez-Bernal, C.; Schvartz, D.; Calvo, J.J.; Sanchez, J.C.; Sanchez-Yague, J. A tandem mass tag (TMT) proteomic analysis during the early phase of experimental pancreatitis reveals new insights in the disease pathogenesis. *J. Proteom.* **2018**, *181*, 190–200. [CrossRef]
19. Wang, C.; Zhang, Y.; Tan, J.; Chen, B.; Sun, L. Improved Integrated Whole Proteomic and Phosphoproteomic Profiles of Severe Acute Pancreatitis. *J. Proteome Res.* **2020**, *19*, 2471–2482. [CrossRef]
20. Papachristou, G.I.; Malehorn, D.E.; Lamb, J.; Slivka, A.; Bigbee, W.L.; Whitcomb, D.C. Serum proteomic patterns as a predictor of severity in acute pancreatitis. *Pancreatology* **2007**, *7*, 317–324. [CrossRef]
21. Peng, Y.; Hong, J.; Raftery, D.; Xia, Q.; Du, D. Metabolomic-based clinical studies and murine models for acute pancreatitis disease: A review. *Biochim. Biophys. Acta Mol. Basis Dis.* **2021**, *1867*, 166123. [CrossRef] [PubMed]
22. Silva-Vaz, P.; Jarak, I.; Rato, L.; Oliveira, P.F.; Morgado-Nunes, S.; Paulino, A.; Castelo-Branco, M.; Botelho, M.F.; Tralhão, J.G.; Alves, M.G.; et al. Plasmatic Oxidative and Metabonomic Profile of Patients with Different Degrees of Biliary Acute Pancreatitis Severity. *Antioxidants* **2021**, *10*, 988. [CrossRef] [PubMed]
23. Neyton, L.P.A.; Zheng, X.; Skouras, C.; Doeschl-Wilson, A.; Gutmann, M.U.; Uings, I.; Rao, F.V.; Nicolas, A.; Marshall, C.; Wilson, L.M.; et al. Molecular Patterns in Acute Pancreatitis Reflect Generalizable Endotypes of the Host Response to Systemic Injury in Humans. *Ann. Surg.* **2022**, *275*, e453–e462. [CrossRef] [PubMed]
24. Rajkomar, A.; Dean, J.; Kohane, I. Machine Learning in Medicine. *N. Engl. J. Med.* **2019**, *380*, 1347–1358. [CrossRef]
25. Deo, R.C. Machine Learning in Medicine. *Circulation* **2015**, *132*, 1920–1930. [CrossRef]
26. DeGregory, K.W.; Kuiper, P.; DeSilvio, T.; Pleuss, J.D.; Miller, R.; Roginski, J.W.; Fisher, C.B.; Harness, D.; Viswanath, S.; Heymsfield, S.B.; et al. A review of machine learning in obesity. *Obes. Rev.* **2018**, *19*, 668–685. [CrossRef]

27. Connor, C.W. Artificial Intelligence and Machine Learning in Anesthesiology. *Anesthesiology* **2019**, *131*, 1346–1359. [CrossRef]
28. Bleidorn, W.; Hopwood, C.J. Using Machine Learning to Advance Personality Assessment and Theory. *Personal. Soc. Psychol. Rev.* **2019**, *23*, 190–203. [CrossRef]
29. Le Berre, C.; Sandborn, W.J.; Aridhi, S.; Devignes, M.D.; Fournier, L.; Smail-Tabbone, M.; Danese, S.; Peyrin-Biroulet, L. Application of Artificial Intelligence to Gastroenterology and Hepatology. *Gastroenterology* **2020**, *158*, 76–94.e2. [CrossRef]
30. Qiu, Q.; Nian, Y.J.; Guo, Y.; Tang, L.; Lu, N.; Wen, L.Z.; Wang, B.; Chen, D.F.; Liu, K.J. Development and validation of three machine-learning models for predicting multiple organ failure in moderately severe and severe acute pancreatitis. *BMC Gastroenterol.* **2019**, *19*, 118. [CrossRef]
31. Qu, C.; Gao, L.; Yu, X.Q.; Wei, M.; Fang, G.Q.; He, J.; Cao, L.X.; Ke, L.; Tong, Z.H.; Li, W.Q. Machine Learning Models of Acute Kidney Injury Prediction in Acute Pancreatitis Patients. *Gastroenterol. Res. Pract.* **2020**, *2020*, 3431290. [CrossRef] [PubMed]
32. Xu, F.; Chen, X.; Li, C.; Liu, J.; Qiu, Q.; He, M.; Xiao, J.; Liu, Z.; Ji, B.; Chen, D.; et al. Prediction of Multiple Organ Failure Complicated by Moderately Severe or Severe Acute Pancreatitis Based on Machine Learning: A Multicenter Cohort Study. *Mediat. Inflamm.* **2021**, *2021*, 5525118. [CrossRef] [PubMed]
33. Pearce, C.B.; Gunn, S.R.; Ahmed, A.; Johnson, C.D. Machine learning can improve prediction of severity in acute pancreatitis using admission values of APACHE II score and C-reactive protein. *Pancreatology* **2006**, *6*, 123–131. [CrossRef] [PubMed]
34. Sun, H.W.; Lu, J.Y.; Weng, Y.X.; Chen, H.; He, Q.Y.; Liu, R.; Li, H.P.; Pan, J.Y.; Shi, K.Q. Accurate prediction of acute pancreatitis severity with integrative blood molecular measurements. *Aging* **2021**, *13*, 8817–8834. [CrossRef]
35. Jin, X.; Ding, Z.; Li, T.; Xiong, J.; Tian, G.; Liu, J. Comparison of MPL-ANN and PLS-DA models for predicting the severity of patients with acute pancreatitis: An exploratory study. *Am. J. Emerg. Med.* **2021**, *44*, 85–91. [CrossRef]
36. Liu, N.; He, J.; Hu, X.; Xu, S.F.; Su, W.; Luo, J.F.; Wang, Q.F.; Guo, F. Acute necrotising pancreatitis: Measurements of necrosis volume and mean CT attenuation help early prediction of organ failure and need for intervention. *Eur. Radiol.* **2021**, *31*, 7705–7714. [CrossRef]
37. Banks, P.A.; Bollen, T.L.; Dervenis, C.; Gooszen, H.G.; Johnson, C.D.; Sarr, M.G.; Tsiotos, G.G.; Vege, S.S. Classification of acute pancreatitis–2012: Revision of the Atlanta classification and definitions by international consensus. *Gut* **2013**, *62*, 102–111. [CrossRef]
38. Working Group IAPAPAAPG. IAP/APA evidence-based guidelines for the management of acute pancreatitis. *Pancreatology* **2013**, *13*, e1–e15. [CrossRef]
39. Von Elm, E.; Altman, D.G.; Egger, M.; Pocock, S.J.; Gotzsche, P.C.; Vandenbroucke, J.P. STROBE Initiative. Strengthening the Reporting of Observational Studies in Epidemiology (STROBE) statement: Guidelines for reporting observational studies. *BMJ* **2007**, *335*, 806–808. [CrossRef]
40. Halonen, K.I.; Pettilä, V.; Leppäniemi, A.K.; Kemppainen, E.A.; Puolakkainen, P.A.; Haapiainen, R.K. Multiple organ dysfunction associated with severe acute pancreatitis. *Crit. Care Med.* **2002**, *30*, 1274–1279. [CrossRef]
41. Mofidi, R.; Duff, M.D.; Wigmore, S.J.; Madhavan, K.K.; Garden, O.J.; Parks, R.W. Association between early systemic inflammatory response, severity of multiorgan dysfunction and death in acute pancreatitis. *Br. J. Surg.* **2006**, *93*, 738–744. [CrossRef] [PubMed]
42. Wu, B.U.; Johannes, R.S.; Sun, X.; Tabak, Y.; Conwell, D.L.; Banks, P.A. The early prediction of mortality in acute pancreatitis: A large population-based study. *Gut* **2008**, *57*, 1698–1703. [CrossRef] [PubMed]
43. Larvin, M.; McMahon, M.J. APACHE-II score for assessment and monitoring of acute pancreatitis. *Lancet* **1989**, *2*, 201–205. [CrossRef]
44. Bollen, T.L.; Singh, V.K.; Maurer, R.; Repas, K.; van Es, H.W.; Banks, P.A.; Mortele, K.J. A comparative evaluation of radiologic and clinical scoring systems in the early prediction of severity in acute pancreatitis. *Am. J. Gastroenterol.* **2012**, *107*, 612–619. [CrossRef] [PubMed]
45. Breiman, L. Random Forests. *Mach. Learn.* **2001**, *45*, 5–32. [CrossRef]
46. Windsor, J.A. A better way to predict the outcome in acute pancreatitis? *Am. J. Gastroenterol.* **2010**, *105*, 1671–1673. [CrossRef]
47. Knight, S.R.; Ots, R.; Maimbo, M.; Drake, T.M.; Fairfield, C.J.; Harrison, E.M. Systematic review of the use of big data to improve surgery in low- and middle-income countries. *Br. J. Surg.* **2019**, *106*, e62–e72. [CrossRef]
48. Murdoch, T.B.; Detsky, A.S. The inevitable application of big data to health care. *JAMA* **2013**, *309*, 1351–1352. [CrossRef]
49. Belle, A.; Thiagarajan, R.; Soroushmehr, S.M.; Navidi, F.; Beard, D.A.; Najarian, K. Big Data Analytics in Healthcare. *Biomed. Res. Int.* **2015**, *2015*, 370194. [CrossRef]
50. Adkins, D.E. Machine Learning and Electronic Health Records: A Paradigm Shift. *Am. J. Psychiatry* **2017**, *174*, 93–94. [CrossRef]
51. Van Santvoort, H.C.; Besselink, M.G.; Bakker, O.J.; Hofker, H.S.; Boermeester, M.A.; Dejong, C.H.; van Goor, H.; Schaapherder, A.F.; van Eijck, C.H.; Bollen, T.L.; et al. A step-up approach or open necrosectomy for necrotizing pancreatitis. *N. Engl. J. Med.* **2010**, *362*, 1491–1502. [CrossRef] [PubMed]
52. Raraty, M.G.; Halloran, C.M.; Dodd, S.; Ghaneh, P.; Connor, S.; Evans, J.; Sutton, R.; Neoptolemos, J.P. Minimal access retroperitoneal pancreatic necrosectomy: Improvement in morbidity and mortality with a less invasive approach. *Ann. Surg.* **2010**, *251*, 787–793. [CrossRef] [PubMed]
53. Gomatos, I.P.; Halloran, C.M.; Ghaneh, P.; Raraty, M.G.; Polydoros, F.; Evans, J.C.; Smart, H.L.; Yagati-Satchidanand, R.; Garry, J.M.; Whelan, P.A.; et al. Outcomes From Minimal Access Retroperitoneal and Open Pancreatic Necrosectomy in 394 Patients With Necrotizing Pancreatitis. *Ann. Surg.* **2016**, *263*, 992–1001. [CrossRef] [PubMed]

54. Bang, J.Y.; Arnoletti, J.P.; Holt, B.A.; Sutton, B.; Hasan, M.K.; Navaneethan, U.; Feranec, N.; Wilcox, C.M.; Tharian, B.; Hawes, R.H.; et al. An Endoscopic Transluminal Approach, Compared With Minimally Invasive Surgery, Reduces Complications and Costs for Patients With Necrotizing Pancreatitis. *Gastroenterology* **2019**, *156*, 1027–1040.e3. [CrossRef]
55. Hollemans, R.A.; Bakker, O.J.; Boermeester, M.A.; Bollen, T.L.; Bosscha, K.; Bruno, M.J.; Buskens, E.; Dejong, C.H.; van Duijvendijk, P.; van Eijck, C.H.; et al. Superiority of Step-up Approach vs Open Necrosectomy in Long-term Follow-up of Patients With Necrotizing Pancreatitis. *Gastroenterology* **2019**, *156*, 1016–1026. [CrossRef]
56. Van Brunschot, S.; Hollemans, R.A.; Bakker, O.J.; Besselink, M.G.; Baron, T.H.; Beger, H.G.; Boermeester, M.A.; Bollen, T.L.; Bruno, M.J.; Carter, R.; et al. Minimally invasive and endoscopic versus open necrosectomy for necrotising pancreatitis: A pooled analysis of individual data for 1980 patients. *Gut* **2018**, *67*, 697–706. [CrossRef]
57. Van Grinsven, J.; van Dijk, S.M.; Dijkgraaf, M.G.; Boermeester, M.A.; Bollen, T.L.; Bruno, M.J.; van Brunschot, S.; Dejong, C.H.; van Eijck, C.H.; van Lienden, K.P.; et al. Postponed or immediate drainage of infected necrotizing pancreatitis (POINTER trial): Study protocol for a randomized controlled trial. *Trials* **2019**, *20*, 239. [CrossRef]
58. Tenner, S.; Baillie, J.; DeWitt, J.; Vege, S.S. American College of Gastroenterology guideline: Management of acute pancreatitis. *Am. J. Gastroenterol.* **2013**, *108*, 1400–1416. [CrossRef]
59. Yokoe, M.; Takada, T.; Mayumi, T.; Yoshida, M.; Isaji, S.; Wada, K.; Itoi, T.; Sata, N.; Gabata, T.; Igarashi, H.; et al. Japanese guidelines for the management of acute pancreatitis: Japanese Guidelines 2015. *J. Hepatobiliary Pancreat. Sci.* **2015**, *22*, 405–432. [CrossRef]
60. Italian Association for the Study of the Pancreas (AISP); Pezzilli, R.; Zerbi, A.; Campra, D.; Capurso, G.; Golfieri, R.; Arcidiacono, P.G.; Billi, P.; Butturini, G.; Calculli, L.; et al. Consensus guidelines on severe acute pancreatitis. *Dig. Liver Dis.* **2015**, *47*, 532–543. [CrossRef]
61. Schepers, N.J.; Bakker, O.J.; Besselink, M.G.; Ahmed Ali, U.; Bollen, T.L.; Gooszen, H.G.; Van Santvoort, H.C.; Bruno, M.J. Impact of characteristics of organ failure and infected necrosis on mortality in necrotising pancreatitis. *Gut* **2019**, *68*, 1044–1051. [CrossRef] [PubMed]
62. Guo, Q.; Li, A.; Xia, Q.; Liu, X.; Tian, B.; Mai, G.; Huang, Z.; Chen, G.; Tang, W.; Jin, X.; et al. The role of organ failure and infection in necrotizing pancreatitis: A prospective study. *Ann. Surg.* **2014**, *259*, 1201–1207. [CrossRef] [PubMed]
63. Shi, N.; Liu, T.; de la Iglesia-Garcia, D.; Deng, L.; Jin, T.; Lan, L.; Zhu, P.; Hu, W.; Zhou, Z.; Singh, V.; et al. Duration of organ failure impacts mortality in acute pancreatitis. *Gut* **2020**, *69*, 604–605. [CrossRef] [PubMed]
64. Lan, L.; Guo, Q.; Zhang, Z.; Zhao, W.; Yang, X.; Lu, H.; Zhou, Z.; Zhou, X. Classification of Infected Necrotizing Pancreatitis for Surgery Within or Beyond 4 Weeks Using Machine Learning. *Front. Bioeng. Biotechnol.* **2020**, *8*, 541. [CrossRef]
65. Mofidi, R.; Duff, M.D.; Madhavan, K.K.; Garden, O.J.; Parks, R.W. Identification of Severe Acute Pancreatitis Using an Artificial Neural Network. *Surgery* **2007**, *141*, 59–66. [CrossRef]
66. Ding, N.; Guo, C.; Li, C.; Zhou, Y.; Chai, X. An Artificial Neural Networks Model for Early Predicting in-Hospital Mortality in Acute Pancreatitis in Mimic-Iii. *Biomed. Res. Int.* **2021**, *202*, 6638919. [CrossRef]

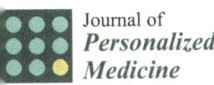

Article

Integrating Coronary Plaque Information from CCTA by ML Predicts MACE in Patients with Suspected CAD

Guanhua Dou [1], Dongkai Shan [2], Kai Wang [3], Xi Wang [4], Zinuan Liu [4], Wei Zhang [4], Dandan Li [2], Bai He [4], Jing Jing [4], Sicong Wang [5], Yundai Chen [2,†] and Junjie Yang [2,*,†]

1. Department of Cardiology, The Second Medical Center & National Clinical Research Center for Geriatric Diseases, Chinese PLA General Hospital, Beijing 100853, China; guanhuadou@163.com
2. Department of Cardiology, Sixth Medical Center, Chinese PLA General Hospital, Beijing 100048, China; shandongkai1234@163.com (D.S.); lidandan5564@163.com (D.L.); cyundai@vip.163.com (Y.C.)
3. Department of Cardiology, Yongchuan Hospital of Chongqing Medical University, Chongqing 402160, China; nkuwangkai@163.com
4. Department of Cardiology, First Medical Center, Chinese PLA General Hospital, Beijing 100853, China; plaghwangxi@163.com (X.W.); liuzinuan1995@163.com (Z.L.); zw77125@Hotmail.com (W.Z.); jsycbhhbqw@163.com (B.H.); jjing301@126.com (J.J.)
5. General Electric Healthcare China, Beijing 100176, China; sicong.wang@ge.com
* Correspondence: fearlessyang@126.com
† These authors contributed equally to this work.

Abstract: Conventional prognostic risk analysis in patients undergoing noninvasive imaging is based upon a limited selection of clinical and imaging findings, whereas machine learning (ML) algorithms include a greater number and complexity of variables. Therefore, this paper aimed to explore the predictive value of integrating coronary plaque information from coronary computed tomographic angiography (CCTA) with ML to predict major adverse cardiovascular events (MACEs) in patients with suspected coronary artery disease (CAD). Patients who underwent CCTA due to suspected coronary artery disease with a 30-month follow-up for MACEs were included. We collected demographic characteristics, cardiovascular risk factors, and information on coronary plaques by analyzing CCTA information (plaque length, plaque composition and coronary artery stenosis of 18 coronary artery segments, coronary dominance, myocardial bridge (MB), and patients with vulnerable plaque) and follow-up information (cardiac death, nonfatal myocardial infarction and unstable angina requiring hospitalization). An ML algorithm was used for survival analysis (CoxBoost). This analysis showed that chest symptoms, the stenosis severity of the proximal anterior descending branch, and the stenosis severity of the middle right coronary artery were among the top three variables in the ML model. After the 22nd month of follow-up, in the testing dataset, ML showed the largest C-index and AUC compared with Cox regression, SIS, SIS score + clinical factors, and clinical factors. The DCA of all the models showed that the net benefit of the ML model was the highest when the treatment threshold probability was between 1% and 9%. Integrating coronary plaque information from CCTA based on ML technology provides a feasible and superior method to assess prognosis in patients with suspected coronary artery disease over an approximately three-year period.

Keywords: coronary plaque; machine learning; major adverse cardiovascular events; coronary artery disease; coronary computed tomographic angiography

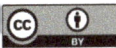

1. Introduction

Coronary computed tomography angiography (CCTA) is increasingly accepted as a first-line noninvasive imaging examination that has shown high accuracy for diagnosing and excluding coronary artery disease (CAD) [1,2]. Furthermore, CCTA examination was used to evaluate various stages of atherosclerosis ranging from plaque formation (length, composition, and morphology) to plaque progression, aiding in risk stratification for future major adverse cardiovascular events (MACE) and medical decision-making for patients with CAD [3–7].

Conventional CCTA risk scores were used to stratify the patients with CAD mainly based on the presence, length, composition, and luminal stenosis of 16-segment coronary plaque [8–10]. This plaque information was integrated into a single score, assuming a linear relationship between the atherosclerosis extent and outcomes [8,11,12]. Machine learning (ML) is a field of computer science that uses advanced algorithms including a great number of variables to optimize prediction, and this methodology has the potential to maximize the utilization of the coronary plaque information derived from CCTA without prior assumptions for independent variables. Previous studies have demonstrated that ML showed improves predictive values for death, myocardial ischemia and myocardial infarction compared with conventional risk scores [13–15]. The aim of the present study was to explore whether ML based on survival data with a time-dependent outcome integrating plaque information from CCTA exhibits better predictive values for MACEs over an approximately three-year follow-up period than the conventional CCTA risk score in patients with suspected coronary artery disease.

2. Materials and Methods

2.1. Study Population

This is a single-center prospective observational study that was approved by the institutional review board of PLA General Hospital. All patients provided written informed consent. A total of 5526 patients with suspected coronary artery disease who sequentially underwent CCTA at the Department of Cardiology of PLA General Hospital were included from January 2015 to December 2016. The inclusion criteria were complete CCTA and clinical data. The exclusion criteria were prior known CAD (defined as prior myocardial infarction or revascularization) or those with early revascularization after CCTA (defined as within 3 months), incomplete CCTA, motion artifacts, poor-quality images, or severe coronary artery calcification that was unable to be interpreted (Figure 1). In total, 4017 patients were included.

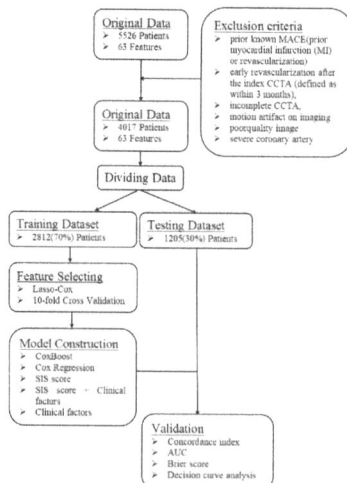

Figure 1. A flowchart about the framework of this study. The data were randomly divided into a training dataset and a testing dataset at a ratio of 7:3. The training dataset was used to build the prediction model, whereas the testing dataset was independently used to verify the effectiveness of the prediction model generated by the training dataset by computing C-index, AUC, Brier score and DCA.

2.2. Clinical Data

Demographic characteristics (age, male sex, and body mass index [BMI]) and conventional cardiovascular risk factors (dyslipidemia, hypertension, diabetes, current smoking, and family history of CAD) were collected by checking the medical record system. Hypertension was defined as a history of blood pressure >140 mmHg or treatment with antihypertensive medications. Diabetes mellitus was defined by a diagnosis made previously and/or use of insulin or oral hypoglycemic agents. Smoking was defined as current smoking or cessation of smoking within the last 3 months. A family history of premature CAD was defined as MI in a first-degree relative <55 years (male) or <65 years (female). Dyslipidemia was defined as known but untreated dyslipidemia or current treatment with lipid-lowering medications.

2.3. Image Acquisition and Analysis

A second-generation dual-source CT (Simens CT SOMATOM Definition Flash, SIEMENS AG, Munich, Germany) was used for the CCTA scanning. The acquisition protocols were performed in accordance with the Society of Cardiovascular Computed Tomography guidelines [16]. A detailed methodology has been previously published [17].

All images were analyzed by three radiologists or cardiologists using the 16-segment coronary artery tree model for the segment involvement score (SIS score) and the 18-segment coronary artery tree model for ML [10,16]. Plaque was defined as a tissue structure > 1 mm^2 within or adjacent to the coronary artery lumen that could be distinguished from surrounding pericardial tissue, epicardial fat, or the vessel lumen [8]. The presence of plaque was evaluated with the corresponding stenosis severity in each segment. The coronary plaques in each segment were classified as noncalcified, mixed, and calcified plaques. The corresponding stenosis severity of the plaques was classified as 0%, 1–24%, 25–49%, 50–69%, 70–99%, and 100%. Lengths of coronary plaque were classified as 0 mm, <10 mm, 10–20 mm, and >20 mm. Coronary dominance was divided into left dominant, right dominant, and balanced types. Myocardial bridge was defined as a coronary artery segment that was surrounded by myocardium and led to systolic compression of a part of the myocardium covering the epicardial vessels [18]. Plaques with two or more characteristics (positive remodeling, spotty calcification, low attenuation plaque, and napkin-ring sign) at the same time were defined as vulnerable plaques [19]. Positive remodeling was assessed as the cross-sectional area at the site of maximal stenosis divided by an average of the proximal and distal reference segment cross-sectional areas [20]. Spotty calcification was defined by calcium deposits (>130 HU) that were <3 mm within an atheroma [21]. A low attenuation plaque was defined as a plaque with an average attenuation <30 HU, and the size of the necrotic core was >1 mm^2 [19]. The napkin-ring sign was defined as a ring of attenuation of <130 HU that formed an arc of higher attenuation around a low attenuating plaque [22].

2.4. Outcome

The survival status of the patient was obtained by reviewing the electronic medical record system or patient interviews at least 90 days after CCTA examination from 1 January 2015 to 31 August 2020. MACEs, including nonfatal myocardial infarction, unstable angina requiring hospitalization, and cardiac death, were recorded as the outcome of the present study. Two physicians judged each event independently. In the case of divergence, a third physician was consulted.

2.5. Machine Learning Algorithm with Survival Times

Fifty-seven CCTA variables (including plaque length, plaque composition and stenosis severity of 18 coronary artery segments, coronary artery dominance, myocardial bridge, and vulnerable plaque) and nine clinical factors (including male, age, BMI, diabetes, hypertension, dyslipidemia, family history of CAD, current smoking, and chest symptoms) were available (Table 1). Machine learning involved automated feature selection, model building, and 10-fold stratified cross-validation for the entire process [23,24]. Machine learning techniques were implemented using R version 4.0.2.

Table 1. Features Selected by Lasso-Cox.

Features	Definition	Category
\multicolumn{3}{c}{Demographic characteristics}		
Age	Age of the patient	continuous variable
BMI	Body mass index	continuous variable
Male	Are they male?	1/0 = yes/no
Cardiovascular risk factors		
Symptom	Types of chest pain	0/1/2 = no/atypical/typical
Hyperlipemia	Is there hyperlipemia	1/0 = yes/no
Hypertension	Is there hypertension	1/0 = yes/no
Diabetes	Is there diabetes	1/0 = yes/no
Currently smoking	Are they currently smoking	1/0 = yes/no
Family history of CAD	Is there family history for CAD	1/0 = yes/no
CCTA Features		
Coronary dominance	Is there left/right/balanced dominance?	1/2/3 = left/right/balanced
Myocardial bridge	Is there myocardial bridge?	1/0 = yes/no
Vulnerable plaque	Are there two or more characteristics of vulnerable plaque?	1/0 = yes/no
RCAp_composition	Composition of plaque in proximal RCA	0/1/2/3 = normal/calcified/non-calcified/mix
RCAm_composition	Composition of plaque in middle RCA	0/1/2/3 = normal/calcified/non-calcified/mix
RCAd_composition	Composition of plaque in distal RCA	0/1/2/3 = normal/calcified/non-calcified/mix
P-PDA_composition	Composition of plaque in PDA of RCA origin	0/1/2/3 = normal/calcified/non-calcified/mix
LM_composition	Composition of plaque in LM	0/1/2/3 = normal/calcified/non-calcified/mix
LADp_composition	Composition of plaque in proximal LAD	0/1/2/3 = normal/calcified/non-calcified/mix
LADm_composition	Composition of plaque in middle LAD	0/1/2/3 = normal/calcified/non-calcified/mix
LADd_composition	Composition of plaque in distal LAD	0/1/2/3 = normal/calcified/non-calcified/mix
D1_composition	Composition of plaque in D1	0/1/2/3 = normal/calcified/non-calcified/mix
D2_composition	Composition of plaque in D2	0/1/2/3 = normal/calcified/non-calcified/mix
LCXp_composition	Composition of plaque in proximal LCX	0/1/2/3 = normal/calcified/non-calcified/mix
OM1_composition	Composition of plaque in OM1	0/1/2/3 = normal/calcified/non-calcified/mix
LCXd_composition	Composition of plaque in distal LCX	0/1/2/3 = normal/calcified/non-calcified/mix
OM2_composition	Composition of plaque in OM2	0/1/2/3 = normal/calcified/non-calcified/mix
L-PDA_composition	Composition of plaque in PDA of LAD origin	0/1/2/3 = normal/calcified/non-calcified/mix
R-PLB_composition	Composition of plaque in PLB of RCA origin	0/1/2/3 = normal/calcified/non-calcified/mix
RI_composition	Composition of plaque in RI	0/1/2/3 = normal/calcified/non-calcified/mix
L-PLB_composition	Composition of plaque in PLB of LAD origin	0/1/2/3 = normal/calcified/non-calcified/mix
RCAp_length	Length of plaque in proximal RCA	0/1/2/3 = normal/localized/segmental/diffuse
RCAm_length	Length of plaque in middle RCA	0/1/2/3 = normal/localized/segmental/diffuse
RCAd_length	Length of plaque in distal RCA	0/1/2/3 = normal/localized/segmental/diffuse
P-PDA_length	Length of plaque in PDA of RCA origin	0/1/2/3 = normal/localized/segmental/diffuse
LM_length	Length of plaque in LM	0/1/2/3 = normal/localized/segmental/diffuse
LADp_length	Length of plaque in proximal LAD	0/1/2/3 = normal/localized/segmental/diffuse
LADm_length	Length of plaque in middle LAD	0/1/2/3 = normal/localized/segmental/diffuse
LADd_length	Length of plaque in distal LAD	0/1/2/3 = normal/localized/segmental/diffuse
D1_length	Length of plaque in D1	0/1/2/3 = normal/localized/segmental/diffuse
D2_length	Length of plaque in D2	0/1/2/3 = normal/localized/segmental/diffuse
LCXp_length	Length of plaque in proximal LCX	0/1/2/3 = normal/localized/segmental/diffuse
OM1_length	Length of plaque in OM1	0/1/2/3 = normal/localized/segmental/diffuse
LCXd_length	Length of plaque in distal LCX	0/1/2/3 = normal/localized/segmental/diffuse
OM2_length	Length of plaque in OM2	0/1/2/3 = normal/localized/segmental/diffuse
L-PDA_length	Length of plaque in PDA of LAD origin	0/1/2/3 = normal/localized/segmental/diffuse
R-PLB_length	Length of plaque in PLB of RCA origin	0/1/2/3 = normal/localized/segmental/diffuse
RI_length	Length of plaque in RI	0/1/2/3 = normal/localized/segmental/diffuse
L-PLB_length	Length of plaque in PLB of LAD origin	0/1/2/3 = normal/localized/segmental/diffuse
RCAp_stenosis	Stenosis of plaque in proximal RCA	0/1/2/3/4 = normal/mininal/mild/moderate/severe
RCAm_stenosis	Stenosis of plaque in middle RCA	0/1/2/3/4 = normal/mininal/mild/moderate/severe

Table 1. *Cont.*

Features	Definition	Category
	Demographic characteristics	
RCAd_stenosis	Stenosis of plaque in distal RCA	0/1/2/3/4 = normal/mininal/mild/moderate/severe
P-PDA_stenosis	Stenosis of plaque in PDA of RCA origin	0/1/2/3/4 = normal/mininal/mild/moderate/severe
LM_stenosis	Stenosis of plaque in LM	0/1/2/3/4 = normal/mininal/mild/moderate/severe
LADp_stenosis	Stenosis of plaque in proximal LAD	0/1/2/3/4 = normal/mininal/mild/moderate/severe
LADm_stenosis	Stenosis of plaque in middle LAD	0/1/2/3/4 = normal/mininal/mild/moderate/severe
LADd_stenosis	Stenosis of plaque in distal LAD	0/1/2/3/4 = normal/mininal/mild/moderate/severe
D1_stenosis	Stenosis of plaque in D1	0/1/2/3/4 = normal/mininal/mild/moderate/severe
D2_stenosis	Stenosis of plaque in D2	0/1/2/3/4 = normal/mininal/mild/moderate/severe
LCXp_stenosis	Stenosis of plaque in proximal LCX	0/1/2/3/4 = normal/mininal/mild/moderate/severe
OM1_stenosis	Stenosis of plaque in OM1	0/1/2/3/4 = normal/mininal/mild/moderate/severe
LCXd_stenosis	Stenosis of plaque in distal LCX	0/1/2/3/4 = normal/mininal/mild/moderate/severe
OM2_stenosis	Stenosis of plaque in OM2	0/1/2/3/4 = normal/mininal/mild/moderate/severe
L-PDA_stenosis	Stenosis of plaque in PDA of LCX origin	0/1/2/3/4 = normal/mininal/mild/moderate/severe
R-PLB_stenosis	Stenosis of plaque in PLB of RCA origin	0/1/2/3/4 = normal/mininal/mild/moderate/severe
RI_stenosis	Stenosis of plaque in RI	0/1/2/3/4 = normal/mininal/mild/moderate/severe
L-PLB_stenosis	Stenosis of plaque in PLB of LCX origin	0/1/2/3/4 = normal/mininal/mild/moderate/severe

BMI, body mass index; CAD, coronary artery disease; CCTA, coronary computed tomography angiography; RCA, right coronary artery; PDA, posterior descending artery; LM, left main coronary artery; LAD, left anterior descending branch; D1, first diagonal branches; D2, second diagonal branches; LCX, left circumflex branch; OM1, first obtuse marginal branch; OM2, second obtuse marginal branch; PLB, posterior lateral branch; RI, intermediate ramus.

First, the data were randomly divided into a training dataset and a testing dataset at a 7:3 ratio. The training dataset was used to build the prediction model, and the testing dataset was independently used to verify the effectiveness of the prediction model generated by the training dataset.

Second, automated feature selection for fifty-seven CCTA variables and nine clinical factors was performed in the training dataset using least absolute shrinkage and selection operator regression for Cox regression (LASSO-COX), which minimizes the log partial likelihood subject to the sum of the absolute values of the parameters being bounded by a constant, shrinks coefficients, and produces some coefficients that are zero, allowing for efficient variable selection (Table 1) [23].

Then, filtered CCTA variables were included for model generation. The model for MACE prediction was constructed using 'CoxBoost', an algorithm used to fit a Cox proportional hazards model by componentwise likelihood based on the offset-based boosting approach. This algorithm is especially suited for models with a large number of variables and allows for mandatory covariates with unpenalized parameter estimates [25–28].

The model building procedure using the training dataset included two steps, as follows. First, the hyperparameters of CoxBoost (penalty, optimal step, and numbers of estimators) were automatically calculated by the training dataset. The penalty value was calculated using a coarse line search that lead to an optimal number of boosting steps for CoxBoost, as determined by 10-fold cross-validation [29]. The optimal step of the model was confirmed using a coarse line search considering the connections between parameters to identify a potential combination of tuned hyperparameters (a penalty updating scheme was helped by an optimum step-size modification for CoxBoost), which results in an optimal model in terms of cross-validated partial log-likelihood [26]. Second, after tuning the hyperparameters from 10-fold stratified cross validation, the model was refitted on the entire training dataset for the training model. Then, the trained model was validated on the independent testing dataset (30% of entire data) to show the prediction probabilities. Compared with other models, the performance of the ML model was derived from the testing dataset.

2.6. The Reference Models

First, Cox proportional hazard regression (Cox regression), including the same variables as the ML model and the conventional CCTA risk score (SIS score) assessing overall plaque burden, was used in this study. The SIS score was calculated as a measure of overall coronary segments with plaque by summation of the absolute number of coronary segments with plaques (0–16) [30]. Second, the clinical factors were added to the SIS score (SIS score + clinical factors), and only clinical factors were used in this study as reference models.

2.7. Statistical Analysis

Continuous variables are presented as the mean ± standard deviation, and categorical variables are presented as counts (%). We assessed the performance of each prediction model (including CoxBoost, Cox regression, SIS score, SIS score + clinical factors, and clinical factors) to discriminate outcomes on the testing dataset using the C-index and AUC [31]. We evaluated the calibration of each prediction model using the Brier score [32]. The Cox regression model included the variables used in the ML model. The Brier score calculates the mean squared distance between the predicted probabilities and actual outcomes, and a smaller value indicates better calibration (<0.25 indicates significant) [32]. Decision curve analysis (DCA) of all models revealed the preferred model with the best net benefit at any given threshold. The statistical analysis was implemented in R version 4.0.2. A two-sided p value < 0.05 was considered statistically significant.

3. Results

3.1. Study Population

A total of 4017 patients were included in this study. The mean age was 57.76 ± 10.98 years, and 54.29% were male (Table 2). Patients without CAD, patients with nonobstructive CAD, and patients with obstructive CAD represented 37.27%, 33.06%, and 29.67% of the study population, respectively. During a mean follow-up of 29 months, 176 events (14 cardiac deaths (0.3%), 9 nonfatal myocardial infarctions (0.2%), and 190 cases of unstable angina requiring hospitalization (4.7%)) were recorded.

Table 2. Demographic and Clinical Characteristics of Patients at Baseline.

Characteristics	Total (n = 4017)	Training Dataset (n = 2812)	Testing Dataset (n = 1205)
Age (y)	57.76 ± 10.98	57.43 ± 10.94	57.71 ± 10.86
Male (n, %)	2181 (54.29)	1544 (54.91)	637 (52.86)
BMI (kg/m^2)	25.47 ± 3.41	25.50 ± 3.43	25.40 ± 3.34
SIS score	1.80 ± 4.17	1.82 ± 2.05	1.74 ± 2.03
Follow-up time (months)	29.56 ± 5.94	29.51 ± 6.09	29.68 ± 5.57
Chest symptom			
No chest pain (n, %)	1935 (48.17)	1338 (47.58)	597 (49.54)
Atypical chest pain (n, %)	1692 (42.12)	1192 (42.39)	500 (41.49)
Typical chest pain (n, %)	390 (9.71)	282 (10.03)	108 (8.96)
Cardiovascular risk factors			
Hyperlipemia (n, %)	1311 (32.64)	912 (32.43)	399 (33.11)
Hypertension (n, %)	1916 (47.70)	1333 (47.40)	583 (48.38)
Diabetes (n, %)	660 (16.43)	451 (16.04)	209 (17.34)
Currently smoking (n, %)	1023 (25.47)	716 (25.46)	307 (25.48)
Family history of CAD (n, %)	845 (21.04)	593 (21.09)	252 (20.91)
CCTA Finding			
No CAD (n, %)	1497 (37.27)	1029 (36.6)	468 (38.8)
Non-obstructive CAD (n, %)	1328 (33.06)	917 (32.6)	411 (34.1)
Obstructive CAD (n, %)	1192 (29.67)	866 (30.8)	326 (27.1)
Vulnerable plaque (n, %)	35 (0.87)	24 (0.85)	11 (0.91)
Myocardial bridge (n, %)	332 (8.26)	221 (7.86)	111 (9.21)

Table 2. Cont.

Characteristics	Total (n = 4017)	Training Dataset (n = 2812)	Testing Dataset (n = 1205)
	Coronary dominance		
Left dominant (n, %)	3736 (93.00)	2613 (92.92)	1123 (93.20)
Right dominant (n, %)	198 (4.93)	138 (4.91)	60 (4.98)
Balanced type (n, %)	83 (2.07)	61 (2.17)	22 (1.83)

Values are means ± SD or counts (%). BMI, body mass index; CAD, coronary artery disease; CCTA, coronary computed tomography angiography.

3.2. Feature Selection and Model Generation

In this study, feature selection was performed by LASSO-COX (Figure 2). When the hyperparameter of feature selection were determined (partial likelihood deviance is minimum), the algorithm output filtered variables with non-zero coefficients (chest symptoms (symptom); MB; plaque composition of the middle right coronary, the left main coronary artery, the proximal, middle and distal anterior descending branch, the first obtuse marginal branch, and the ramus intermedius artery (RCAm_composition, LM_composition, LADp_composition, LADm_composition, LADd_composition, OM1_composition, RI_composition); plaque length of the distal right coronary, the proximal anterior descending branch, and the proximal circumflex branch (RCAd_length, LADp_length, LCXp_length); and stenosis of the proximal and middle right coronary, the left main coronary artery, the proximal, middle and distal anterior descending branch, the first and second diagonal branch, and the proximal circumflex branch (RCAp_stenosis, RCAm_stenosis, LM_stenosis, LADp_stenosis, LADm_stenosis, LADd_stenosis, D1_stenosis, D2_stenosis, LCXp_stenosis)) (Figure 2).

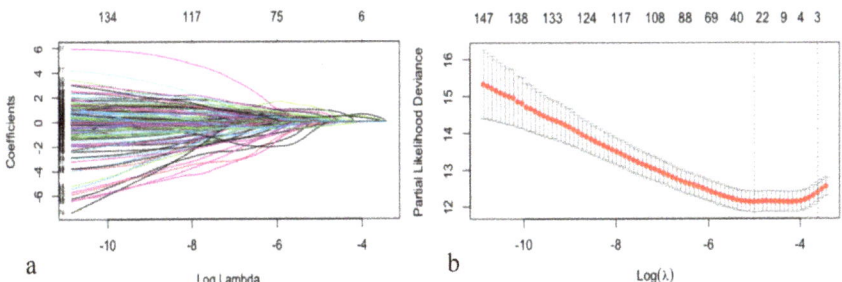

Figure 2. Selecting process for features by Lasso-Cox. Automated feature selection for fifty-seven CCTA variables and nine clinical factors was performed using LASSO-COX, which minimizes the log partial likelihood subject to the sum of the absolute values of the parameters being bounded by a constant, shrinks coefficients, and produces some coefficients that are zero, allowing efficient variable selection (**a**). When the hyperparameters of feature selection were determined (partial likelihood deviance is minimum) (**b**), the algorithm outputted 21 filtered variables with non-zero coefficients (the filtered variables were included in model generation subsequently).

After feature selection, the filtered variables were included in model generation (Figure 3). When the hyperparameters of the ML model were determined (the penalty was 1116, and the step was 74), the optimal model (the logplik of the 10-fold stratified cross validation was the largest) was identified in the training dataset (Figure 3a). In the ML model, chest symptoms, stenosis of the proximal anterior descending branch, and stenosis of the middle right coronary artery were among the top three variables (Figure 3b).

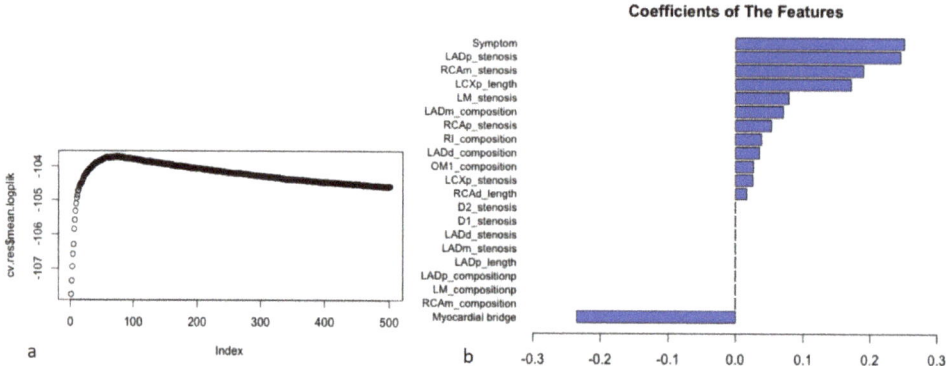

Figure 3. The process of model construction and coefficients of the features in the ML model. Filtered CCTA variables were included in model generation. The 21 filtered variables with non-zero coefficients in the results of LASSO-COX were included in ML model generation. The hyperparameters of ML model were automatically calculated on the training dataset. After tuning the hyperparameters (the penalty was 1116, and the step was 74) from 10-fold stratified cross validation, the model was refitted on the entire training dataset for training model. When the logplik of the 10-fold stratified cross validation was the largest (cv.res$mean.logplik = −103.723), it showed the optimal model in the training dataset and the coefficients of features (**a**). In the ML model, chest symptoms (symptom), the stenosis severity of the proximal anterior descending branch (LADp_stenosis), and the stenosis severity of the middle right coronary artery (RCAm_stenosis) were among the top three variables (coefficients: 0.251, 0.245, and 0.190, respectively) (**b**).

3.3. Assessment of the Performance of Each Prediction Model

After the 22nd month of follow-up, compared to other models (Cox regression, SIS score, SIS score + clinical factors, and clinical factors), the C-index of the ML model for prediction of the MACE in the testing dataset (30% of the data not used for model building) was significantly increased (C-index: 0.770–0.782, 0.723–0.752, 0.706–0.742, 0.686–0.712, 0.639–0.653, $p < 0.05$) (Figure 4 and Table 3), whereas the AUC of the ML model for the prediction of the MACE was also significantly increased in approximately three years [AUC (CI): 0.780 (0.726, 0.834), 0.738 (0.667, 0.809), 0.725 (0.669, 0.782), 0.702 (0.643, 0.762), 0.656 (0.581, 0.730), $p < 0.05$] (Figure 5 and Table 4).

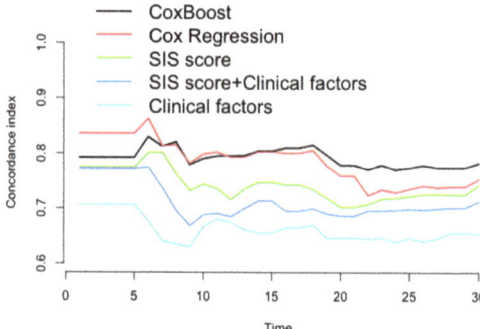

Figure 4. The concordance index for each model in testing dataset every month. After 22nd month in follow-up, compared to other models (Cox regression, SIS score, SIS score + clinical factors, and clinical factors), the C-index of ML model for prediction of the MACE in the testing dataset was significantly increased (C-index: 0.770–0.782, 0.723–0.752, 0.706–0.742, 0.786–0.712, 0.639–0.653, $p < 0.05$).

Table 3. The performance (concordance-index) for each model validated at each half year of follow-up.

Model	6th Month C-Index	12th Month C-Index	18th Month C-Index	24th Month C-Index	30th Month C-Index
CoxBoost	83.0	79.5	81.5	77.0	78.2
Cox regression	86.3	79.3	80.5	72.8	75.2
SIS score	80.0	71.5	73.3	71.8	74.2
SIS score + clinical factors	77.4	68.4	69.9	69.6	71.2
Clinical factors	67.6	67.4	67.0	63.9	65.3

Cox regression, Cox proportional hazard regression; SIS score, segment involvement score; SIS score + clinical factors, clinical factors added to segment involvement score.

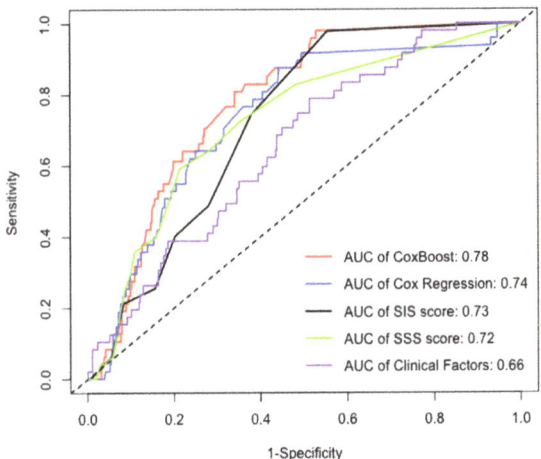

Figure 5. The AUC of each model in testing dataset over 30 months. Over an approximately three-year period, compared to the AUC of other models (Cox regression, SIS score, SIS score + clinical factors, and clinical factors), the AUC of ML model for prediction of MACE was significantly increased [AUC(CI): 0.780 (0.726, 0.834), 0.738 (0.667, 0.809), 0.725 (0.669, 0.782), 0.702 (0.643, 0.762), 0.656 (0.581, 0.730), $p < 0.05$].

Table 4. Comparison of AUC for each model validated at 30 months of follow-up.

Model	AUC	95%CI	p (CoxBoost vs.)
CoxBoost	0.780	0.726, 0.834	\
Cox regression	0.738	0.667, 0.809	0.048
SIS score	0.725	0.669, 0.782	0.010
SIS score + clinical factors	0.702	0.643, 0.762	0.003
Clinical factors	0.656	0.581, 0.730	0.005

AUC, area under the receiver operator characteristic curve; Cox regression, Cox proportional hazard regression; SIS score, segment involvement score; SIS score + clinical factors, clinical factors added to segment involvement score.

3.4. Model Evaluation Using Calibration and DCA

In this study, we evaluated each model through calibration and DCA. In the model calibration, this study shows that the Brier score for each model to predict the MACE was less than 0.040 in approximately three years (<0.25 means significant) (Table 5). The DCA of all the models showed that the proportion of the benefit for the population each year was the highest when the risk assessment of the ML model was used for treatment, while the treatment threshold probability was between 1% and 9% over a period of approximately three years. (Figure 6).

Table 5. The calibration (Brier score) for each model validated at each half year of follow-up.

Model	6th Month BS	12th Month BS	18th Month BS	24th Month BS	30th Month BS
CoxBoost	0.004	0.006	0.020	0.033	0.039
Cox regression	0.004	0.012	0.021	0.033	0.039
SIS score	0.006	0.012	0.021	0.033	0.039
SIS score + clinical factors	0.004	0.011	0.020	0.033	0.039
Clinical factors	0.004	0.011	0.020	0.033	0.039

BS, Brier score; Cox regression, Cox proportional hazard regression; SIS score, segment involvement score; SIS score + clinical factors, clinical factors added to segment involvement score.

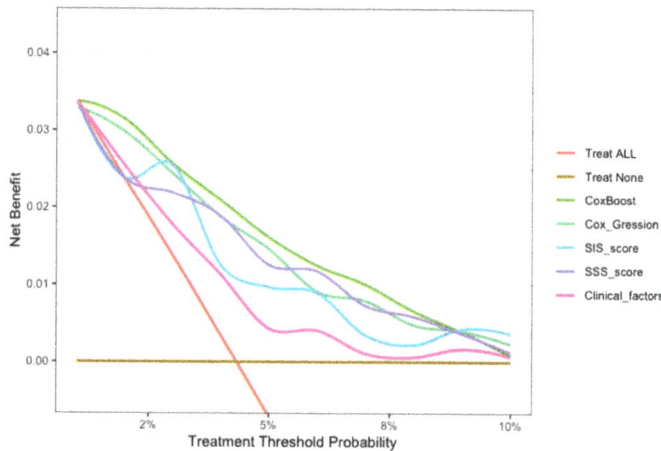

Figure 6. The decision curve analysis of all models for patients over 30 months. The brown transverse line = net benefit when all patients are considered as not having the outcome (MACEs); red oblique line = net benefit when all patients are considered as having the outcome (MACEs). The decision curve analysis of all models showed that the proportion of the benefit for the population each year was the highest when the risk assessment of the ML model was used for treatment, while the treatment threshold probability was between 1% and 9% over a period of approximately three years.

4. Discussion

In this study, we used ML integrating numerous coronary plaque factors (stenosis severity, lesion length, plaque location and composition considering the 18 coronary segments, coronary dominance, myocardial bridge (MB), and patient with vulnerable plaque) and clinical and demographic information to predict MACEs after an approximately three-year period in a cohort study that accounts for time to event. The results of this study suggest that a newly generated model based on ML, accounting for nonlinearities, provided better event prediction. This study, integrating coronary plaque information from CCTA and clinical factors based on ML technology, provides a feasible and superior method to assess prognosis in patients with suspected coronary artery disease over an approximately three-year period.

4.1. Risk Stratification with CCTA

Until recently, cardiac imaging studies were more inclined to use clinical and coronary plaque features (presence, extent, location, and composition) of CCTA for risk stratification of future events [33,34]. Cheruvu C showed that the maximal severity of CAD is related to major cardiovascular events [35]. The number of segments with plaque, location, and composition also improve risk assessment [36,37]. Currently, the use of CCTA information is far from insufficient, whereas the resolution of CCTA can provide massive information for mining. The conventional CCTA risk score, linear assumptions, and conventional statistical approaches may be insufficient to complete this study [38].

4.2. Machine Learning Algorithms Improve the Integration of Coronary Plaque Information for Survival Analysis

ML, a subset of artificial intelligence accounting for nonlinearities, is able to integrate a number of variables [11]. Cox regression is often limited for data mining purposes due to the correlation between variables, nonlinearity of variables (including potential complex interactions among them), and the possibility of overfitting.

The feasibility of ML has been demonstrated previously in CAD risk reclassification analysis. Using 25 clinical and 44 CCTA features, Motwani et al. showed that ML significantly improved the prediction of death compared with the Framinghan risk score, SSS, SIS, and the Duke prognostic index [13]. Moreover, Dey et al. showed that an ML model incorporating semiautomatically quantified measures of coronary plaque (plaque volumes, stenosis severity, lesion length, and contrast density difference) identified vessels with hemodynamically significant CAD (fractional flow reserve ≤ 0.80) with high accuracy (AUC = 0.84) [14]. Specifically, the ML model showed greater diagnostic accuracy than a conventional statistical model that utilized the exact same data. The findings above suggest that ML improves the integration of the available data for the prediction of a certain outcome.

However, these studies are similar to a cross-sectional study (as opposed to a cohort study) because the follow-up outcomes of these studies do not include survival time and only showed dichotomous outcomes (not time-dependent).

This study accounted for time to event to obtain a more appropriate risk estimation. In the ML model, chest symptoms, stenosis of the proximal anterior descending branch, and stenosis of the middle right coronary artery were among the top three factors (Figure 3), suggesting that we need to pay more attention to these characteristics in patients with suspected coronary disease. In the assessment of the model's performance, this study shows that the ML model significantly improved the prediction of MACEs compared with other models (Cox-Boost vs. SIS score, SIS score + clinical factors, and clinical factors: C-index: 0.770–0.782, 0.706–0.742, 0.686–0.712, 0.639–0.653, $p < 0.05$; AUC (CI): 0.780 (0.726, 0.834), 0.725 (0.669, 0.782), 0.702 (0.643, 0.762), 0.656 (0.581, 0.730), $p < 0.05$) (Figures 4 and 5 and Tables 2 and 3). Specifically, the ML model showed better predicted values than a conventional statistical model (Cox regression) that utilized the exact same variables after the 22nd month of follow-up (Cox-Boost vs. Cox regression: C-index: 0.770–0.782, 0.723–0.752, $p < 0.05$; 30-month AUC (CI): 0.780 (0.726, 0.834), 0.738 (0.667, 0.809), $p < 0.05$) (Figures 4 and 5 and Tables 2 and 3).

In the model evaluation, the ML model showed great calibration for approximately three years (Brier score < 0.040), demonstrating a low difference between the predicted risk and the actual observed risk for events, and a good prediction performance (<0.25 indicates significant) (Table 5). The decision curve analysis of all models showed that the ML model was the preferred model, with the best net benefit when the treatment threshold probability was between 1% and 9% in approximately three years (Figure 6).

This ML model can potentially translate the detailed 18-segment CCTA reads and clinical factors into an individualized risk report that might help physicians tailor preventive medical therapy. The present study established an integrated machine-learning model to predict clinical outcomes and compared it to currently available tools including SIS score, SIS score with clinical factors, and clinical factors models. The results demonstrated that the machine-learning model was feasible and easily-obtainable. Furthermore, the machine-learning model demonstrated the best performance in discrimination and calibration. The ML model could directly output MACE risk assessment within three years based on 13 non-zero variables and their coefficients in Figure 3b (symptom, LADp_stenosis, RCAm_stenosis, LCXp_length, LM_stenosis, LADm_composition, RCAp_stenosis, RI_composition, LADd_composition, OM1_composition, LCXp_stenosis, RCAd_length). For individualized preventive therapy, as is shown in present study, the proportion of the benefit for the population each year was between 0% and 3% when the risk assessment of the ML model was used for treatment, while the treatment threshold probability was between 1% and 9% over a period of approximately three years (Figure 6). Considering the incidence of MACE events (4.4%), the proportion of the benefit for the population each year of 3% is relatively better.

4.3. Study Limitations

This study, which was designed as a respective single-center cohort study, was performed in a middle-aged population with suspected coronary artery disease. Therefore, the results of this study may not be generalizable to other study populations. This study was lacking in medication history and only followed up after nearly three years. Further research may follow up for longer, add follow-up medication history, include genetic data, and identify the image feature-genome interaction, wihle combined prediction ability may potentially improve the risk estimation.

5. Conclusions

Integrating coronary plaque information from CCTA based on machine learning technology provides a feasible and superior method to assess prognosis in patients with suspected coronary artery disease over an approximately three-year period.

Author Contributions: G.D. and D.S. contributed equally to this work. Conceptualization, G.D. and J.Y.; methodology, G.D. and D.S.; software, G.D., K.W. and S.W.; validation, G.D. and K.W.; formal analysis, G.D., D.S. and K.W.; investigation, J.Y., W.Z., G.D., D.S., D.L., X.W., Z.L., B.H. and J.J.; resources, J.Y., W.Z. and Y.C.; data curation, G.D.; writing—original draft preparation, G.D.; writing—review and editing, G.D., D.S., Y.C. and J.Y.; visualization, G.D. and K.W.; supervision, Y.C.; project administration, J.Y.; funding acquisition, Y.C. All authors have read and agreed to the published version of the manuscript.

Funding: This work was supported by grants from the National Key R&D Program of China (2016YFC1300304 and 2021YFC2500505), and Medical Big Data Program of PLAGH (2019MBD-035).

Institutional Review Board Statement: The study was conducted in accordance with the Declaration of Helsinki, and approved by the Ethics Committee of Chinese PLA General Hospital (protocol code S2020-255-01 and 23 June 2020).

Informed Consent Statement: Written informed consent has been obtained from the patient(s) to publish this paper.

Data Availability Statement: Not applicable.

Acknowledgments: We acknowledge all the investigators and subjects in the study. This work was supported by grants from the National Key R&D Program of China (2016YFC1300304 and 2021YFC2500505), and Medical Big Data Program of PLAGH (2019MBD-035).

Conflicts of Interest: The authors declare no conflict of interest.

References

1. Danad, I.; Szymonifka, J.; Twisk, J.W.; Nørgaard, B.; Zarins, C.K.; Knaapen, P.; Min, J.K. Diagnostic performance of cardiac imaging methods to diagnose ischaemia-causing coronary artery disease when directly compared with fractional flow reserve as a reference standard: A meta-analysis. *Eur. Heart J.* **2016**, *38*, 991–998. [CrossRef] [PubMed]
2. Moss, A.J.; Williams, M.C.; Newby, D.E.; Nicol, E.D. The Updated NICE Guidelines: Cardiac CT as the First-Line Test for Coronary Artery Disease. *Curr. Cardiovasc. Imaging Rep.* **2017**, *10*, 15. [CrossRef] [PubMed]

3. Abdelrahman, K.M.; Chen, M.Y.; Dey, A.K.; Virmani, R.; Finn, A.V.; Khamis, R.Y.; Choi, A.D.; Min, J.K.; Williams, M.C.; Buckler, A.J.; et al. Coronary Computed Tomography Angiography From Clinical Uses to Emerging Technologies. *J. Am. Coll. Cardiol.* **2020**, *76*, 1226–1243. [CrossRef] [PubMed]
4. Hoffmann, U.; Ferencik, M.; Udelson, J.E.; Picard, M.H.; Truong, Q.A.; Patel, M.R.; Huang, M.; Pencina, M.; Mark, D.B.; Heitner, J.F.; et al. Prognostic Value of Noninvasive Cardiovascular Testing in Patients With Stable Chest Pain: Insights From the PROMISE Trial (Prospective Multicenter Imaging Study for Evaluation of Chest Pain). *Circulation* **2017**, *135*, 2320–2332. [CrossRef]
5. Schulman-Marcus, J.; ó Hartaigh, B.; Gransar, H.; Lin, F.; Valenti, V.; Cho, I.; Berman, D.; Callister, T.; DeLago, A.; Hadamitzky, M.; et al. Sex-Specific Associations Between Coronary Artery Plaque Extent and Risk of Major Adverse Cardiovascular Events: The CONFIRM Long-Term Registry. *JACC Cardiovasc. Imaging* **2016**, *9*, 364–372. [CrossRef]
6. Williams, M.C.; Hunter, A.; Shah, A.S.V.; Assi, V.; Lewis, S.; Smith, J.; Berry, C.; Boon, N.A.; Clark, E.; Flather, M.; et al. Use of Coronary Computed Tomographic Angiography to Guide Management of Patients With Coronary Disease. *J. Am. Coll. Cardiol.* **2016**, *67*, 1759–1768. [CrossRef]
7. Knuuti, J.; Wijns, W.; Saraste, A.; Capodanno, D.; Barbato, E.; Funck-Brentano, C.; Prescott, E.; Storey, R.F.; Deaton, C.; Cuisset, T.; et al. 2019 ESC Guidelines for the diagnosis and management of chronic coronary syndromes. *Eur. Heart J.* **2020**, *41*, 407–477. [CrossRef]
8. Min, J.K.; Shaw, L.J.; Devereux, R.B.; Okin, P.M.; Weinsaft, J.W.; Russo, D.J.; Lippolis, N.J.; Berman, D.S.; Callister, T.Q. Prognostic Value of Multidetector Coronary Computed Tomographic Angiography for Prediction of All-Cause Mortality. *J. Am. Coll. Cardiol.* **2007**, *50*, 1161–1170. [CrossRef]
9. Andreini, D.; Pontone, G.; Mushtaq, S.; Gransar, H.; Conte, E.; Bartorelli, A.L.; Pepi, M.; Opolski, M.P.; Hartaigh, B.Ó.; Berman, D.S.; et al. Long-term prognostic impact of CT-Leaman score in patients with non-obstructive CAD: Results from the COronary CT Angiography EvaluatioN For Clinical Outcomes InteRnational Multicenter (CONFIRM) study. *Int. J. Cardiol.* **2017**, *231*, 18–25. [CrossRef]
10. Cury, R.C.; Abbara, S.; Achenbach, S.; Agatston, A.; Berman, D.S.; Budoff, M.J.; Dill, K.E.; Jacobs, J.E.; Maroules, C.D.; Rubin, G.D.; et al. CAD-RADSTM Coronary Artery Disease—Reporting and Data System. An expert consensus document of the Society of Cardiovascular Computed Tomography (SCCT), the American College of Radiology (ACR) and the North American Society for Cardiovascular Imaging (NASCI). Endorsed by the American College of Cardiology. *J. Cardiovasc. Comput. Tomogr.* **2016**, *10*, 269–281. [CrossRef]
11. Bzdok, D.; Altman, N.; Krzywinski, M. Statistics versus machine learning. *Nat. Methods* **2018**, *15*, 233–234. [CrossRef] [PubMed]
12. Van Rosendael, A.R.; Shaw, L.J.; Xie, J.X.; Dimitriu-Leen, A.C.; Smit, J.M.; Scholte, A.J.; van Werkhoven, J.M.; Callister, T.Q.; DeLago, A.; Berman, D.S.; et al. Superior Risk Stratification With Coronary Computed Tomography Angiography Using a Comprehensive Atherosclerotic Risk Score. *JACC Cardiovasc. Imaging* **2019**, *12*, 1987–1997. [CrossRef] [PubMed]
13. Motwani, M.; Dey, D.; Berman, D.S.; Germano, G.; Achenbach, S.; Al-Mallah, M.H.; Andreini, D.; Budoff, M.J.; Cademartiri, F.; Callister, T.Q.; et al. Machine learning for prediction of all-cause mortality in patients with suspected coronary artery disease: A 5-year multicentre prospective registry analysis. *Eur. Heart J.* **2017**, *38*, 500–507. [CrossRef] [PubMed]
14. Dey, D.; Gaur, S.; Ovrehus, K.A.; Slomka, P.J.; Betancur, J.; Goeller, M.; Hell, M.M.; Gransar, H.; Berman, D.S.; Achenbach, S.; et al. Integrated prediction of lesion-specific ischaemia from quantitative coronary CT angiography using machine learning: A multicentre study. *Eur. Radiol.* **2018**, *28*, 2655–2664. [CrossRef] [PubMed]
15. Van Rosendael, A.R.; Maliakal, G.; Kolli, K.K.; Beecy, A.; Al'Aref, S.J.; Dwivedi, A.; Singh, G.; Panday, M.; Kumar, A.; Ma, X.; et al. Maximization of the usage of coronary CTA derived plaque information using a machine learning based algorithm to improve risk stratification; insights from the CONFIRM registry. *J. Cardiovasc. Comput. Tomogr.* **2018**, *12*, 204–209. [CrossRef]
16. Abbara, S.; Arbab-Zadeh, A.; Callister, T.Q.; Desai, M.Y.; Mamuya, W.; Thomson, L.; Weigold, W.G. SCCT guidelines for performance of coronary computed tomographic angiography: A report of the Society of Cardiovascular Computed Tomography Guidelines Committee. *J. Cardiovasc. Comput. Tomogr.* **2009**, *3*, 190–204. [CrossRef]
17. Kalaria, V.G.; Koradia, N.; Breall, J.A. Myocardial bridge: A clinical review. *Catheter. Cardiovasc. Interv.* **2002**, *57*, 552–556. [CrossRef]
18. Small, G.R.; Chow, B.J.W. CT Imaging of the Vulnerable Plaque. *Curr. Treat. Options Cardiovasc. Med.* **2017**, *19*, 92. [CrossRef]
19. Smits, P.C.; Pasterkamp, G.; Ufford, M.A.Q.V.; Eefting, F.D.; Stella, P.R.; De Jaegere, P.P.T.; Borst, C. Coronary artery disease: Arterial remodelling and clinical presentation. *Heart* **1999**, *82*, 461–464. [CrossRef]
20. Maurovich-Horvat, P.; Ferencik, M.; Voros, S.; Merkely, B.; Hoffmann, U. Comprehensive plaque assessment by coronary CT angiography. *Nat. Rev. Cardiol.* **2014**, *11*, 390–402. [CrossRef]
21. Tanaka, A.; Shimada, K.; Yoshida, K.; Jissyo, S.; Tanaka, H.; Sakamoto, M.; Matsuba, K.; Imanishi, T.; Akasaka, T.; Yoshikawa, J. Non-invasive assessment of plaque rupture by 64-slice multidetector computed tomography comparison with intravascular ultrasound. *Circ. J.* **2008**, *72*, 1276–1281. [CrossRef] [PubMed]
22. Yin, P.; Dou, G.; Yang, X.; Wang, X.; Shan, D.; He, B.; Jing, J.; Jin, Q.; Chen, Y.; Yang, J. Noninvasive Quantitative Plaque Analysis Identifies Hemodynamically Significant Coronary Arteries Disease. *J. Thorac. Imaging* **2021**, *36*, 102–107. [CrossRef] [PubMed]
23. Tibshirani, R. The lasso method for variable selection in the Cox model. *Stat. Med.* **1997**, *16*, 385–395. [CrossRef]
24. Harald Binder. CoxBoost, Cox Models by Likelihood Based Boosting for a Single Survival Endpoint or Competing Risks. R Package Version 1.4. Available online: https://cran/R-project.org/package=CoxBoost.2013 (accessed on 2 March 2022).

25. Binder, H.; Allignol, A.; Schumacher, M.; Beyersmann, J. Boosting for high-dimensional time-to-event data with competing risks. *Bioinformatics* **2009**, *25*, 890–896. [CrossRef] [PubMed]
26. Binder, H.; Schumacher, M. Incorporating pathway information into boosting estimation of high-dimensional risk prediction models. *BMC Bioinform.* **2009**, *10*, 18. [CrossRef] [PubMed]
27. Hadamitzky, M.; Achenbach, S.; Al-Mallah, M.; Berman, D.; Budoff, M.; Cademartiri, F.; Callister, T.; Chang, H.J.; Cheng, V.; Chinnaiyan, K.; et al. Optimized prognostic score for coronary computed tomographic angiography: Results from the CONFIRM registry (COronary CT Angiography EvaluatioN For Clinical Outcomes: An InteRnational Multicenter Registry). *J. Am. Coll. Cardiol.* **2013**, *62*, 468–476. [CrossRef]
28. Binder, H.; Schumacher, M. Allowing for mandatory covariates in boosting estimation of sparse high-dimensional survival models. *BMC Bioinform.* **2008**, *9*, 14. [CrossRef]
29. Tutz, G.; Binder, H. Boosting ridge regression. *Comput. Stat. Data Anal.* **2007**, *51*, 6044–6059. [CrossRef]
30. Tutz, G.; Binder, H. Generalized Additive Modeling with Implicit Variable Selection by Likelihood-Based Boosting. *Biometrics* **2006**, *62*, 961–971. [CrossRef]
31. Harrell, F.E.; Califf, R.M.; Pryor, D.B.; Lee, K.L.; Rosati, R.A. Evaluating the yield of medical tests. *JAMA* **1982**, *247*, 2543–2546. [CrossRef]
32. Brier, G.W. Verification of forecasts expressed in terms of probability. *Mon. Weather Rev.* **1950**, *78*, 1–3. [CrossRef]
33. Chow, B.J.; Small, G.; Yam, Y.; Chen, L.; Achenbach, S.; Al-Mallah, M.; Berman, D.S.; Budoff, M.J.; Cademartiri, F.; Callister, T.Q.; et al. Incremental prognostic value of cardiac computed tomography in coronary artery disease using CONFIRM: COroNary computed tomography angiography evaluation for clinical outcomes: An InteRnational Mul-ticenter registry. *Circ. Cardiovasc. Imaging* **2011**, *4*, 463–472. [CrossRef] [PubMed]
34. Deseive, S.; Shaw, L.J.; Min, J.K.; Achenbach, S.; Andreini, D.; Al-Mallah, M.H.; Berman, D.S.; Budoff, M.J.; Callister, T.Q.; Cademartiri, F.; et al. Improved 5-year prediction of all-cause mortality by coronary CT angiography applying the CONFIRM score. *Eur. Heart J. Cardiovasc. Imaging* **2016**, *18*, 286–293. [CrossRef] [PubMed]
35. Cheruvu, C.; Precious, B.; Naoum, C.; Blanke, P.; Ahmadi, A.; Soon, J.; Arepalli, C.; Gransar, H.; Achenbach, S.; Berman, D.S.; et al. Long term prognostic utility of coronary CT angiography in patients with no modifiable coronary artery disease risk factors: Results from the 5 year follow-up of the CONFIRM International Multicenter Registry. *J. Cardiovasc. Comput. Tomogr.* **2016**, *10*, 22–27. [CrossRef]
36. Hadamitzky, M.; Täubert, S.; Deseive, S.; Byrne, R.A.; Martinoff, S.; Schömig, A.; Hausleiter, J. Prognostic value of coronary computed tomography angiography during 5 years of follow-up in patients with suspected coronary artery disease. *Eur. Heart J.* **2013**, *34*, 3277–3285. [CrossRef]
37. Ahmadi, A.; Stone, G.W.; Leipsic, J.; Shaw, L.J.; Villines, T.C.; Kern, M.J.; Hecht, H.; Erlinge, D.; Ben-Yehuda, O.; Maehara, A.; et al. Prognostic Determinants of Coronary Atherosclerosis in Stable Ischemic Heart Disease: Anatomy, Physiology, or Morphology? *Circ. Res.* **2016**, *119*, 317–329. [CrossRef]
38. Kolossváry, M.; Kellermayer, M.; Merkely, B.; Maurovich-Horvat, P. Cardiac Computed Tomography Radiomics: A Comprehensive Review on Radiomic Techniques. *J. Thorac. Imaging* **2018**, *33*, 26–34. [CrossRef]

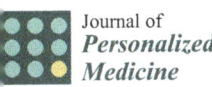

Article

Development and Evaluation of a Machine Learning Prediction Model for Small-for-Gestational-Age Births in Women Exposed to Radiation before Pregnancy

Xi Bai, Zhibo Zhou, Yunyun Luo, Hongbo Yang, Huijuan Zhu, Shi Chen and Hui Pan *

Key Laboratory of Endocrinology of National Health Commission, Department of Endocrinology, State Key Laboratory of Complex Severe and Rare Diseases, Peking Union Medical College Hospital, Chinese Academy of Medical Science and Peking Union Medical College, Beijing 100730, China; baixi199532@163.com (X.B.); pumc_zhouzhibo@student.pumc.edu.cn (Z.Z.); pumc_luoyunyun@student.pumc.edu.cn (Y.L.); yanghb@pumch.cn (H.Y.); shengxin2004@163.com (H.Z.); cspumch@163.com (S.C.)
* Correspondence: panhui20111111@163.com; Tel.: +86-10-6915-4211

Abstract: Exposure to radiation has been associated with increased risk of delivering small-for-gestational-age (SGA) newborns. There are no tools to predict SGA newborns in pregnant women exposed to radiation before pregnancy. Here, we aimed to develop an array of machine learning (ML) models to predict SGA newborns in women exposed to radiation before pregnancy. Patients' data was obtained from the National Free Preconception Health Examination Project from 2010 to 2012. The data were randomly divided into a training dataset ($n = 364$) and a testing dataset ($n = 91$). Eight various ML models were compared for solving the binary classification of SGA prediction, followed by a post hoc explainability based on the SHAP model to identify and interpret the most important features that contribute to the prediction outcome. A total of 455 newborns were included, with the occurrence of 60 SGA births (13.2%). Overall, the model obtained by extreme gradient boosting (XGBoost) achieved the highest area under the receiver-operating-characteristic curve (AUC) in the testing set (0.844, 95% confidence interval (CI): 0.713–0.974). All models showed satisfied AUCs, except for the logistic regression model (AUC: 0.561, 95% CI: 0.355–0.768). After feature selection by recursive feature elimination (RFE), 15 features were included in the final prediction model using the XGBoost algorithm, with an AUC of 0.821 (95% CI: 0.650–0.993). ML algorithms can generate robust models to predict SGA newborns in pregnant women exposed to radiation before pregnancy, which may thus be used as a prediction tool for SGA newborns in high-risk pregnant women.

Keywords: small for gestational age; exposure to radiation; machine learning; prediction

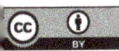

1. Introduction

Small-for-gestational-age (SGA) neonate is defined as a birth weight below a distribution-based gestational age threshold, usually the 10th percentile [1]. SGA newborns are at increased risk of perinatal morbidity and mortality [2,3]. The main risk factor related to stillbirth is unrecognized SGA before birth [4]. However, if the condition is identified before delivery, the risk can be substantially reduced, even a four-fold reduction, because antenatal prediction of SGA allows for closer monitoring and timely delivery to reduce adverse fetal outcomes [2].

Environmental pollutants have been associated with adverse pregnancy outcomes and a reduction in birth weight [5–7]. Human and animal studies have shown that the proportion of SGA increases with exposure to radiation [8,9]. High-level radiation exposure produced SGA neonates in the offspring of pregnant atomic bomb survivors [10]. Additionally, it has been reported that the radiation exposure rate in mothers with low-birth-weight newborns was higher than those with normal weight newborns [11]. Even data from studies has demonstrated that each cGy radiation reduced the birth weight of newborns by 37.6 g [12]. The causes have been reported to be the effects of radiation on the function of the ovary and uterus, as well as the effect on the hypothalamus–pituitary–thyroid axis [13,14]. However, no study has established a predictive model for SGA newborns in women exposed to radiation before pregnancy.

Risk predictive models relying on conventional statistical methods affect their application and performance in large datasets with multiple variables due to the inherent limitations of not considering the potential interactions between risk factors [15,16]. However, these limitations can be solved by machine learning (ML) approaches which can model complex interactions and maximize prediction accuracy from complex data [17]. In terms of SGA risk prediction, ML algorithms have been introduced into a few studies to obtain predictive models for SGA in the general population [18–20]. Unfortunately, these models performed poorly, with the maximum area under the receiver operating characteristic (ROC) curve (AUC) value as high as only 0.7+. In addition, paternal risk factors and maternal PM2.5 exposure during pregnancy have been confirmed as risk factors for SGA newborns [21–23]. Although these independent risk factors are identified, they have not been included in previous predictive models.

In this report, we aimed to develop and validate models using different ML algorithms to predict SGA newborns in pregnant women exposed to radiation in a living or working environment before pregnancy, based on data from a nationwide, prospective cohort study in China. In addition, paternal risk factors and pregnancy PM2.5 exposure were innovatively included in the models as predictive features.

2. Materials and Methods

2.1. Data Source

Data were obtained from the National Free Preconception Health Examination Project (NFPHEP), a 3-year project from 1 January 2010 to 31 December 2012, which was carried out in 220 counties from 31 provinces or municipalities and initiated by the National Health Commission of the People's Republic of China [24–26]. In short, the NFPHEP aimed to investigate risk factors for adverse pregnancy outcomes and improve the health of pregnant women and newborns. All data were uploaded to the nationwide electronic data acquisition system, and quality control was carried out by the National Quality Inspection Center for Family Planning Techniques. This study was approved by the Institutional Review Committee of the National Research Institute for Family Planning in Beijing, China, and informed consent was obtained from all participants.

2.2. Study Participants and Features

All singleton live newborns with complete birth records and gestational age of more than 24 weeks were included in the study, and then we selected newborns whose mothers were exposed to radiation in their living or working environment before pregnancy, involving 985 cases. After removing records with missing and extreme data of baseline characteristics, 455 births were included in the final analysis.

A pre-pregnancy examination was conducted, and follow-up was performed during pregnancy and postpartum. Information of 153 features regarding parents' social demographic characteristics, lifestyle, family history, pre-existing medical conditions, laboratory examinations and neonatal birth information were collected through face-to-face investigation and examination performed by trained and qualified staff. PM2.5 concentrations for all included counties were provided by the Chinese Center for Disease Control and Prevention, using a hindcast model specific to historical PM2.5 estimation provided by satellite-retrieved aerosol optical depth [27]. The definition of SGA was newborns with a birth weight below the 10th percentile for the gestational age and sex according to the Chinese Neonatal Network [28].

2.3. Study Design

The data processing flow is shown in Figure 1. All analyses were developed in Python (version 3.8.5). The dataset was divided randomly into the training set (80%, $n = 364$) and the testing sets (20%, $n = 91$) for the development and validation of the ML algorithms, respectively. Initially, 153 related features (Table S1) were included in ML as candidate variables for predictors. In the current study, eight ML algorithms were applied to develop the predictive models. The performances of the eight ML algorithms were evaluated by sensitivity, specificity, positive predictive value (PPV), negative predictive value (NPV) and AUC. Another measure of the quality of binary classification, Matthew's correlation coefficient (MCC), was also evaluated, which is not affected by heavily imbalanced classes. Its value ranges from −1 to 1, where the random classification has a value of 0, the perfect classification has a value of 1, and the "completely wrong" classification has a value of −1. Furthermore, Cohen's kappa was evaluated, which is another metric estimating the overall model performance. The AUC metric results were taken as the main index to measure the performances of the ML algorithms.

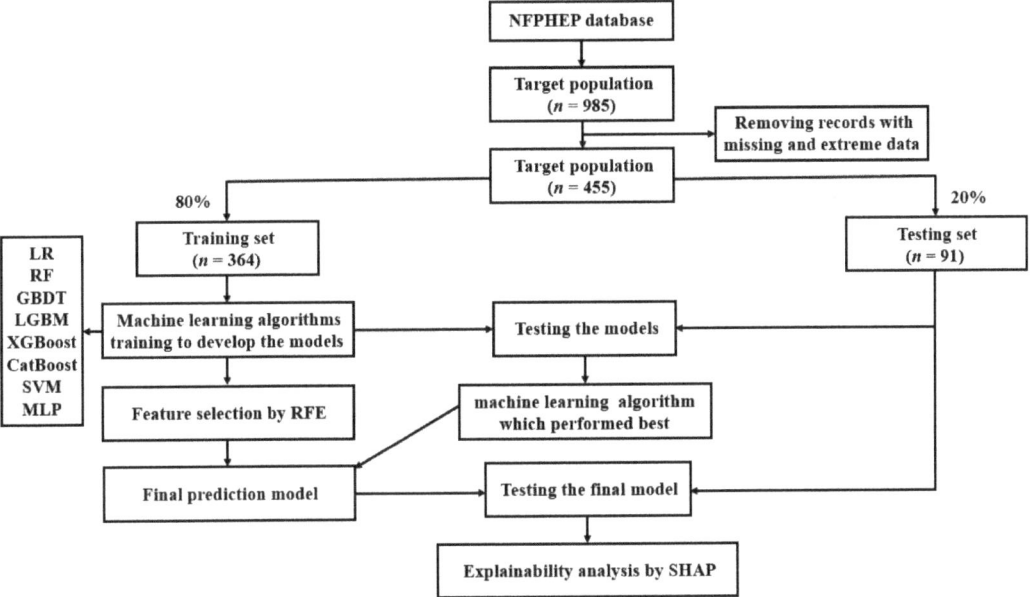

Figure 1. A flow chart of the methods used for data extraction, training, and testing. NFPHEP = National Free Preconception Health Examination Project, LR = logistic regression, RF = random forest, GBDT = gradient boosting decision tree, LGBM = light gradient boosting machine, XGBoost = extreme gradient boosting, CatBoost = category boosting, SVM = support vector machine, MLP = multi-layer perceptron, RFE = recursive feature elimination, SHAP = Shapley Additive Explanation.

Being the best performing model, the extreme gradient boosting (XGBoost) algorithm was chosen for the final prediction model. In order to reduce the computational cost of modeling, 15 features which contributed greatly to the prediction were selected from 153 features by recursive feature elimination (RFE) to reduce the number of variables in the prediction model, incorporating a XGBoost classifier as the estimator. The effectiveness of RFE approach has been proven in various medical data [29–31]. A 5-fold cross-validation was performed to select the 15 most important features. These 15 features were included in the final prediction model using the ML algorithm which performed best among the eight algorithms. Grid search was employed for the hyperparameter tunning, and the employed hyperparameters of the best performed ML algorithm (XGBoost) were max depth = [(2, 3, 4, 5, 6, 7, 8), min child weight = (1, 2, 3, 4, 5, 6) and gamma = (0.5, 1, 1.5, 2, 5). The characteristics of the final model used in the hyperparameter tunning were booster = gbtree, gamma = 1, importance type = gain, learning rate = 0.01, max depth = 6, min child weight = 1, random state = 0, reg alpha = 0, reg lambda = 1.

Furthermore, in order to correctly interpret the ML prediction model, we applied post hoc explainability on the final model using the XGBoost algorithm, based on the Shapley Additive Explanation (SHAP) model, to explain the influence of all features included for model prediction. SHAP is a game theory approach which can evaluate the importance of individual input features to the prediction of a given model [32].

2.4. ML Algorithms

A conventional logistic regression (LR) method and seven popular ML classification algorithms, including random forest (RF), gradient boosting decision tree (GBDT), XGBoost, light gradient boosting machine (LGBM), category boosting (CatBoost), support vector machine (SVM) and multi-layer perceptron (MLP), were applied in the current study to model the data. All these algorithms are the most popular and up-to-date supervised ML methods for the problem of classification. The LR model is used to predict the probability of the binary dependent variable using a sigmoid function to determine the logistic transformation of the probability [33]. RF is an ensemble classification algorithm that combines multiple decision trees by majority voting [34,35]. GBDT is based on the ensembles of decision trees, which is popular for its accuracy, efficiency and interpretability. A new decision tree is trained at each step to fit the residual between ground truth and current prediction [36]. Many improvements have been made on the basis of GBDT. LGBM aggregates gradient information in the form of a histogram, which significantly improves the training efficiency [37]. CatBoost proposes a new strategy to deal with categorical features, which can solve the problems of gradient bias and prediction shift [38]. XGBoost is an optimized distributed gradient boosting library designed for speed and performance. It uses the second-order gradient, which is improved in the aspects of the approximate greedy search, parallel learning and hyperparameters [39]. SVM is a supervised learning model which targets to create a hyperplane. The hyperplane is a decision boundary between two classes, enabling the prediction of labels from one or more feature vectors. The main goal of SVM is to maximize the distance between the closest points of each class, called support vectors [40,41]. MLP is based on a supervised training process to generate a nonlinear predictive model, which belongs to the category of artificial neural network (ANN) and is the most common neural network. It consists of multiple layers such as input layer, output layer and hidden layer. Therefore, MLP is a hierarchical feed-forward neural network, where the information is unidirectionally passed from the input layer to the output layer through the hidden layer [42].

2.5. Statistical Analyses

Categorical variables were described as number (%) and compared by Chi-square or Fisher's exact test where appropriate. Continuous variables that satisfy normal distribution were described as mean (standard deviation [SD]) and compared by the 2-tailed Student's t-test; otherwise, median (interquartile range [IQR]) and Wilcoxon Mann–Whitney U test were used. The sensitivity, specificity, PPV, NPV, MCC and kappa of the models were calculated. The predictive power of the ML models was measured by AUC in the training and testing datasets. A two-sided p value < 0.05 was considered statistically significant. All statistical analyses were performed with Python (version 3.8.5).

3. Results

3.1. Baseline Characteristics

Of the 455 newborns whose mothers had been exposed to radiation in their living or working environment before pregnancy from 1 January 2010 to 31 December 2012 in the

NFPHEP database, a total of 60 SGA births occurred (13.2%). Demographic characteristics of the study population are shown in Table 1. Supplementary Table S1 lists the results comparing the 153 candidate variables for predictors in the study cohort. Overall, the median gestational age of the newborns in the cohort was 40.0 weeks (IQR, 39.0–40.0). The birth weight of SGA newborns (2.6 kg [2.2–2.8]) was significantly lower than that of non-SGA newborns (3.4 kg [3.1–3.6]). Maternal height was significantly lower in the SGA newborns compared to the non-SGA newborns (158.0 cm [155.0–160.0] versus 160.0 cm [157.0–163.0]). The mothers of SGA newborns had a significantly higher incidence of adnexitis before pregnancy (15.0% vs. 3.5%) compared to the mothers of non-SGA newborns. In addition, the number of previous pregnancies in the mothers of SGA newborns was significantly higher than those of non-SGA newborns. Furthermore, the fathers of SGA newborns had a significantly higher incidence of anemia (8.3% vs. 1.3%) compared with those of non-SGA newborns.

Table 1. Demographic characteristics of the subjects included in analysis.

Parameters	Overall (n = 455)	Not SGA (n = 395)	SGA (n = 60)	p Value
Gestational at birth, week	40.0 (39.0–40.0)	40.0 (39.0–40.0)	40.0 (39.0–40.0)	0.013
Birth weight, kg	3.3 (3.0–3.6)	3.4 (3.1–3.6)	2.6 (2.2–2.8)	<0.001
Maternal age, year	24.0 (23.0–27.0)	24.0 (23.0–27.0)	24.5 (22.0–26.0)	0.184
Maternal height, cm	160.0 (156.0–163.0)	160.0 (157.0–163.0)	158.0 (155.0–160.0)	0.014
Maternal BMI, kg/m^2	20.2 (18.8–22.0)	20.2 (18.8–22.0)	20.0 (18.6–22.2)	0.332
Maternal education level				0.635
Below junior high school	168 (36.9%)	149 (37.7%)	19 (31.7%)	
Senior high school	146 (32.1%)	126 (31.9%)	20 (33.3%)	
Bachelor's degrees and above	141 (31.0%)	120 (30.4%)	21 (35.0%)	
Mother adnexitis before pregnancy	23 (5.1%)	14 (3.5%)	9 (15.0%)	0.001
Number of previous pregnancies	0.0 (0.0–1.0)	0.0 (0.0–1.0)	1.0 (0.0–1.0)	0.003
Paternal age, year	26.0 (24.0–29.0)	26.0 (24.0–28.0)	26.0 (24.0–29.0)	0.328
Paternal height, cm	171.4 ± 5.3	171.6 ± 5.2	170.2 ± 5.6	0.055
Paternal education level				0.810
Below junior high school	174 (38.2%)	153 (38.7%)	21 (35.0%)	
Senior high school	151 (33.2%)	131 (33.2%)	20 (33.3%)	
Bachelor's degrees and above	130 (28.6%)	111 (28.1%)	19 (31.7%)	
Father anemia before pregnancy	10 (2.2%)	5 (1.3%)	5 (8.3%)	0.003

SGA = small for gestational age, BMI = body mass index. Data are presented as median (interquartile range), mean (standard deviation) or number (%). Categorical variables are compared by Chi-square or Fisher's exact test where appropriate. Continuous variables that satisfy normal distribution are compared by the 2-tailed Student's t-test; otherwise, Wilcoxon Mann–Whitney U test are used.

3.2. ML Algorithms' Performance Comparison

LR, RF, GBDT, XGBoost, LGBM, CatBoost, SVM and MLP were developed in the training dataset (n = 364), and their SGA prediction performance was compared in the testing dataset (n = 91). Figure 2 shows the ROC curve comparison of the developed models in the testing dataset for SGA prediction. Overall, the model obtained by XGBoost achieved the highest AUC value in the testing set, 0.844 [95% confidence interval (CI): 0.713–0.974]. All models showed a good AUC for predicting SGA: XGBoost (AUC: 0.844, 95% CI: 0.713–0.974), RF (AUC: 0.835, 95% CI: 0.682–0.988), GBDT (AUC: 0.821, 95% CI: 0.699–0.944), CatBoost (AUC: 0.801, 95% CI: 0.698–0.904), LGBM (AUC: 0.768, 95% CI: 0.566–0.970), MLP (AUC: 0.723, 95% CI: 0.492–0.953) and SVM (AUC: 0.673, 95% CI: 0.474–0.873), except for LR (AUC: 0.561, 95% CI: 0.355–0.768). In addition, the AUC values in the training set and testing set, sensitivity, specificity, PPV, NPV, MCC and kappa values of each model are listed in Table 2. Model sensitivity, specificity, PPV, NPV, MCC and kappa ranged from 0.714 to 1.000, 0.333 to 0.869, 0.111 to 0.312, 0.970 to 1.000, 0.161 to 0.408 and 0.071 to 0.367, respectively.

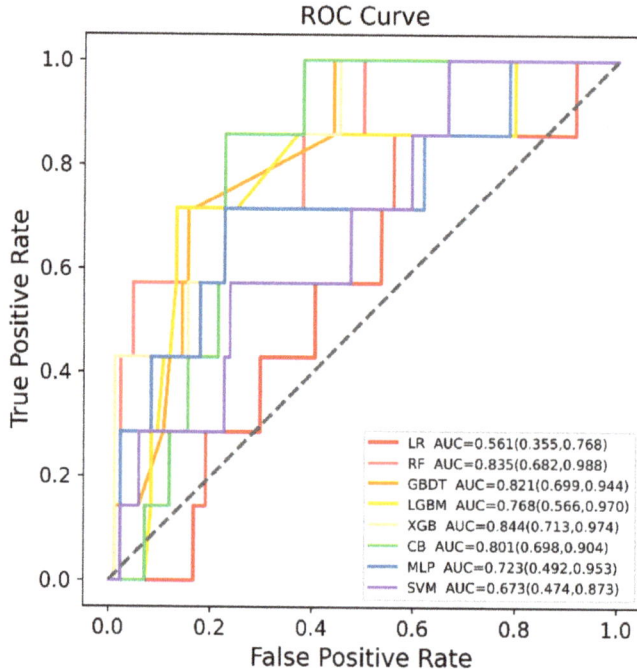

Figure 2. Receiver operating characteristic (ROC) curves of the eight machine learning (ML) models in predicting small for gestational age (SGA) in the testing dataset. LR = logistic regression, RF = random forest, GBDT = gradient boosting decision tree, LGBM = light gradient boosting machine, XGB = extreme gradient boosting, CB = category boosting, MLP = multi-layer perceptron, SVM = support vector machine.

Table 2. Performance of models by different algorithms in predicting small for gestational age (SGA) neonates.

Model	AUC Training	AUC Testing	Sensitivity	Specificity	PPV	NPV	MCC	Kappa
LR	0.620	0.561	0.857	0.440	0.113	0.974	0.161	0.074
RF	0.897	0.835	0.714	0.845	0.278	0.973	0.374	0.325
GBDT	0.850	0.821	0.714	0.845	0.278	0.973	0.374	0.325
XGBoost	0.958	0.844	0.857	0.774	0.240	0.985	0.377	0.290
LGBM	0.844	0.768	0.714	0.869	0.312	0.973	0.408	0.367
CatBoost	0.853	0.801	0.857	0.774	0.240	0.985	0.377	0.290
SVM	0.836	0.673	1.000	0.333	0.111	1.000	0.192	0.071
MLP	0.902	0.723	0.714	0.774	0.208	0.970	0.295	0.231

AUC = area under the receiver-operating-characteristic curve, PPV = positive predictive value, NPV = negative predictive value, MCC = Matthews correlation coefficient, LR = logistic regression, RF = random forest, GBDT = gradient boosting decision tree, XGBoost = extreme gradient boosting, LGBM = light gradient boosting machine, CatBoost = category boosting, SVM = support vector machine, MLP = multi-layer perceptron.

3.3. Feature Selection and Final Prediction Model

In order to reduce the computational cost of modeling, 15 features which contributed greatly to the prediction were selected from 153 features by the RFE method. These features were maternal adnexitis before pregnancy, maternal body mass index (BMI) before pregnancy, maternal systolic blood pressure before pregnancy, maternal education level, maternal platelet count (PLT) before pregnancy, maternal blood glucose before pregnancy, maternal alanine aminotransferase (ALT) before pregnancy, maternal creatinine before pregnancy, paternal drinking before pregnancy, paternal economic pressure before pregnancy, paternal systolic blood pressure before pregnancy, paternal diastolic blood pressure before pregnancy, paternal ALT before pregnancy, maternal PM2.5 exposure in the first trimester and maternal PM2.5 exposure in the last trimester. These 15 features were included in the final prediction model using the XGBoost algorithm which exhibited the highest AUC value in the previous model comparison. Figure 3 shows the ROC curve of the final prediction model in the training and testing dataset for SGA prediction. The AUC values in the training set and testing set, sensitivity, specificity, PPV, NPV, MCC and kappa values of the final model were 0.953 (95% CI: 0.918–0.988), 0.821 (95% CI: 0.650–0.993), 0.714, 0.881, 0.333, 0.974, 0.427 and 0.391, respectively, proving the superiority of the feature selection approach and the employed ML algorithm.

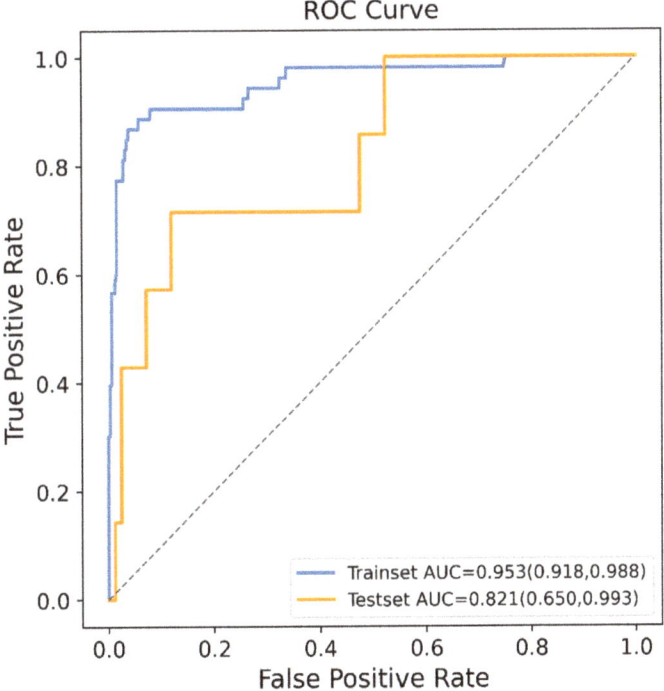

Figure 3. Receiver operating characteristic (ROC) curves of the final machine learning (ML) model generated after recursive feature elimination (RFE) in predicting small for gestational age (SGA).

3.4. Assessment of Variable Importance

In order to identify the features that had the greatest impact on the final prediction model (XGBoost), we drew the SHAP summary diagram of the final prediction model (Figure 4). The feature names were plotted on the *y*-axis from top to bottom according to their importance, while the *x*-axis represented the mean SHAP values. Each dot represented a sample. Plot was colored red (blue) if the value of the feature was high (low). The 6 most important features for the SGA prediction were maternal ALT before pregnancy, maternal PLT before pregnancy, maternal adnexitis before pregnancy, maternal blood glucose before pregnancy, maternal PM2.5 exposure in the last trimester and maternal BMI before pregnancy. In addition, Figure 5 shows two examples for newborns that were classified correctly as non-SGA and SGA, respectively.

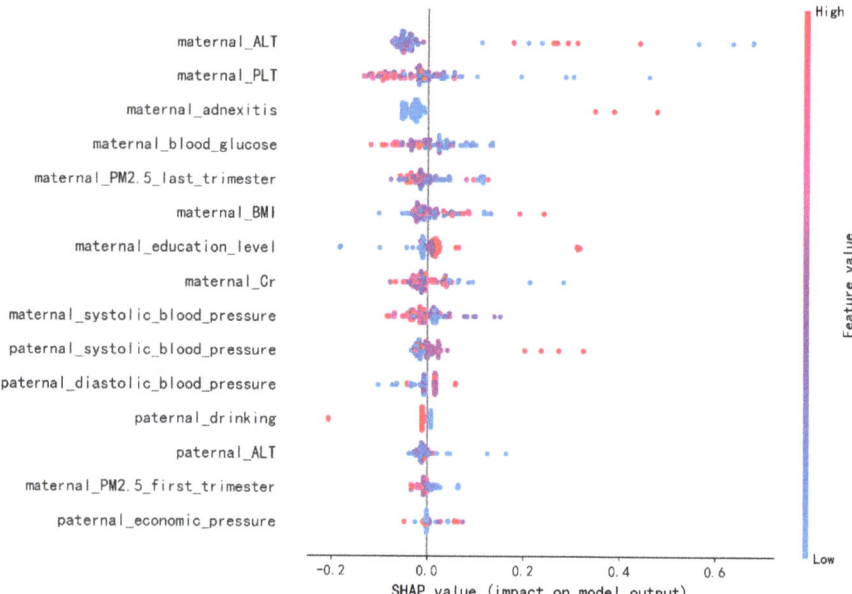

Figure 4. The Shapley Additive Explanation (SHAP) values for most important predictors of small for gestational age (SGA) in the final model. ALT = alanine aminotransferase, PLT = platelet count, BMI = body mass index, Cr = creatinine. Each line represents a feature, and the abscissa is the SHAP value, which represents the degree of influence on the outcome. Each dot represents a sample. Plot is colored red (blue) if the value of the feature is high (low).

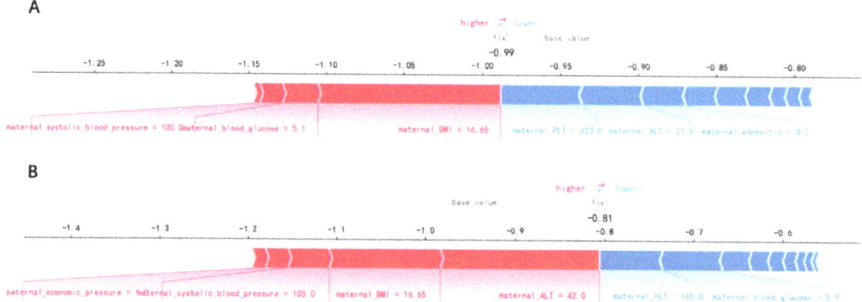

Figure 5. Newborns correctly classified as non-small-for-gestational-age (**A**) and small-for-gestational-age (**B**).

4. Discussion

This study represents the first report using ML algorithms in the development and validation of a risk prediction model for SGA newborns in pregnant women exposed to radiation before pregnancy. Additionally, paternal risk factors and maternal PM2.5 exposure during pregnancy were innovatively included in our ML models as predictive features. Our study demonstrates that ML algorithms can yield more effective prediction models than the conventional logistic regression, and the XGBoost model exhibited the best performance for SGA prediction (AUC: 0.844), suggesting that ML is a promising approach in predicting SGA newborns. With our models, the antenatal prediction of SGA could be made to monitor at-risk fetuses more closely and improve perinatal outcomes.

Evidence indicated that the SGA proportions increased with the radiation exposure [8,9]. Females who have received abdominal or pelvic radiation, radiation for their childhood cancer and diagnostic radiography for idiopathic scoliosis experienced an increased risk of low birth weight among their offspring [12,43–45]. Low birth weight has been considered to be an indicator of genetic damage caused by mutations in humans exposed to radiation [46]. However, to our knowledge, no study has established a prediction model for SGA newborns in women exposed to radiation before pregnancy. In our study, eight ML models were used for a comparative evaluation (Table 2). Among these models, XGBoost, RF, GBDT and CatBoost showed similar performance based on the AUC value, with XGBoost having the highest AUC value (0.844). However, the LR model had the lowest AUC value of 0.561. This might be due to the fact that the LR algorithm is sensitive to outliers and requires a large dataset to work well. Additionally, the imbalanced dataset may affect the performance of the LR model. The results of our study indicated that the ML algorithm was a promising approach to predict SGA newborns in women exposed to radiation before pregnancy, with superior discrimination than the conventional LR (AUC: 0.844 versus 0.561).

Only based on 15 features including the demographic characteristics of parents, simple and feasible clinical test indexes and regional PM2.5 exposure, an effective SGA prediction model could be established (AUC: 0.821, Figure 3), indicating that the appropriate features were selected from 153 features by RFE approach. The RFE algorithm is a wrapper-based backward elimination process by recursively computing the learning function, performing a recursive ranking of a given feature set [47]. Its effectiveness has been extensively proven in various medical data [29–31,48]. Recently, a new ensemble feature selection methodology has been proposed, which aggregates the outcomes of several feature selection algorithms (filter, wrapper and embedded ones) to avoid bias [49,50]. The robust feature selection methodology can be applied in future work. Additionally, advanced ML algorithms provided great potential for improving SGA prediction. The reason was that the interactions between predictors might exist but were not detected by conventional modeling methods. Such weakness could be remedied with the advanced ML algorithms explored in our current study. The ability of ML algorithms to automatically process multidimensional and multivariate data could eventually reveal novel associations between specific features and the SGA outcome and identify trends that would be unobvious to researchers otherwise [51].

Paternal risk factors and maternal PM2.5 exposure during pregnancy were included in the ML prediction models for SGA newborns for the first time. Mounting studies have been devoted to identifying maternal risk factors for the adverse birth outcomes. Little attention has been paid to the fact that paternal factors could also predict adverse birth outcomes. Several paternal factors have been confirmed as risk factors for SGA newborns, such as paternal age, height, ethnicity, education level and smoking during pregnancy [21,22,52–54]. Moreover, women exposed to excessive PM2.5 during pregnancy also had an increased risk of delivering SGA offspring [23]. However, these factors have not been considered in the previous SGA prediction models established in the general population. The results of our study demonstrated that paternal drinking, economic pressure, blood pressure and ALT, maternal PM2.5 exposure in the first trimester and last trimester were all included in the top 15 most contributing features, suggesting that the paternal factor and maternal PM2.5 exposure during pregnancy were involved in the risk prediction for SGA in the study population.

Figure 4 showed the features' impact on the output of the final model (XGBoost). The SHAP values were used to represent the impact distribution of each feature on the model output. For instance, a low maternal PLT level increased the predicted status of the subjects. The features maternal blood glucose, creatinine and systolic blood pressure presented a similar behavior. In contrast to that, maternal adnexitis, high education level and high paternal blood pressure had a positive effect on the prediction outcome. The top 6 most influential features in the SHAP summary plot of the final prediction model were maternal ALT, PLT, adnexitis, blood glucose, PM2.5 exposure in the last trimester and BMI before pregnancy. In addition to the known risk factor maternal PM2.5 exposure, recent studies showed that reduced fetal growth was associated with increased maternal ALT [55]. The significant association between maternal PLT and adverse perinatal outcome has been reported [56]. Additionally, pelvic inflammatory diseases have been linked to adverse perinatal outcomes including SGA [57,58]. In addition, maternal blood glucose and pre-pregnancy BMI have been reported to be associated with increased risk of delivering SGA infants [59–61], which is consistent with our findings. Changes in these features caused by radiation exposure also have been reported in previous studies [62–65]. In addition, using SHAP force plots, two examples that were classified correctly as non-SGA and SGA were selected to explain the effects of the features on the prediction outcome (Figure 5). The contribution of each feature to the output result was represented by an arrow, the force of which was related to the Shapley value. They showed how each feature contributed to push the model output from the baseline prediction to the corresponding model output. The red arrows represented features increasing the predicted results. The blue arrows represented features decreasing the predicted results. It was observed that lower values of maternal BMI, blood glucose, systolic blood pressure and higher values of maternal ALT pushed the output prediction to the SGA class.

This study has several limitations. Firstly, although the data were collected nationally, the sample size was small which may indicate bias. With a larger sample size in the future work, a stratified k-fold cross validation can be used to improve the accuracy of the results. Secondly, there was a lack of the type and average daily exposure of the radiation in mothers' living or working environment before pregnancy in the dataset. Moreover, ultrasound biometrics measurements were lacking in the dataset, and their inclusion in the prediction model may further improve the accuracy and applicability of the model. Further validation and application of ML into the daily clinical practice is still necessary to better understand its real value in predicting SGA newborns.

5. Conclusions

In this work, a comprehensive analysis of SGA newborns prediction in pregnant women exposed to radiation in their living or working environment before pregnancy was carried out, with the help of feature selection and optimization techniques. It is concluded that ML algorithms show good performances on the classification of SGA newborns. The final model using the XGBoost algorithm achieves effective SGA prediction (AUC: 0.821) only based on 15 features, including the demographic characteristics of parents, simple and feasible clinical test indexes and regional PM2.5 exposure. Furthermore, the post hoc analysis complemented the prediction results by enhancing the understanding of the contribution of the selected features to the classification of SGA newborns. ML models may be a potential assistant approach for the early prediction of delivering SGA newborns in high-risk populations. Future work aims to work with other ensemble feature selection methodologies and apply the proposed methodology to other high-risk populations for delivering SGA newborns.

Supplementary Materials: The following supporting information can be downloaded at: https://www.mdpi.com/article/10.3390/jpm12040550/s1, Table S1: 153 features included in machine learning models as candidate variables for predictors.

Author Contributions: Conceptualization, X.B., S.C. and H.P.; methodology, X.B., H.Z. and H.Y.; software, X.B. and Z.Z.; validation, X.B. and Y.L.; resources, H.P.; data curation, X.B. and S.C.; writing—original draft preparation, X.B.; writing—review and editing, S.C. and H.P.; visualization, H.Z.; supervision, H.P.; project administration, X.B. and H.P.; funding acquisition, H.P. All authors have read and agreed to the published version of the manuscript.

Funding: This research received no external funding.

Institutional Review Board Statement: The study was conducted in accordance with the Declaration of Helsinki, and approved by the Institutional Review Board of the National Research Institute for Family Planning, Beijing, China (protocol code 2017101702).

Informed Consent Statement: Informed consent was obtained from all subjects involved in the study.

Data Availability Statement: Our research data were derived from the National Free Preconception Health Examination Project (NFPHEP). Requests to access these datasets should be directed to Hui Pan, panhui20111111@163.com.

Conflicts of Interest: The authors declare no conflict of interest.

References

1. McCowan, L.M.; Figueras, F.; Anderson, N.H. Evidence-based national guidelines for the management of suspected fetal growth restriction: Comparison, consensus, and controversy. *Am. J. Obstet. Gynecol.* **2018**, *218*, S855–S868. [CrossRef] [PubMed]
2. Lindqvist, P.G.; Molin, J. Does antenatal identification of small-for-gestational age fetuses significantly improve their outcome? *Ultrasound. Obstet. Gynecol.* **2005**, *25*, 258–264. [CrossRef] [PubMed]
3. Frøen, J.F.; Gardosi, J.O.; Thurmann, A.; Francis, A.; Stray-Pedersen, B. Restricted fetal growth in sudden intrauterine unexplained death. *Acta Obstet. Et. Gynecol. Scand.* **2004**, *83*, 801–807. [CrossRef]
4. Gardosi, J.; Madurasinghe, V.; Williams, M.; Malik, A.; Francis, A. Maternal and fetal risk factors for stillbirth: Population based study. *BMJ* **2013**, *346*, f108. [CrossRef] [PubMed]
5. Dugandzic, R.; Dodds, L.; Stieb, D.; Smith-Doiron, M. The association between low level exposures to ambient air pollution and term low birth weight: A retrospective cohort study. *Environ. Health* **2006**, *5*, 3. [CrossRef] [PubMed]
6. Grazuleviciene, R.; Nieuwenhuijsen, M.J.; Vencloviene, J.; Kostopoulou-Karadanelli, M.; Krasner, S.W.; Danileviciute, A.; Balcius, G.; Kapustinskiene, V. Individual exposures to drinking water trihalomethanes, low birth weight and small for gestational age risk: A prospective Kaunas cohort study. *Environ. Health* **2011**, *10*, 32. [CrossRef] [PubMed]
7. Morello-Frosch, R.; Jesdale, B.M.; Sadd, J.L.; Pastor, M. Ambient air pollution exposure and full-term birth weight in California. *Environ. Health* **2010**, *9*, 44. [CrossRef] [PubMed]
8. Yoshimoto, Y.; Schull, W.J.; Kato, H.; Neel, J.V. Mortality among the offspring (F1) of atomic bomb survivors, 1946–1985. *J. Radiat. Res.* **1991**, *32*, 327–351. [CrossRef] [PubMed]
9. Tang, F.R.; Loke, W.K.; Khoo, B.C. Low-dose or low-dose-rate ionizing radiation-induced bioeffects in animal models. *J. Radiat. Res.* **2017**, *58*, 165–182. [CrossRef]
10. Otake, M.; Fujikoshi, Y.; Funamoto, S.; Schull, W.J. Evidence of radiation-induced reduction of height and body weight from repeated measurements of adults exposed in childhood to the atomic bombs. *Radiat. Res.* **1994**, *140*, 112–122. [CrossRef]
11. Hamilton, P.M.; Roney, P.L.; Keppel, K.G.; Placek, P.J. Radiation procedures performed on U.S. women during pregnancy: Findings from two 1980 surveys. *Public Health Rep.* **1984**, *99*, 146–151. [PubMed]
12. Goldberg, M.S.; Mayo, N.E.; Levy, A.R.; Scott, S.C.; Poîtras, B. Adverse reproductive outcomes among women exposed to low levels of ionizing radiation from diagnostic radiography for adolescent idiopathic scoliosis. *Epidemiology* **1998**, *9*, 271–278. [CrossRef] [PubMed]
13. Hudson, M.M. Reproductive outcomes for survivors of childhood cancer. *Obstet. Gynecol.* **2010**, *116*, 1171–1183. [CrossRef] [PubMed]
14. Hujoel, P.P.; Bollen, A.M.; Noonan, C.J.; del Aguila, M.A. Antepartum dental radiography and infant low birth weight. *JAMA* **2004**, *291*, 1987–1993. [CrossRef] [PubMed]
15. Shouval, R.; Bondi, O.; Mishan, H.; Shimoni, A.; Unger, R.; Nagler, A. Application of machine learning algorithms for clinical predictive modeling: A data-mining approach in SCT. *Bone Marrow Transplant.* **2014**, *49*, 332–337. [CrossRef]
16. Wu, Q.; Nasoz, F.; Jung, J.; Bhattarai, B.; Han, M.V. Machine Learning Approaches for Fracture Risk Assessment: A Comparative Analysis of Genomic and Phenotypic Data in 5130 Older Men. *Calcif. Tissue Int.* **2020**, *107*, 353–361. [CrossRef]
17. Deo, R.C. Machine Learning in Medicine. *Circulation* **2015**, *132*, 1920–1930. [CrossRef]
18. Kuhle, S.; Maguire, B.; Zhang, H.; Hamilton, D.; Allen, A.C.; Joseph, K.S.; Allen, V.M. Comparison of logistic regression with machine learning methods for the prediction of fetal growth abnormalities: A retrospective cohort study. *BMC Pregnancy Childbirth* **2018**, *18*, 333. [CrossRef]
19. Papastefanou, I.; Wright, D.; Nicolaides, K.H. Competing-risks model for prediction of small-for-gestational-age neonate from maternal characteristics and medical history. *Ultrasound Obstet. Gynecol.* **2020**, *56*, 196–205. [CrossRef]
20. Saw, S.N.; Biswas, A.; Mattar, C.N.Z.; Lee, H.K.; Yap, C.H. Machine learning improves early prediction of small-for-gestational-age births and reveals nuchal fold thickness as unexpected predictor. *Prenat. Diagn.* **2021**, *41*, 505–516. [CrossRef]
21. Shah, P.S. Paternal factors and low birthweight, preterm, and small for gestational age births: A systematic review. *Am. J. Obstet. Gynecol.* **2010**, *202*, 103–123. [CrossRef] [PubMed]
22. Shapiro, G.D.; Bushnik, T.; Sheppard, A.J.; Kramer, M.S.; Kaufman, J.S.; Yang, S. Paternal education and adverse birth outcomes in Canada. *J. Epidemiol. Community Health* **2017**, *71*, 67–72. [CrossRef] [PubMed]
23. Kloog, I.; Melly, S.J.; Ridgway, W.L.; Coull, B.A.; Schwartz, J. Using new satellite based exposure methods to study the association between pregnancy $PM_{2.5}$ exposure, premature birth and birth weight in Massachusetts. *Environ. Health* **2012**, *11*, 40. [CrossRef] [PubMed]

24. Pan, Y.; Zhang, S.; Wang, Q.; Shen, H.; Zhang, Y.; Li, Y.; Yan, D.; Sun, L. Investigating the association between prepregnancy body mass index and adverse pregnancy outcomes: A large cohort study of 536 098 Chinese pregnant women in rural China. *BMJ Open* **2016**, *6*, e011227. [CrossRef] [PubMed]
25. Wang, Y.Y.; Li, Q.; Guo, Y.; Zhou, H.; Wang, X.; Wang, Q.; Shen, H.; Zhang, Y.; Yan, D.; Zhang, Y.; et al. Association of Long-term Exposure to Airborne Particulate Matter of 1 μm or Less With Preterm Birth in China. *JAMA Pediatr.* **2018**, *172*, e174872. [CrossRef]
26. Zhang, S.; Wang, Q.; Shen, H. Design of the National Free Preconception Health Examination Project in China. *Natl. Med. J. China* **2015**, *95*, 162–165.
27. Xiao, Q.; Chang, H.H.; Geng, G.; Liu, Y. An Ensemble Machine-Learning Model To Predict Historical PM(2.5) Concentrations in China from Satellite Data. *Environ. Sci. Technol.* **2018**, *52*, 13260–13269. [CrossRef]
28. Zhu, L.; Zhang, R.; Zhang, S.; Shi, W.; Yan, W.; Wang, X.; Lyu, Q.; Liu, L.; Zhou, Q.; Qiu, Q.; et al. Chinese neonatal birth weight curve for different gestational age. *Zhonghua Er Ke Za Zhi* **2015**, *53*, 97–103.
29. Gong, J.; Bao, X.; Wang, T.; Liu, J.; Peng, W.; Shi, J.; Wu, F.; Gu, Y. A short-term follow-up CT based radiomics approach to predict response to immunotherapy in advanced non-small-cell lung cancer. *Oncoimmunology* **2022**, *11*, 2028962. [CrossRef]
30. Lim, L.J.; Lim, A.J.W.; Ooi, B.N.S.; Tan, J.W.L.; Koh, E.T.; Chong, S.S.; Khor, C.C.; Tucker-Kellogg, L.; Lee, C.G.; Leong, K.P. Machine Learning using Genetic and Clinical Data Identifies a Signature that Robustly Predicts Methotrexate Response in Rheumatoid Arthritis. *Rheumatology* **2022**. [CrossRef]
31. Lu, C.; Song, J.; Li, H.; Yu, W.; Hao, Y.; Xu, K.; Xu, P. Predicting Venous Thrombosis in Osteoarthritis Using a Machine Learning Algorithm: A Population-Based Cohort Study. *J. Pers. Med.* **2022**, *12*, 114. [CrossRef] [PubMed]
32. Bloch, L.; Friedrich, C.M. Data analysis with Shapley values for automatic subject selection in Alzheimer's disease data sets using interpretable machine learning. *Alzheimer's. Res. Ther.* **2021**, *13*, 155. [CrossRef] [PubMed]
33. Le Cessie, S.; Van Houwelingen, J.C. Ridge estimators in logistic regression. *Appl. Stat.* **1992**, *41*, 191–201. [CrossRef]
34. Kulkarni, V.Y.; Sinha, P.K.; Petare, M.C. Weighted hybrid decision tree model for random forest classifier. *J. Inst. Eng. Ser. B.* **2016**, *97*, 209–217. [CrossRef]
35. Breiman, L. Random forests. *Mach. Learn.* **2001**, *45*, 5–32. [CrossRef]
36. Zhang, Z.; Jung, C. GBDT-MO: Gradient-Boosted Decision Trees for Multiple Outputs. *IEEE. Trans. Neural Netw. Learn. Syst.* **2021**, *32*, 3156–3167. [CrossRef]
37. Kobayashi, Y.; Yoshida, K. Quantitative structure-property relationships for the calculation of the soil adsorption coefficient using machine learning algorithms with calculated chemical properties from open-source software. *Environ. Res.* **2021**, *196*, 110363. [CrossRef]
38. Hancock, J.T.; Khoshgoftaar, T.M. CatBoost for big data: An interdisciplinary review. *J. Big Data* **2020**, *7*, 94. [CrossRef]
39. Li, Y.; Li, M.; Li, C.; Liu, Z. Forest aboveground biomass estimation using Landsat 8 and Sentinel-1A data with machine learning algorithms. *Sci. Rep.* **2020**, *10*, 9952. [CrossRef]
40. Huang, S.; Cai, N.; Pacheco, P.P.; Narrandes, S.; Wang, Y.; Xu, W. Applications of Support Vector Machine (SVM) Learning in Cancer Genomics. *Cancer Genom. Proteom.* **2018**, *15*, 41–51. [CrossRef]
41. Long, Z.; Jing, B.; Yan, H.; Dong, J.; Liu, H.; Mo, X.; Han, Y.; Li, H. A support vector machine-based method to identify mild cognitive impairment with multi-level characteristics of magnetic resonance imaging. *Neuroscience* **2016**, *331*, 169–176. [CrossRef] [PubMed]
42. Prout, T.A.; Zilcha-Mano, S.; Aafjes-van Doorn, K.; Békés, V.; Christman-Cohen, I.; Whistler, K.; Kui, T.; Di Giuseppe, M. Identifying Predictors of Psychological Distress During COVID-19: A Machine Learning Approach. *Front. Psychol.* **2020**, *11*, 586202. [CrossRef] [PubMed]
43. Reulen, R.C.; Zeegers, M.P.; Wallace, W.H.; Frobisher, C.; Taylor, A.J.; Lancashire, E.R.; Winter, D.L.; Hawkins, M.M. Pregnancy outcomes among adult survivors of childhood cancer in the British Childhood Cancer Survivor Study. *Cancer Epidemiol. Prev. Biomark.* **2009**, *18*, 2239–2247. [CrossRef]
44. Green, D.M.; Whitton, J.A.; Stovall, M.; Mertens, A.C.; Donaldson, S.S.; Ruymann, F.B.; Pendergrass, T.W.; Robison, L.L. Pregnancy outcome of female survivors of childhood cancer: A report from the Childhood Cancer Survivor Study. *Am. J. Obstet. Gynecol.* **2002**, *187*, 1070–1080. [CrossRef] [PubMed]
45. Signorello, L.B.; Cohen, S.S.; Bosetti, C.; Stovall, M.; Kasper, C.E.; Weathers, R.E.; Whitton, J.A.; Green, D.M.; Donaldson, S.S.; Mertens, A.C.; et al. Female survivors of childhood cancer: Preterm birth and low birth weight among their children. *J. Natl. Cancer Inst.* **2006**, *98*, 1453–1461. [CrossRef] [PubMed]
46. Scherb, H.; Hayashi, K. Spatiotemporal association of low birth weight with Cs-137 deposition at the prefecture level in Japan after the Fukushima nuclear power plant accidents: An analytical-ecologic epidemiological study. *Environ. Health* **2020**, *19*, 82. [CrossRef]
47. Dasgupta, S.; Goldberg, Y.; Kosorok, M.R. Feature elimination in kernel machines in moderately high dimensions. *Ann. Stat.* **2019**, *47*, 497–526. [CrossRef] [PubMed]
48. Lim, A.J.W.; Lim, L.J.; Ooi, B.N.S.; Koh, E.T.; Tan, J.W.L.; Chong, S.S.; Khor, C.C.; Tucker-Kellogg, L.; Leong, K.P.; Lee, C.G. Functional coding haplotypes and machine-learning feature elimination identifies predictors of Methotrexate Response in Rheumatoid Arthritis patients. *EBioMedicine* **2022**, *75*, 103800. [CrossRef]

49. Ntakolia, C.; Kokkotis, C.; Moustakidis, S.; Tsaopoulos, D. Identification of most important features based on a fuzzy ensemble technique: Evaluation on joint space narrowing progression in knee osteoarthritis patients. *Int. J. Med. Inform.* **2021**, *156*, 104614. [CrossRef] [PubMed]
50. Ntakolia, C.; Kokkotis, C.; Moustakidis, S.; Tsaopoulos, D. Prediction of Joint Space Narrowing Progression in Knee Osteoarthritis Patients. *Diagnostics* **2021**, *11*, 285. [CrossRef] [PubMed]
51. Hernandez-Suarez, D.F.; Kim, Y.; Villablanca, P.; Gupta, T.; Wiley, J.; Nieves-Rodriguez, B.G.; Rodriguez-Maldonado, J.; Feliu Maldonado, R.; da Luz Sant'Ana, I.; Sanina, C.; et al. Machine Learning Prediction Models for In-Hospital Mortality After Transcatheter Aortic Valve Replacement. *JACC Cardiovasc. Interv.* **2019**, *12*, 1328–1338. [CrossRef] [PubMed]
52. Miletić, T.; Stoini, E.; Mikulandra, F.; Tadin, I.; Roje, D.; Milić, N. Effect of parental anthropometric parameters on neonatal birth weight and birth length. *Coll. Antropol.* **2007**, *31*, 993–997. [PubMed]
53. Myklestad, K.; Vatten, L.J.; Magnussen, E.B.; Salvesen, K.; Romundstad, P.R. Do parental heights influence pregnancy length?: A population-based prospective study, HUNT 2. *BMC Pregnancy Childbirth* **2013**, *13*, 33. [CrossRef] [PubMed]
54. Meng, Y.; Groth, S.W. Fathers Count: The Impact of Paternal Risk Factors on Birth Outcomes. *Matern. Child. Health J.* **2018**, *22*, 401–408. [CrossRef] [PubMed]
55. Harville, E.W.; Chen, W.; Bazzano, L.; Oikonen, M.; Hutri-Kähönen, N.; Raitakari, O. Indicators of fetal growth and adult liver enzymes: The Bogalusa Heart Study and the Cardiovascular Risk in Young Finns Study. *J. Dev. Orig. Health Dis.* **2017**, *8*, 226–235. [CrossRef] [PubMed]
56. Larroca, S.G.; Arevalo-Serrano, J.; Abad, V.O.; Recarte, P.P.; Carreras, A.G.; Pastor, G.N.; Hernandez, C.R.; Pacheco, R.P.; Luis, J.L. Platelet Count in First Trimester of Pregnancy as a Predictor of Perinatal Outcome. *Maced. J. Med. Sci.* **2017**, *5*, 27–32. [CrossRef]
57. Heumann, C.L.; Quilter, L.A.; Eastment, M.C.; Heffron, R.; Hawes, S.E. Adverse Birth Outcomes and Maternal Neisseria gonorrhoeae Infection: A Population-Based Cohort Study in Washington State. *Sex. Transm. Dis.* **2017**, *44*, 266–271. [CrossRef]
58. Johnson, H.L.; Ghanem, K.G.; Zenilman, J.M.; Erbelding, E.J. Sexually transmitted infections and adverse pregnancy outcomes among women attending inner city public sexually transmitted diseases clinics. *Sex. Transm. Dis.* **2011**, *38*, 167–171. [CrossRef]
59. Leng, J.; Hay, J.; Liu, G.; Zhang, J.; Wang, J.; Liu, H.; Yang, X.; Liu, J. Small-for-gestational age and its association with maternal blood glucose, body mass index and stature: A perinatal cohort study among Chinese women. *BMJ Open* **2016**, *6*, e010984. [CrossRef]
60. Siega-Riz, A.M.; Viswanathan, M.; Moos, M.K.; Deierlein, A.; Mumford, S.; Knaack, J.; Thieda, P.; Lux, L.J.; Lohr, K.N. A systematic review of outcomes of maternal weight gain according to the Institute of Medicine recommendations: Birthweight, fetal growth, and postpartum weight retention. *Am. J. Obstet. Gynecol.* **2009**, *201*, 339.e1–339.e14. [CrossRef]
61. Lederman, S.A. Pregnancy weight gain and postpartum loss: Avoiding obesity while optimizing the growth and development of the fetus. *J. Am. Med. Women's Assoc.* **2001**, *56*, 53–58.
62. Nadi, S.; Elahi, M.; Moradi, S.; Banaei, A.; Ataei, G.; Abedi-Firouzjah, R. Radioprotective Effect of Arbutin in Megavoltage Therapeutic X-irradiated Mice using Liver Enzymes Assessment. *J. Biomed. Phys. Eng.* **2019**, *9*, 533–540. [CrossRef] [PubMed]
63. Singh, V.K.; Seed, T.M. A review of radiation countermeasures focusing on injury-specific medicinals and regulatory approval status: Part I. Radiation sub-syndromes, animal models and FDA-approved countermeasures. *Int. J. Radiat. Biol.* **2017**, *93*, 851–869. [CrossRef] [PubMed]
64. Fan, Z.B.; Zou, J.F.; Bai, J.; Yu, G.C.; Zhang, X.X.; Ma, H.H.; Cheng, Q.M.; Wang, S.P.; Ji, F.L.; Yu, W.L. The occupational and procreation health of immigrant female workers in electron factory. *Zhonghua Lao Dong Wei Sheng Zhi Ye Bing Za Zhi* **2011**, *29*, 661–664. [CrossRef] [PubMed]
65. Meo, S.A.; Alsubaie, Y.; Almubarak, Z.; Almutawa, H.; AlQasem, Y.; Hasanato, R.M. Association of Exposure to Radio-Frequency Electromagnetic Field Radiation (RF-EMFR) Generated by Mobile Phone Base Stations with Glycated Hemoglobin (HbA1c) and Risk of Type 2 Diabetes Mellitus. *Int. J. Environ. Res. Public Health* **2015**, *12*, 14519–14528. [CrossRef]

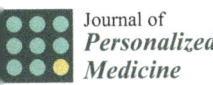

Article

Physical Activity Is Associated with a Lower Risk of Osteoporotic Fractures in Osteoporosis: A Longitudinal Study

Chan-Yang Min [1], Jung-Woo Lee [2], Bong-Cheol Kwon [3], Mi-Jung Kwon [4], Ji-Hee Kim [5], Joo-Hee Kim [6], Woo-Jin Bang [7] and Hyo-Geun Choi [1,8,*]

1. Hallym Data Science Laboratory, Hallym University College of Medicine, Anyang 14066, Korea; joicemin@naver.com
2. Department of Orthopaedic Surgery, Yonsei University Wonju College of Medicine, Wonju 26426, Korea; berrybearlee@gmail.com
3. Department of Orthopaedic Surgery, Hallym University College of Medicine, Anyang 14068, Korea; bckwon@hallym.or.kr
4. Department of Pathology, Hallym Sacred Heart Hospital, Hallym University College of Medicine, Anyang 14068, Korea; mulank@hanmail.net
5. Department of Neurosurgery, Hallym University College of Medicine, Anyang 14068, Korea; kimjihee.ns@gmail.com
6. Division of Pulmonary, Allergy, and Critical Care Medicine, Department of Medicine, Hallym Sacred Heart Hospital, Hallym University College of Medicine, Anyang 14068, Korea; luxjhee@gmail.com
7. Department of Urology, Hallym Sacred Heart Hospital, Hallym University College of Medicine, Anyang 14068, Korea; yybbang@gmail.com
8. Department of Otorhinolaryngology-Head & Neck Surgery, Hallym University College of Medicine, Anyang 14068, Korea
* Correspondence: pupen@naver.com

Citation: Min, C.-Y.; Lee, J.-W.; Kwon, B.-C.; Kwon, M.-J.; Kim, J.-H.; Kim, J.-H.; Bang, W.-J.; Choi, H.-G. Physical Activity Is Associated with a Lower Risk of Osteoporotic Fractures in Osteoporosis: A Longitudinal Study. J. Pers. Med. **2022**, 12, 491. https://doi.org/10.3390/jpm12030491

Academic Editor: Youxin Wang

Received: 3 February 2022
Accepted: 16 March 2022
Published: 18 March 2022

Publisher's Note: MDPI stays neutral with regard to jurisdictional claims in published maps and institutional affiliations.

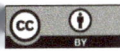

Copyright: © 2022 by the authors. Licensee MDPI, Basel, Switzerland. This article is an open access article distributed under the terms and conditions of the Creative Commons Attribution (CC BY) license (https://creativecommons.org/licenses/by/4.0/).

Abstract: The purpose of our study was to examine the occurrence of osteoporotic fractures (fxs) according to the level of physical activity (PA) among osteoporosis using the Korean National Health Insurance Service (NHIS) customized database. From NHIS data from 2009 to 2017, osteoporosis was selected as requested. PA was classified into 'high PA' (n = 58,620), 'moderate PA' (n = 58,620), and 'low PA' (n = 58,620) and were matched in a 1:1:1 ratio by gender, age, income within the household unit, and region of residence. A stratified Cox proportional hazard model was used to calculate hazard ratios (HRs) for each type of fx comparing PA groups. The 'low PA' group was the reference group. For vertebral fx, the adjusted HR (95% confidence intervals (CIs)) was 0.27 (0.26–0.28) for the 'high PA' group and 0.43 (0.42–0.44) for the 'moderate PA' group. For hip fx, the adjusted HR (95% CIs) was 0.37 (0.34–0.40) for the 'high PA' group and 0.51 (0.47–0.55) for the 'moderate PA' group. For distal radius fx, the adjusted HR (95% CIs) was 0.32 (0.30–0.33) for the 'high PA' group and 0.46 (0.45–0.48) for the 'moderate PA' group. The results of this study suggest that a higher intensity of PA is associated with a lower risk of osteoporotic fxs, including vertebral fx, hip fx, and distal radius fx.

Keywords: physical activity; osteoporosis; osteoporotic fracture; vertebral fracture; hip fracture; distal radius fracture

1. Introduction

The negative health effects of physical inactivity are already well known [1]. The problem of physical inactivity is expected to worsen due to the novel coronavirus pandemic (COVID-19) [2]. A study from the United States reported that among study subjects, 30% responded that they engaged in less physical activity (PA) during the pandemic [3]. Likewise, among the population of England, the rate of physical activity declined by 30% in 2020 compared to that in the period from 2016 to 2019 [4]. In Korea, the time spent in high-intensity PA decreased in all age and gender groups in 2020 compared to that of 2019 according to the Korean Community Health Survey data [5]. World Health Organization

(WHO) reported that lack of physical activity (PA) is one of the risk factors for chronic diseases such as cancers, cardiovascular disease burden, and even death [6]. In other words, PA is crucial to maintain and improve one's health.

One of the goals of PA is improving osteoporosis, one of the major musculoskeletal diseases [7]. Osteoporosis is characterized by a decrease in bone mineral density (BMD) [8]. Although osteoporosis has no outward symptoms, osteoporotic patients are at critical risk of osteoporotic fractures (fxs), including vertebral fx, hip fx, and distal radius fx [9]. Fxs is a critical concern for older adults and can even lead to death. A previous study from Ontario, Canada reported that the absolute mortality risk within 1 year among participants ≥ 66 years old was 19.5% and 12.5% for men and women with fx, respectively, whereas it was 13.5% and 7.4% for men and women without fx, respectively [10]. Another study from Korea reported that the standardized mortality ratios (SMRs) 2 years after vertebral fracture were 2.53 in men and 1.86 in women compared to the general population [11].

Increasing evidence has demonstrated that PA can increase BMD and lower the risk of osteoporosis, hence reducing the risk of some osteoporotic complications. Several randomized controlled trials (RCTs) evaluated if PA could improve bone strength, including BMD, in osteoporotic postmenopausal women [12]. Specifically, resistance training, impact loading and balance exercise increased total hip BMD [13], maximal strength training, including squat exercise showed higher femoral neck and lumbar spine bone mineral contents (BMC) [14], and aerobic dance improved femoral neck BMD [15]. Moreover, several previous cohort studies confirmed that PA could lower the risk of hip fx in each cohort regardless of osteoporosis [16,17].

However, although several RCT studies demonstrated that PA could increase BMD in osteoporotic patients, few RCT studies have included osteoporotic fx as the primary endpoint because of the limited length of the typical study period. Moreover, in RCT studies, few men were recruited as study participants due to the low frequency of osteoporosis in men. In addition, although several cohort studies have demonstrated that PA could prevent hip fx in the certain cohort, few cohort studies have selected osteoporotic patients as a subject population because of insufficient data. In other words, we could not find a study regarding the association between PA and osteoporotic fx in osteoporosis, although osteoporosis increases the risk of osteoporotic fxs. Moreover, the association between PA and vertebral/distal radius fx was not evident in previous studies.

The purpose of our study was to confirm whether a higher intensity of PA could lower the rate of occurrence of osteoporotic fx at each specific site in osteoporotic men and women. We used the Korean National Health Insurance Service (NHIS) customized database to identify the osteoporotic patients.

2. Materials and Methods

2.1. Study Population and Participant Selection

Hallym University ethics committee (HALLYM 2019-08-029) approved this study according to the Institutional Review Board (IRB) guidelines.

The Korean National Health Insurance Sharing Service (NHISS) provided the customized database as requested. Among the Korean population who are holding the national health insurance from 2009 to 2017, 948,390 were selected as having osteoporosis according to our definition. Among them, we excluded participants who had insufficient socioeconomic status information ($n = 4329$) or who were diagnosed with osteoporotic fx before osteoporosis diagnosis ($n = 145,039$). Participants were also excluded who had no information on PA after osteoporosis diagnosis and before osteoporotic fx onset ($n = 286,865$). In addition, participants were removed if health-check information was insufficient ($n = 58$) or if they were <50 years old ($n = 1161$). In total, 510,938 participants ($n = 71,060$ with 'high PA'; $n = 262,136$ with 'moderate PA'; $n = 177,742$ with 'low PA') were included in the study. The 'high PA', 'moderate PA', and 'low PA' groups were matched at a 1:1:1 ratio for gender, age, income within household unit, and region of residence using a random number. The index date was assigned on the day that the PA was first collected before the first diagnosis of osteoporosis. After matching those PA groups, 335,078 participants were removed due to a lack of availability of matched controls. Finally, 58,620 'high PA' subjects, 58,620 'moderate PA' subjects, and 58,620 'low PA' subjects were selected as study participants (Figure 1).

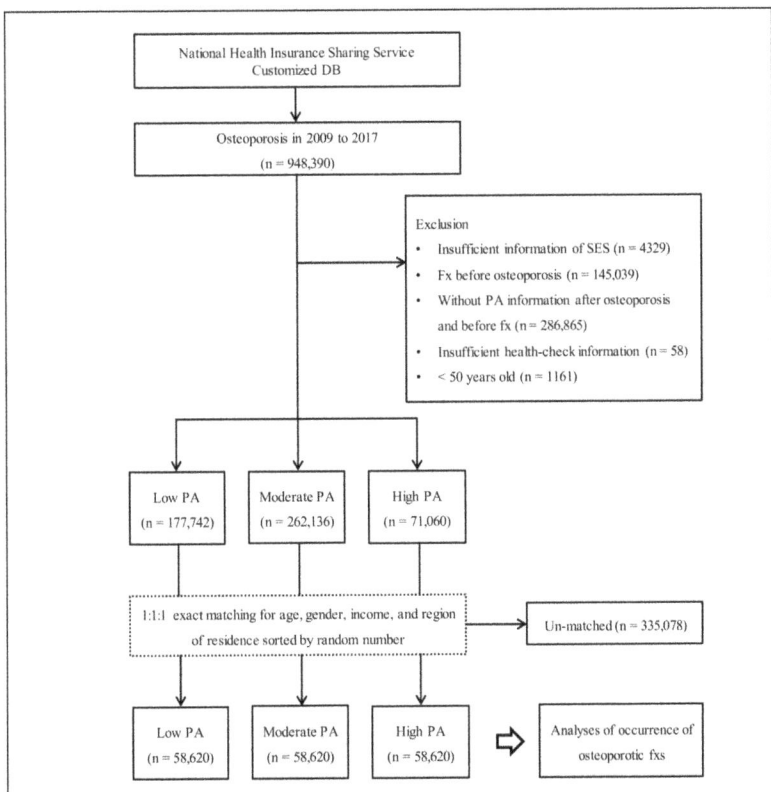

Figure 1. The participant selection flow. Out of a total of 948,390 participants with osteoporosis, 'high PA' (*n* = 58,620), 'moderate PA' (*n* = 58,620), and 'low PA' (*n* = 58,620) were matched by a ratio of 1:1:1 by age, gender, income, and region of residence. Abbreviation: fxs, fractures; PA, physical activity; SES, socioeconomic status.

2.2. Definition of Osteoporosis (Participants)

We used International Classification of Disease 10th edition (ICD-10) codes and examination insurance claim codes to identify cases of osteoporosis. The definition of osteoporosis cases included participants who were diagnosed or treated with osteoporosis with pathological fx (M80), osteoporosis without pathological fx (M81), or osteoporosis in diseases classified elsewhere (M82) ≥ 2 times and with BMD test using dual energy X-ray absorptiometry (DXA), computed tomography (CT) scans or others [18].

2.3. Exposure (Physical Activity)

Information on PA was surveyed according to the International Physical Activity Questionnaire (IPAQ) [19]. The first record of PA information after the first diagnosis of osteoporosis was used. PA groups were defined based on the IPAQ classification. Participants who did vigorous-intensity activity on ≥3 days with ≥1500 metabolic equivalent task (MET)-minutes/week or any combination of moderate- or vigorous-intensity activities or walking ≥7 days with ≥3000 MET-minutes/week were classified in the 'high PA' group. Participants who performed moderate-intensity activity or walking ≥5 days with

≥30 min/day, performed vigorous-intensity activity ≥3 days with ≥20 min/day, or any combination of moderate- or vigorous-intensity activities or walking ≥600 MET-minutes/week were classified in the 'moderate PA' group. The rest of the participants were classified into the 'low PA' group.

2.4. Outcome (Time to Event (Osteoporotic Fractures))

The time to event (osteoporotic fxs) was calculated as the month from the date of PA to the censored date or event date. The date of fxs was assigned as the first-time diagnosis of each fx. Osteoporotic fxs were vertebral fx, hip fx, and distal radius fx. The vertebral fx included participants who were diagnosed with fx of thoracic vertebra (S220) or fx of lumbar vertebra (S320) using ICD-10 codes [20]. The hip fx group included participants who were diagnosed with fx of the neck or the femur (S720), pertrochanteric fx (S721), or subtrochanteric fx (S722) using ICD-10 codes [20]. The distal radius fx group included participants who were diagnosed with fx of the lower end of the radius (S525) using ICD-10 codes [21].

2.5. Covariates

Age was categorized from 50 years old to ≥85 years old with 5-year intervals (a total of 8 groups). Income within household units and regions of residence were classified based on our previous studies [22,23]. Categories of smoking status, alcohol consumption, and obesity based on body mass index (BMI) were defined as described in our previous studies [22,23]. Blood pressure (BP, including systolic BP (SBP) and diastolic BP (DBP)), fasting blood glucose, and total cholesterol were also collected. The Charlson Comorbidity Index (CCI) score was assigned to each participant to assess the burden of comorbidities [24].

2.6. Statistical Analyses

The Kruskal–Wallis test was used to compare the percentage of each characteristic among the PA groups. To compare the cumulative occurrence of each osteoporotic fx among the PA groups, Kaplan–Meier failure analysis and the log-rank test were performed. To analyze the hazard ratios (HRs) with 95% CIs for each osteoporotic fx, including vertebral fx, hip fx, and distal radius fx in the PA groups, a stratified Cox proportional hazard model was used. In this analysis, the crude and adjusted models (adjusted for fasting blood glucose, SBP, DBP, total cholesterol, alcohol consumption, smoking status, obesity, and CCI scores) were fit. The analysis was stratified by gender, age, income within household unit, and region of residence. For the subgroup analyses, age groups (<65 years old and ≥65 years old) and gender (men and women) were recategorized, and the crude and adjusted models were implemented with a stratified Cox model. Other subgroup analyses were performed (Tables S1–S3).

Two-tailed testing was performed, and significance was defined as a p value < 0.05. A Bonferroni correction was used to control type 1 errors when calculating the p value for three outcomes of osteoporotic fxs ($\alpha = 0.05/3$). For statistical analyses, SAS Enterprise Guide version 7.13 (SAS Institute Inc., Cary, NC, USA) was used.

3. Results

PA groups were exactly matched by a 1:1:1 ratio according to age, gender, income within household unit, and region of residence (all $p = 1.000$). The percentage of obesity, smoking status, alcohol consumption, and CCI score and mean of total cholesterol, BP, and fasting blood glucose were significantly different among the PA groups (all $p < 0.005$). The percentage of subjects with vertebral fx (no. of subjects with vertebral fx/total participants) in the 'high PA', 'moderate PA', and 'low PA' groups was 6.9% (4042/58,620), 10.6% (6233/58,620), and 21.8% (12,787/58,620), respectively ($p < 0.001$). The percentage of subjects with hip fx (no. of subjects with hip fx/total participants) in the 'high PA', 'moderate PA', and 'low PA' groups was 1.2% (687/58,620), 1.7% (984/58,620), and 3.5% (2048/58,620), respectively ($p < 0.001$). The percentage of subjects with distal radius fx (no. of subjects with distal radius fx/total participants) in the 'high PA', 'moderate PA', and 'low PA' groups was 5.1% (2991/58,620), 7.2% (4229/58,620), and 13.9% (8119/58,620), respectively ($p < 0.001$, Table 1).

Cumulative rate of each fx was higher in order of the 'low PA', 'moderate PA', and 'high PA' groups (log-rank test, each $p < 0.001$, Figure 2).

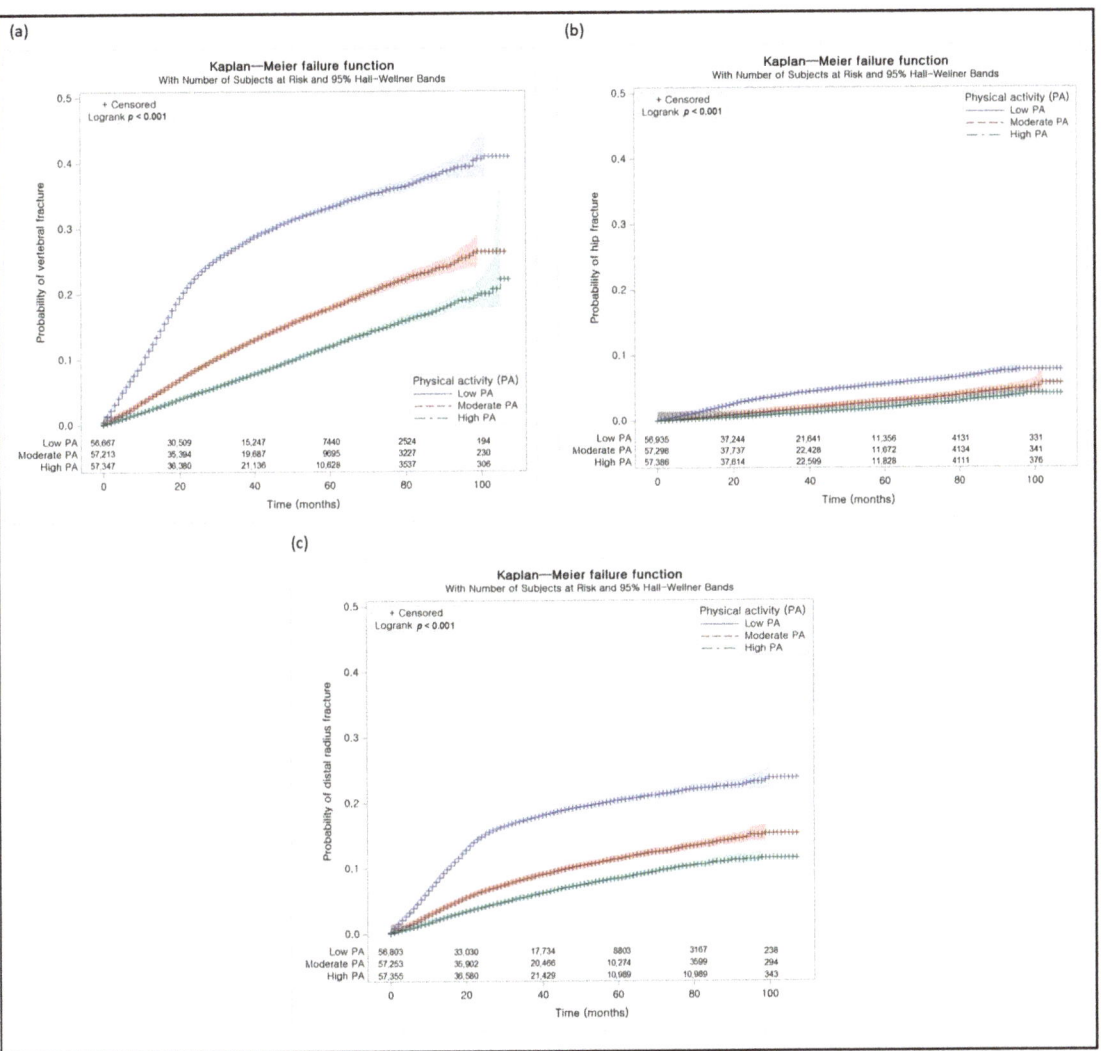

Figure 2. Kaplan–Meier failure analyses. (**a**) The cumulative proportion of vertebral fracture was low in the order of 'high PA', 'moderate PA', and 'low PA'. (**b**) The cumulative proportion of hip fracture was low in the order of 'high PA', 'moderate PA', and 'low PA'. (**c**) The cumulative proportion of distal radius fracture was low in the order of 'high PA', 'moderate PA', and 'low PA'.

Table 1. General characteristics of participants.

Characteristics	Total Participants			
	Low PA (n = 58,620)	Moderate PA (n = 58,620)	High PA (n = 58,620)	p-Value
Age (years old, n, %)				1.000
50–54	4370 (7.5)	4370 (7.5)	4370 (7.5)	
55–59	8419 (14.4)	8419 (14.4)	8419 (14.4)	
60–64	12,257 (20.9)	12,257 (20.9)	12,257 (20.9)	
65–69	11,545 (19.7)	11,545 (19.7)	11,545 (19.7)	
70–74	14,223 (24.3)	14,223 (24.3)	14,223 (24.3)	
75–79	5241 (8.9)	5241 (8.9)	5241 (8.9)	
80–84	2275 (3.9)	2275 (3.9)	2275 (3.9)	
85+	290 (0.5)	290 (0.5)	290 (0.5)	
Gender (n, %)				1.000
Men	7046 (12.0)	7046 (12.0)	7046 (12.0)	
Women	51,574 (88.0)	51,574 (88.0)	51,574 (88.0)	
Income within household unit (n, %)				1.000
1 (lowest)	11,563 (19.7)	11,563 (19.7)	11,563 (19.7)	
2	10,873 (18.6)	10,873 (18.6)	10,873 (18.6)	
3	13,467 (23.0)	13,467 (23.0)	13,467 (23.0)	
4	12,522 (21.4)	12,522 (21.4)	12,522 (21.4)	
5 (highest)	10,195 (17.4)	10,195 (17.4)	10,195 (17.4)	
Region of residence (n, %)				1.000
Urban	25,523 (43.5)	25,523 (43.5)	25,523 (43.5)	
Rural	33,097 (56.5)	33,097 (56.5)	33,097 (56.5)	
Total cholesterol level (mg/dL, mean, SD)	197.9 (44.1)	197.2 (40.1)	196.8 (39.0)	0.002 *
SBP (mmHg, mean, SD)	126.5 (16.0)	125.7 (15.3)	125.6 (15.1)	<0.001 *
DBP (mmHg, mean, SD)	76.5 (9.9)	76.1 (9.6)	75.9 (9.5)	<0.001 *
Fasting blood glucose level (mg/dL, mean, SD)	102.4 (27.3)	100.7 (22.8)	100.6 (22.4)	<0.001 *
Obesity [1] (n, %)				<0.001 *
Underweight	2433 (4.2)	2022 (3.5)	1526 (2.6)	
Normal	21,127 (36.0)	22,246 (38.0)	22,883 (39.0)	
Overweight	13,857 (23.6)	15,003 (25.6)	15,651 (26.7)	
Obese I	18,274 (31.2)	17,275 (29.5)	16,898 (28.8)	
Obese II	2929 (5.0)	2074 (3.5)	1662 (2.8)	
Smoking status (n, %)				<0.001 *
Nonsmoker	52,333 (89.3)	52,950 (90.3)	53,580 (91.4)	
Past smoker	3000 (5.1)	3372 (5.8)	3327 (5.7)	
Current smoker	3287 (5.6)	2298 (3.9)	1713 (2.9)	
Alcohol consumption (n, %)				<0.001 *
<1 time a week	51,745 (88.3)	51,022 (87.0)	50,725 (86.5)	
≥1 time a week	6875 (11.7)	7598 (13.0)	7895 (13.5)	
CCI score (n, %)				<0.001 *
0	35,109 (59.9)	38,616 (65.9)	39,930 (68.1)	
1	9807 (16.7)	9107 (15.5)	8552 (14.6)	
≥2	13,704 (23.4)	10,897 (18.6)	10,138 (17.3)	
Osteoporotic fxs (n, %)				
Vertebral fx	12,787 (21.8)	6233 (10.6)	4042 (6.9)	<0.001 *
Hip fx	2048 (3.5)	984 (1.7)	687 (1.2)	<0.001 *
Distal radius fx	8119 (13.9)	4229 (7.2)	2991 (5.1)	<0.001 *

CCI, Charlson comorbidity index; DBP, diastolic blood pressure; fx, fracture; PA, physical activity; SBP, systolic blood pressure. * Kruskal–Wallis test. Significance at <0.05 with Bonferroni correction (α = 0.05/3). [1] Obesity (BMI, body mass index, kg/m^2) was categorized as <18.5 (underweight), ≥18.5 to <23 (normal), ≥23 to <25 (overweight), ≥25 to <30 (obese I), and ≥30 (obese II).

The adjusted HR (95% CIs) for vertebral fx in the 'high PA' group was 0.27 (0.26–0.28) and in the 'moderate PA' group was 0.43 (0.42–0.44) as compared to the 'low PA' group. In analyses of subgroups defined by age and gender, the findings were consistent with the above findings (Table 2).

Table 2. HR (95% CIs) for vertebral fx in the PA groups with subgroup analyses according to age and gender.

Characteristics	No. of Vertebral fx/ No. of Participants	Follow-Up Duration, PY	Incidence Rate, per 100 PY	Hazard Ratios for Vertebral fx				p for Interaction
				Crude [1]	p-Value	Adjusted [1,2]	p-Value	
			Total participants (n = 175,860)					
Low PA	12,787/58,620 (21.8)	108,317	11.8	1		1		
Moderate PA	6233/58,620 (10.6)	129,073	4.8	0.43 (0.41–0.44)	<0.001 *	0.43 (0.42–0.44)	<0.001 *	
High PA	4042/58,620 (6.9)	136,100	3.0	0.27 (0.26–0.28)	<0.001 *	0.27 (0.26–0.28)	<0.001 *	
			Age group Age < 65 years old (n = 38,367)					
Low PA	1962/12,789 (15.3)	26,400	7.4	1		1		
Moderate PA	779/12,789 (6.1)	30,351	2.6	0.35 (0.33–0.37)	<0.001 *	0.36 (0.34–0.38)	<0.001 *	
High PA	450/12,789 (3.5)	31,412	1.4	0.19 (0.18–0.20)	<0.001 *	0.20 (0.18–0.21)	<0.001 *	<0.001 *
			Age ≥ 65 years old (n = 137,493)					
Low PA	10,825/45,831 (23.6)	81,917	13.2	1		1		
Moderate PA	5454/45,831 (11.9)	98,722	5.5	0.47 (0.45–0.48)	<0.001 *	0.47 (0.45–0.49)	<0.001 *	
High PA	3592/45,831 (7.8)	104,688	3.4	0.31 (0.30–0.32)	<0.001 *	0.31 (0.30–0.32)	<0.001 *	
			Gender Men (n = 21,138)					
Low PA	1917/7046 (27.2)	12,757	15.0	1		1		
Moderate PA	1112/7046 (15.8)	15,246	7.3	0.51 (0.47–0.55)	<0.001 *	0.51 (0.47–0.55)	<0.001 *	
High PA	754/7046 (10.7)	16,382	4.6	0.33 (0.30–0.36)	<0.001 *	0.33 (0.31–0.36)	<0.001 *	0.093
			Women (n = 154,722)					
Low PA	10,870/51,574 (21.1)	95,560	11.4	1		1		
Moderate PA	5121/51,574 (9.9)	113,827	4.5	0.41 (0.40–0.43)	<0.001 *	0.42 (0.40–0.43)	<0.001 *	
High PA	3288/51,574 (6.4)	119,718	2.7	0.26 (0.25–0.27)	<0.001 *	0.26 (0.25–0.27)	<0.001 *	

CCI, Charlson comorbidity index; CIs, confidence intervals; DBP, diastolic blood pressure; fx, fracture; HR, hazard ratio; PA, physical activity; PY, person–year; SBP, systolic blood pressure. * Stratified Cox proportional hazard model, significance at <0.05 with Bonferroni correction (α = 0.05/3). [1] Stratified by gender, age, income within household unit, and region of residence. [2] Adjusted for total cholesterol, SBP, DBP, fasting blood glucose, obesity, smoking, alcohol consumption, and CCI score.

The adjusted HR (95% CIs) for hip fx in the 'high PA' group was 0.37 (0.34–0.40) and in the 'moderate PA' group was 0.51 (0.47–0.55) compared to 'low PA'. In analyses of subgroups defined by age and gender, the findings were consistent with the above findings in all subgroups (Table 3).

The adjusted HR (95% CIs) for distal radius fx in the 'high PA' group was 0.32 (0.30–0.33) and in the 'moderate PA' group was 0.46 (0.45–0.48) compared to the 'low PA' group. In analyses of subgroups defined by age and gender, the findings were consistent with the above findings in all subgroups (Table 4).

Table 3. HR (95% CIs) for hip fx in the PA groups with subgroup analyses according to age and gender.

Characteristics	No. of Hip fx/ No. of Participants	Follow-up Duration, PY	Incidence Rate, per 100 PY	Hazard Ratios for Hip fx				p for Interaction
				Crude [1]	p-Value	Adjusted [1,2]	p-Value	
			Total participants (n = 175,860)					
Low PA	2048/58,620 (3.5)	139,819	1.5	1		1		
Moderate PA	984/58,620 (1.7)	142,750	0.7	0.47 (0.44–0.51)	<0.001 *	0.51 (0.47–0.55)	<0.001 *	
High PA	687/58,620 (1.2)	143,707	0.5	0.33 (0.30–0.36)	<0.001 *	0.37 (0.34–0.40)	<0.001 *	
			Age group					
			Age < 65 years old (n = 38,367)					
Low PA	230/12,789 (1.8)	31,829	0.7	1		1		
Moderate PA	81/12,789 (0.6)	32,213	0.3	0.33 (0.28–0.39)	<0.001 *	0.35 (0.30–0.42)	<0.001 *	
High PA	53/12,789 (0.4)	32,338	0.2	0.20 (0.17–0.25)	<0.001 *	0.23 (0.18–0.28)	<0.001 *	<0.001 *
			Age ≥ 65 years old (n = 137,493)					
Low PA	1818/45,831 (4.0)	107,990	1.7	1		1		
Moderate PA	903/45,831 (2.0)	110,537	0.8	0.52 (0.47–0.56)	<0.001 *	0.56 (0.51–0.61)	<0.001 *	
High PA	634/45,831 (1.4)	111,369	0.6	0.37 (0.34–0.41)	<0.001 *	0.42 (0.38–0.46)	<0.001 *	
			Gender					
			Men (n = 21,138)					
Low PA	554/7046 (7.9)	16,666	3.3	1		1		
Moderate PA	311/7046 (4.4)	17,311	1.8	0.54 (0.47–0.63)	<0.001 *	0.59 (0.51–0.68)	<0.001 *	
High PA	199/7046 (2.8)	17,630	1.1	0.35 (0.30–0.41)	<0.001 *	0.40 (0.34–0.47)	<0.001 *	0.009 *
			Women (n = 154,722)					
Low PA	1494/51,574 (2.9)	123,153	1.2	1		1		
Moderate PA	673/51,574 (1.3)	125,439	0.5	0.44 (0.40–0.48)	<0.001 *	0.48 (0.43–0.52)	<0.001 *	
High PA	488/51,574 (1.0)	126,077	0.4	0.32 (0.29–0.35)	<0.001 *	0.35 (0.32–0.39)	<0.001 *	

CCI, Charlson comorbidity index; CIs, confidence intervals; DBP, diastolic blood pressure; fx, fracture; HR, hazard ratio; PA, physical activity; PY, person–year; SBP, systolic blood pressure. * Stratified Cox proportional hazard model, significance at <0.05 with Bonferroni correction ($\alpha = 0.05/3$). [1] Stratified by gender, age, income within household unit, and region of residence. [2] Adjusted for total cholesterol, SBP, DBP, fasting blood glucose, obesity, smoking, alcohol consumption, and CCI score.

In other subgroup analyses, the findings were also consistent with the above findings in all subgroups for each fx (Supplementary Tables S1–S3).

Table 4. HR (95% CIs) for distal radius fx in the PA groups with subgroup analyses according to age and gender.

Characteristics	No. of Distal Radius fx/ No. of Participants	Follow-Up Duration, PY	Incidence Rate, per 100 PY	Hazard Ratios for Distal Radius fx				p for Interaction
				Crude [1]	p-Value	Adjusted [1,2]	p-Value	
			Total participants (n = 175,860)					
Low PA	8119/58,620 (13.9)	119,633	6.8	1		1		
Moderate PA	4229/58,620 (7.2)	132,804	3.2	0.48 (0.46–0.50)	<0.001 *	0.46 (0.45–0.48)	<0.001 *	
High PA	2991/58,620 (5.1)	137,923	2.2	0.33 (0.32–0.34)	<0.001 *	0.32 (0.30–0.33)	<0.001 *	
			Age group Age < 65 years old (n = 38,367)					
Low PA	2812/12,789 (22.0)	23,162	12.1	1		1		
Moderate PA	1332/12,789 (10.4)	28,389	4.7	0.42 (0.40–0.44)	<0.001 *	0.41 (0.39–0.43)	<0.001 *	<0.001 *
High PA	898/12,789 (7.0)	30,308	3.0	0.27 (0.26–0.29)	<0.001 *	0.26 (0.25–0.28)	<0.001 *	
			Age ≥ 65 years old (n = 137,493)					
Low PA	5307/45,831 (11.6)	96,471	5.5	1		1		
Moderate PA	2897/45,831 (6.3)	104,415	2.8	0.57 (0.54–0.60)	<0.001 *	0.55 (0.52–0.58)	<0.001 *	
High PA	2093/45,831 (4.6)	107,615	1.9	0.42 (0.39–0.45)	<0.001 *	0.40 (0.38–0.43)	<0.001 *	
			Gender Men (n = 21,138)					
Low PA	403/7046 (5.7)	16,895	2.4	1		1		
Moderate PA	282/7046 (4.0)	17,269	1.6	0.69 (0.59–0.81)	<0.001 *	0.66 (0.57–0.77)	<0.001 *	0.008 *
High PA	212/7046 (3.0)	17,539	1.2	0.52 (0.44–0.61)	<0.001 *	0.49 (0.41–0.58)	<0.001 *	
			Women (n = 154,722)					
Low PA	7716/51,574 (15.0)	102,738	7.5	1		1		
Moderate PA	3947/51,574 (7.7)	115,535	3.4	0.47 (0.45–0.49)	<0.001 *	0.45 (0.44–0.47)	<0.001 *	
High PA	2779/51,574 (5.4)	120,384	2.3	0.32 (0.31–0.33)	<0.001 *	0.31 (0.29–0.32)	<0.001 *	

CCI, Charlson comorbidity index; CIs, confidence intervals; DBP, diastolic blood pressure; fx, fracture; HR, hazard ratio; PA, physical activity; PY, person–year; SBP, systolic blood pressure. * Stratified Cox proportional hazard model, significance at <0.05 with Bonferroni correction (α = 0.05/3). [1] Stratified by gender, age, income within household unit, and region of residence. [2] Adjusted for total cholesterol, SBP, DBP, fasting blood glucose, obesity, smoking, alcohol consumption, and CCI score.

4. Discussion

We confirmed the association between the intensity of PA and the occurrence of each osteoporotic fx in subjects with osteoporosis using the NHIS customized data. Based on our results, the higher the intensity of PA is, the lower the rate of occurrence of each osteoporotic fx. The findings were consistent across all subgroup analyses.

According to previous studies, PA is likely to influence the fx risk. One such study that reviewed randomized controlled trials (RCTs) reported that exercise improved BMD or decreased fall risk to prevent fx risks in postmenopausal women with osteoporosis [12]. Among the RCT studies, one study with 52-week intervention in postmenopausal women with osteoporosis reported that the adjusted mean difference in hip total BMD in the exercise group compared to the control group was 0.012 (95% CI = 0.002 to 0.022, $p < 0.05$) [13]. In another study with a 24-week intervention in postmenopausal women with osteopenia, the change in femoral neck BMD was $-1.3 \pm 2.7\%$ and $3.1 \pm 4.6\%$ in the control group and in the exercise group, respectively ($p = 0.001$) [15]. However, few studies for an association between PA and vertebral fx or distal radius fx in osteoporosis in the RCT study have been performed. Instead, some studies have demonstrated that the type of exercise differently affects BMD in the spine [25,26]. Furthermore, no RCT studies were found with fx as the endpoint.

On the other hand, a meta-analysis study using prospective cohort studies suggested that PA could prevent hip fx (relative risk = 0.62, 95% CI = 0.56–0.69 for women; relative risk = 0.55, 95% CI = 0.44–0.69 for men) [16]. Another meta-analysis of cohort studies also suggested that leisure PA could reduce the risk of hip fx in older women (relative risk = 0.93, 95% CI = 0.91–0.96) [17]. However, no association was found between PA and the risk of distal radius fx or vertebral fx in previous studies. Furthermore, no observational study has used osteoporotic patients as their target study population.

In our study, using the NHIS customized database, we selected osteoporotic men and women who were at risk of osteoporotic fxs, and we examined osteoporotic fxs as the primary endpoint. Due to the large sample size and high statistical power of our study, we found an inverse association between PA intensity and all types of osteoporotic fxs in patients with osteoporosis. Moreover, we found associations according to specific characteristics, such as age and gender due to the large sample size.

Although a high intensity of PA might be considered to be a risk factor for falls and fxs in osteoporosis patients, increasing evidence has demonstrated that increasing PA could prevent fxs, actually reducing falls by resistance and balance training and increased BMD. One review study found that exercise reduced the incidence of one or more fall-related fxs in 10 RCTs (risk ratio = 0.73, 95% CIs = 0.56–0.95). Specifically, the best exercises for reducing falls were balance and functional exercises, such as Tai Chi, and multiple other types of exercise [27]. One of the recommendations of an international panel was that individuals with osteoporosis or osteoporotic vertebral fxs should not perform aerobic PA without resistance and balance PA to prevent falls [28]. Exercises that use body weight or other forms of weight, including resistance training and cycling, are the major reasons why increased PA could lead to higher BMD [29].

We hypothesized that participants might have a higher fx risk if they first started moderate- to high-intensity PA after the onset of osteoporosis. Therefore, additional subgroup analyses were performed for subgroups defined by previous PA intensity before the onset of osteoporosis in subjects for whom previous PA information was available. Surprisingly, the findings were all consistent with the main findings (Supplementary Table S4). Hence, a higher intensity of PA does not seem to be a risk factor for osteoporotic diseases, regardless of whether the participants were not active in PAs prior to the diagnosis of osteoporosis.

Although our study findings show that a higher intensity of PA lowered each osteoporotic fx in osteoporosis, the findings should be cautiously interpreted on the basis of previous studies. Obviously, falls are one of the major risk factors for fxs [9]. In addition, functional impairment is likely to be associated with a high risk of fx [30]. Because data regarding falls or functional impairment was not available in the NHIS customized database, we could not assess the contribution of those factors in our study. Based on the results of previous studies and practical knowledge, the intensity and type of PA should be accounted for depending on the level of functional impairment or risk of falls.

Several limitations of our study mainly regarding using the secondary data should be noted. Some variables were not available, including the history of falls, functional impairment, and dietary intake with supplement intake, including vitamin D and calcium intake. Moreover, in defining the PA groups, the METs were limited because the variable related to time of walking and moderate activity was collected as binary ($\geq$30 min or not), and the variable for vigorous activity was also binary ($\geq$20 min or not). In addition, the association between specific types of PA and fxs in osteoporosis could not be determined from the data. In addition, not only were specific BMD values not available for each participant, but BMD measurements also differed according to the type of instrument in the hospital. We could not confirm whether the actual osteoporotic fx is or not because we defined osteoporotic fxs using only ICD-10 codes. Specific medication regarding protective or affecting bone was not available to adjust in the analysis. Due to the observational study design and based on the above limitations, determination of causality between PA and osteoporotic fxs in osteoporosis should be carefully considered.

The major strength of our study was the use of a national customized database including data from osteoporotic men and women. Because of the large number of subjects, matching by gender, age, income within household unit, and region of residence in a 1:1:1 ratio for each PA group was feasible. Moreover, various lifestyle factors and health indicators, such as alcohol consumption, smoking status, obesity, and CCI scores, were used as covariates. Therefore, the study was uniquely positioned to demonstrate an association between PA and osteoporotic fxs in osteoporosis. In addition, 9 years' worth of follow-up data were available. Therefore, we had sufficient data to use osteoporotic fxs as endpoints in our study.

5. Conclusions

The results suggested that a higher intensity of PA was negatively associated with osteoporotic fxs, including vertebral fx, hip fx, and distal radius fx. In addition, we found that a higher intensity of PA was negatively associated with each osteoporotic fx under various conditions.

Supplementary Materials: The following are available online at https://www.mdpi.com/article/10.3390/jpm12030491/s1, Table S1: Subgroup analyses of hazard ratio (95% confidence interval) for vertebral fx in the PA groups according to income, region of residence, obesity, smoking, alcohol consumption, total cholesterol, blood pressure, and fasting blood glucose, Table S2: Subgroup analyses of hazard ratio (95% confidence interval) for hip fx in the PA groups according to income, region of residence, obesity, smoking, alcohol consumption, total cholesterol, blood pressure, and fasting blood glucose, Table S3: Subgroup analyses of hazard ratio (95% confidence interval) for distal radius fx in the PA groups according to income, region of residence, obesity, smoking, alcohol consumption, total cholesterol, blood pressure, and fasting blood glucose, Table S4: Subgroup analyses of hazard ratios (95% confidence intervals) for each osteoporotic fracture in the PA groups according to previous PA level.

Author Contributions: Conceptualization, J.-W.L. and B.-C.K.; methodology, H.-G.C.; software, C.-Y.M.; validation, M.-J.K. and J.-H.K. (Ji-Hee Kim); formal analysis, C.-Y.M.; investigation, C.-Y.M.; data curation, C.-Y.M.; writing—original draft preparation, C.-Y.M.; writing—review and editing, J.-H.K. (Joo-Hee Kim), W.-J.B. and H.-G.C.; visualization, C.-Y.M.; supervision, H.-G.C.; project administration, H.-G.C.; funding acquisition, H.-G.C. All authors have read and agreed to the published version of the manuscript.

Funding: This research was funded by the Hallym University Research Fund (HURF) and in part by the National Research Foundation (NRF) of Korea, grant numbers "NRF-2019-R1A6A3A01091963" and "NRF-2021-R1C1C1004986".

Institutional Review Board Statement: This study was approved by the ethics committee of Hallym University (HALLYM 2019-08-029, approval date was 19 September 2019) following the guidelines of the IRB.

Informed Consent Statement: Patient consent was waived due to the fact that the study utilized secondary data.

Data Availability Statement: Restrictions apply to the availability of these data. Data were obtained from the Korean National Health Insurance Sharing Service (NHISS) and are available at https://nhiss.nhis.or.kr (accessed on 25 January 2022) with the permission of the NHIS.

Acknowledgments: This study used NHIS—National Health Information Database (NHIS-2021-1-466) made by the NHIS.

Conflicts of Interest: The authors declare no conflict of interest.

References

1. World Health Organization. Physical Inactivity. Available online: https://www.who.int/data/gho/indicator-metadata-registry/imr-details/3416 (accessed on 3 January 2021).
2. Amini, H.; Habibi, S.; Islamoglu, A.H.; Isanejad, E.; Uz, C.; Daniyari, H. COVID-19 pandemic-induced physical inactivity: The necessity of updating the Global Action Plan on Physical Activity 2018–2030. *Environ. Health Prev. Med.* **2021**, *26*, 32. [CrossRef]
3. Watson, K.B.; Whitfield, G.P.; Huntzicker, G.; Omura, J.D.; Ussery, E.; Chen, T.J.; Fanfair, R.N. Cross-sectional study of changes in physical activity behavior during the COVID-19 pandemic among US adults. *Int. J. Behav. Nutr. Phys. Act.* **2021**, *18*, 91. [CrossRef]
4. Strain, T.; Sharp, S.J.; Spiers, A.; Price, H.; Williams, C.; Fraser, C.; Brage, S.; Wijndaele, K.; Kelly, P. Population level physical activity before and during the first national COVID-19 lockdown: A nationally representative repeat cross-sectional study of 5 years of Active Lives data in England. *Lancet Reg. Health Eur.* **2022**, *12*, 100265. [CrossRef]
5. Lee, Y.; Baek, S.; Shin, J. Changes in Physical Activity Compared to the Situation before the Outbreak of COVID-19 in Korea. *Int. J. Environ. Res. Public Health* **2021**, *19*, 126. [CrossRef]
6. World Health Organization. *Global Strategy on Diet, Physical Activity and Health*; WHO: Geneva, Switzerland; Available online: https://www.who.int/dietphysicalactivity/pa/en/ (accessed on 8 May 2020).
7. Zhu, K.; Prince, R.L. Lifestyle and osteoporosis. *Curr. Osteoporos. Rep.* **2015**, *13*, 52–59. [CrossRef]
8. Woolf, A.D.; Pfleger, B. Burden of major musculoskeletal conditions. *Bull. World Health Organ.* **2003**, *81*, 646–656.
9. World Health Organization. *Assessment of Fracture Risk and Its Application to Screening for Postmenopausal Osteoporosis: Report of a WHO Study Group*; WHO: Geneva, Switzerland, 1994.
10. Brown, J.P.; Adachi, J.D.; Schemitsch, E.; Tarride, J.E.; Brown, V.; Bell, A.; Reiner, M.; Oliveira, T.; Motsepe-Ditshego, P.; Burke, N.; et al. Mortality in older adults following a fragility fracture: Real-world retrospective matched-cohort study in Ontario. *BMC Musculoskelet. Disord.* **2021**, *22*, 105. [CrossRef]
11. Lee, Y.K.; Jang, S.; Jang, S.; Lee, H.J.; Park, C.; Ha, Y.C.; Kim, D.Y. Mortality after vertebral fracture in Korea: Analysis of the National Claim Registry. *Osteoporos. Int.* **2012**, *23*, 1859–1865. [CrossRef]
12. Anupama, D.S.; Norohna, J.A.; Acharya, K.K.; Ravishankar; George, A. Effect of exercise on bone mineral density and quality of life among postmenopausal women with osteoporosis without fracture: A systematic review. *Int. J. Orthop. Trauma Nurs.* **2020**, *39*, 100796. [CrossRef]
13. Bolton, K.L.; Egerton, T.; Wark, J.; Wee, E.; Matthews, B.; Kelly, A.; Craven, R.; Kantor, S.; Bennell, K.L. Effects of exercise on bone density and falls risk factors in post-menopausal women with osteopenia: A randomised controlled trial. *J. Sci. Med. Sport* **2012**, *15*, 102–109. [CrossRef]
14. Mosti, M.P.; Kaehler, N.; Stunes, A.K.; Hoff, J.; Syversen, U. Maximal strength training in postmenopausal women with osteoporosis or osteopenia. *J. Strength Cond. Res.* **2013**, *27*, 2879–2886. [CrossRef]
15. Yu, P.A.; Hsu, W.H.; Hsu, W.B.; Kuo, L.T.; Lin, Z.R.; Shen, W.J.; Hsu, R.W. The effects of high impact exercise intervention on bone mineral density, physical fitness, and quality of life in postmenopausal women with osteopenia: A retrospective cohort study. *Medicine (Baltimore)* **2019**, *98*, e14898. [CrossRef]
16. Moayyeri, A. The association between physical activity and osteoporotic fractures: A review of the evidence and implications for future research. *Ann. Epidemiol.* **2008**, *18*, 827–835. [CrossRef]
17. Rong, K.; Liu, X.Y.; Wu, X.H.; Li, X.L.; Xia, Q.Q.; Chen, J.; Yin, X.F. Increasing Level of Leisure Physical Activity Could Reduce the Risk of Hip Fracture in Older Women: A Dose-Response Meta-analysis of Prospective Cohort Studies. *Medicine (Baltimore)* **2016**, *95*, e2984. [CrossRef]
18. Kim, S.Y.; Kim, H.J.; Min, C.; Choi, H.G. Association between benign paroxysmal positional vertigo and osteoporosis: Two nested case-control studies. *Osteoporos. Int.* **2020**, *31*, 2017–2024. [CrossRef]
19. International Physical Activity Questionnaire. International Physical Activity Questionnaire (IPAQ) Scoring Protocol. Available online: https://sites.google.com/site/theipaq/scoring-protocol (accessed on 7 October 2021).
20. Kim, S.Y.; Lee, J.K.; Lim, J.S.; Park, B.; Choi, H.G. Increased risk of dementia after distal radius, hip, and spine fractures. *Medicine (Baltimore)* **2020**, *99*, e19048. [CrossRef]
21. Lee, J.W.; Lee, Y.B.; Kwon, B.C.; Yoo, J.H.; Choi, H.G. Mortality and cause of death in distal radius fracture patients: A longitudinal follow-up study using a national sample cohort. *Medicine (Baltimore)* **2019**, *98*, e18604. [CrossRef]
22. Kim, S.Y.; Oh, D.J.; Park, B.; Choi, H.G. Bell's palsy and obesity, alcohol consumption and smoking: A nested case-control study using a national health screening cohort. *Sci. Rep.* **2020**, *10*, 4248. [CrossRef]
23. Min, C.; Yoo, D.M.; Wee, J.H.; Lee, H.J.; Byun, S.H.; Choi, H.G. Mortality and cause of death in physical activity and insufficient physical activity participants: A longitudinal follow-up study using a national health screening cohort. *BMC Public Health* **2020**, *20*, 1469. [CrossRef]
24. Quan, H.; Li, B.; Couris, C.M.; Fushimi, K.; Graham, P.; Hider, P.; Januel, J.M.; Sundararajan, V. Updating and validating the Charlson comorbidity index and score for risk adjustment in hospital discharge abstracts using data from 6 countries. *Am. J. Epidemiol.* **2011**, *173*, 676–682. [CrossRef]
25. Sinaki, M. Yoga spinal flexion positions and vertebral compression fracture in osteopenia or osteoporosis of spine: Case series. *Pain Pract.* **2013**, *13*, 68–75. [CrossRef] [PubMed]
26. Sinaki, M.; Mikkelsen, B.A. Postmenopausal spinal osteoporosis: Flexion versus extension exercises. *Arch. Phys. Med. Rehabil.* **1984**, *65*, 593–596. [PubMed]

27. Sherrington, C.; Fairhall, N.J.; Wallbank, G.K.; Tiedemann, A.; Michaleff, Z.A.; Howard, K.; Clemson, L.; Hopewell, S.; Lamb, S.E. Exercise for preventing falls in older people living in the community. *Cochrane Database Syst. Rev.* **2019**, *1*, Cd012424. [CrossRef] [PubMed]
28. Giangregorio, L.M.; Papaioannou, A.; Macintyre, N.J.; Ashe, M.C.; Heinonen, A.; Shipp, K.; Wark, J.; McGill, S.; Keller, H.; Jain, R.; et al. Too Fit To Fracture: Exercise recommendations for individuals with osteoporosis or osteoporotic vertebral fracture. *Osteoporos. Int.* **2014**, *25*, 821–835. [CrossRef] [PubMed]
29. Carter, M.I.; Hinton, P.S. Physical activity and bone health. *Mo Med.* **2014**, *111*, 59–64.
30. Lai, J.K.; Lucas, R.M.; Armstrong, M.; Banks, E. Prospective observational study of physical functioning, physical activity, and time outdoors and the risk of hip fracture: A population-based cohort study of 158,057 older adults in the 45 and up study. *J. Bone Miner. Res.* **2013**, *28*, 2222–2231. [CrossRef]

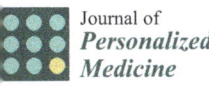

Article

Multi-Task Deep Learning Approach for Simultaneous Objective Response Prediction and Tumor Segmentation in HCC Patients with Transarterial Chemoembolization

Yuze Li [1,†], Ziming Xu [1,†], Chao An [2], Huijun Chen [1,*] and Xiao Li [3,*]

1. Center for Biomedical Imaging Research, School of Medicine, Tsinghua University, Beijing 100084, China; liyz17@mails.tsinghua.edu.cn (Y.L.); xuzm20@mails.tsinghua.edu.cn (Z.X.)
2. Department of Minimal Invasive Intervention, Sun Yat-sen University Cancer Center, Guangzhou 510060, China; anchao@sysucc.org.cn
3. Department of Interventional Therapy, Chinese Academy of Medical Sciences and Peking Union Medical College, Beijing 100021, China
* Correspondence: chenhj_cbir@mail.tsinghua.edu.cn (H.C.); lixiao@cicams.ac.cn (X.L.)
† These authors contributed equally to this work.

Abstract: This study aimed to develop a deep learning-based model to simultaneously perform the objective response (OR) and tumor segmentation for hepatocellular carcinoma (HCC) patients who underwent transarterial chemoembolization (TACE) treatment. A total of 248 patients from two hospitals were retrospectively included and divided into the training, internal validation, and external testing cohort. A network consisting of an encoder pathway, a prediction pathway, and a segmentation pathway was developed, and named multi-DL (multi-task deep learning), using contrast-enhanced CT images as input. We compared multi-DL with other deep learning-based OR prediction and tumor segmentation methods to explore the incremental value of introducing the interconnected task into a unified network. Additionally, the clinical model was developed using multivariate logistic regression to predict OR. Results showed that multi-DL could achieve the highest AUC of 0.871 in OR prediction and the highest dice coefficient of 73.6% in tumor segmentation. Furthermore, multi-DL can successfully perform the risk stratification that the low-risk and high-risk patients showed a significant difference in survival ($p = 0.006$). In conclusion, the proposed method may provide a useful tool for therapeutic regime selection in clinical practice.

Keywords: treatment outcome; liver neoplasms; deep learning

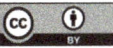

1. Introduction

Hepatocellular carcinoma (HCC) is one of the leading causes of cancer mortality worldwide, with more than 800,000 deaths reported annually [1–4]. HCC patients at an early stage are encouraged to perform curative therapies, such as liver resection, transplantation, and local ablation, observing the prolongation of overall survival (OS) [5,6]. However, more than half of patients with HCC are already in the intermediate and advanced stage for the initial diagnosis, and palliative treatment is the first choice [7]. According to the Barcelona Clinical Liver Cancer (BCLC) staging system, transarterial chemoembolization (TACE) is used as first-line therapy for patients at stage B. Patients with an objective response (OR) after the first session of TACE can obtain the survival benefit [8]. However, some patients still suffer a poor prognosis due to the complex heterogeneity of the tumor microenvironment [9,10]. Therefore, developing a prediction model for OR and OS of HCC patients who underwent TACE may have huge clinically significant for managing patients in this precision medicine era.

At present, several scoring systems have been proposed to predict the outcome of TACE for HCC patients. For example, Sieghart et al. developed the Assessment for Retreatment with transarterial chemoembolization (ART) score [11], which integrated radiologic tumor response, Child–Pugh increase, and aspartate aminotransferase increase to perform the staging. Hucke et al. proposed the selection for TACE treatment (STATE) score [12], measuring the serum-albumin level, tumor load, and C-reactive protein level to identify patients who were suitable or unsuitable for the first TACE. Furthermore, Granito et al. recently demonstrated that the post-TACE increase in transaminases could represent an independent factor for a complete response to TACE in patients with early and intermediate stage HCC [13]. This study may suggest a simple clinical tool associated with TACE's efficacy to improve management and treatment planning. However, these scores are not widely used in clinical and are limited by the unsatisfied predictive accuracy. Moreover, researchers introduced quantitative imaging-based methods, such as radiomics approaches, to predict the OR of the TACE using high-throughput features extracted from computed tomography (CT) or magnetic resonance imaging (MRI) data [14–16]. Though these methods achieved considerable predictive ability, they rely on hand-crafted feature extractors and manual tumor segmentation, where the performance and efficiency can be further improved.

Machine learning, as a big data-driven approach, is widely used in the medical field [17], including liver tumor segmentation [18–23] and outcome prediction after TACE treatment [24–29]. For the former, researchers developed multi-layer convolutional networks, fully convolutional networks, and encoder–decoder structures, with which more and more information contained in images was utilized. For the latter, deeper and deeper neural networks were applied to extract features from the tumor region, aiming to provide more accurate outcome prediction. However, existing methods only utilized the deep neural network to perform a single task, ignoring the combination of these two interconnected tasks: tumor segmentation and outcome prediction. Here, we aimed to develop a tumor-aware deep neural network for multi-task learning towards both the TACE outcome prediction and tumor segmentation. We hypothesized that combining these two interconnected tasks in a unified model could behave better than only doing any single one of them. The network was constructed on a large cohort of HCC patients with TACE treatment and backed by external testing to demonstrate the effeteness and robustness of the proposed method.

2. Materials and Methods

2.1. Study Population

This study retrospectively enrolled patients with HCC who underwent TACE between May 2014 and December 2019 at two hospitals. The whole protocol was approved by the institutional ethics board, and the written informed consent was waived because of the retrospective nature of this study. All procedures involving human participants were performed following the 1975 Helsinki declaration and its later amendments.

In this study, HCC was confirmed by the European Association for the Study of the Liver (EASL) or the American Association for the Study of Liver Disease (AASLD). Specifically, the presence of arterial enhancement on contrast-enhanced CT (CECT) or contrast-enhanced MRI (CEMRI) of a nodule 2 cm or larger with subsequent washout on the portal or delayed phases was considered the HCC. CEMRI was recommended due to its high sensitivity [30]. Biopsy was performed if the nodule did not show typical features in images.

A total of 248 patients have analyzed in this study according to the following inclusion criteria: (1) age of the patient was equal to or older than 18; (2) BCLC stage A or B; (3) the CECT was performed within one month before the first session of the TACE; and (4) follow-up CECT or CEMRI was obtained two months after the treatment to determine the tumor response to TACE. The exclusion criteria were as follows: (1) other treatments such as resection, ablation, or transplantation were conducted before TACE; (2) presence of macrovascular invasion or extrahepatic metastasis; and (3) Child–Pugh C. Patients in hospital 1 were randomly divided into training and internal validation cohorts, and patients in hospital 2 were used as the external testing cohort (Figure 1).

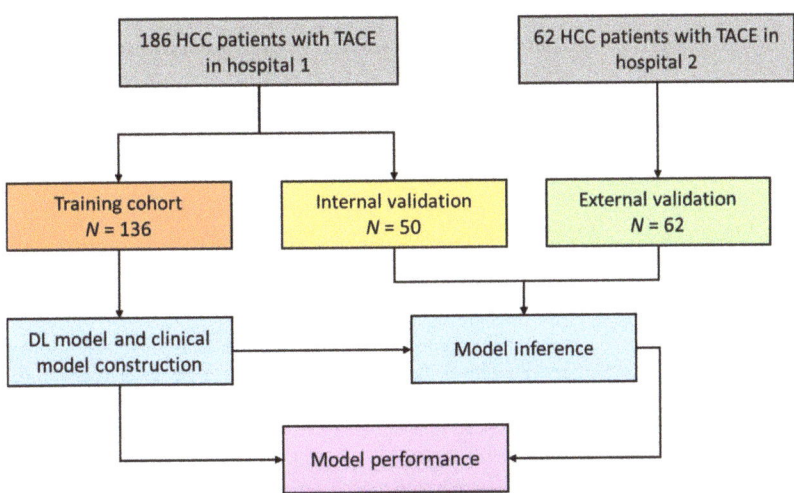

Figure 1. The diagram of the patient inclusion, model construction, and performance evaluation.

Clinical variables for each patient were collected from the medical records, including 4 groups of data: demographics and clinical characteristics variables (sex, age, hepatitis B); laboratory findings (alpha-fetoprotein (AFP), alanine aminotransferase (ALT), aspartate aminotransferase (AST), albumin (ALB), prothrombin time (PT), total bilirubin (TBil), platelet (PLT), Child–Pugh class and BCLC grade); tumor characteristics (tumor number and tumor size); and treatment and follow-up information.

2.2. TACE Procedure and Follow Up

TACE treatment was decided by two experienced interventional radiologists with more than 10 years of TACE experience and approved by the patients. The TACE procedure was guided using digital subtraction angiography (Philips, type FD 20 1250 mA, Amsterdam, Netherlands). A 5-Fr micro-catheter (Terumo, Tokyo, Japan) was used to assess the feeding artery. Superselective embolization of the artery directly supplying the tumor was carried out with a microcatheter whenever necessary. Emulsion, which consisted of 10–20 mL lipiodol, 30–50 mg lobaplatin, and 20–40 mg epirubicin was injected slowly until the offending vessel occluded [31,32].

To determine the subsequent treatment, the CECT or CEMRI were conducted 4–8 weeks after TACE to evaluate the effectiveness and the tumor status. TACE can be discontinued when the residual tumor or new lesions are not found. In comparison, the patient can choose the "on-demand" TACE procedure with the presence of the vital tumor or recurrence.

The OR of TACE was determined by two interventional radiologists with more than 6 years of TACE operation experience according to the post-operative CECT with modified Response Evaluation Criteria in Solid Tumors (mRECIST) criteria, as recommended in [33]. Four categories of outcome were defined, including complete response (CR), partial response (PR), stable disease (SD), and progression disease (PD). CR and PR can be further classified into objective response (OR) group, while SD and PD were classified into non-response (Non-OR) group [34,35]. OS was defined as the period between the initial TACE treatment and all-cause death.

2.3. Image Acquisition and Pre-Processing

The detailed CECT imaging protocol can be found in Supplementary Materials Note S1. The arterial phase (AP) and portal venous phase (PP) of CECT images were used in this study. The normalization of the image was performed using the nearest interpolation method [36] to obtain $1 \times 1 \times 1$ mm^3 spatial resolution and using the Z-score method on the image intensity to 0–1 value. Then, the image was processed by the nnUNet [37] to obtain the initial tumor segmentation. One primary radiologist with 6 years of experience in liver imaging corrected the segmentation faults, while a secondary radiologist with 10 years of experience in liver imaging reviewed and adjusted the delineation. All adjustment was performed on in-house software coded by Python.

2.4. Deep-Learning Model Construction

Here, a tumor-aware deep neural network for multi-task learning was developed to perform the OR prediction and tumor segmentation. The network was named multi-DL (multi-task deep learning) and its structure is shown in Figure 2 and Table 1. Inspired by the previous studies [38,39], we constructed the multi-DL model based on the encoder–decoder network where the encoder part (encoder pathway in the multi-DL) extracted the multi-scale information from the inputted images by down-sampling the resolution with pooling layer. In contrast, the decoder part (segmentation pathway) restored the resolution of feature maps layer by layer and integrated the multi-scale information through the skip connection. This encoder–decoder architecture was widely applied in liver tumor segmentation and showed promising results [18–22]. However, to the best of our knowledge, there is no relevant work to segment the liver tumor and predict the OR after TACE treatment simultaneously, which leaves a technique gap to fill. Therefore, we added the prediction pathway after the encoder pathway in multi-DL to realize the OR prediction in this study. There were two advantages of combining tumor segmentation and OR prediction into a unified network: first, existing OR prediction methods had to delineate the tumor region manually and then ran the algorithm on the image patch, which was time-consuming, while our multi-DL model can automatically locate the tumor area and generate OR prediction at the same time; and second, optimizing the tumor segmentation and OR prediction in the same network can obtain better performance than doing the single task, because these two tasks were interconnected and shared common characteristics which can be learned by the deep neural network. Additionally, the network output of the prediction pathway was a 0–1 value, indicating the probability of OR. The risk score was calculated by 1-OR probability and then used in the survival analysis to perform the risk stratification.

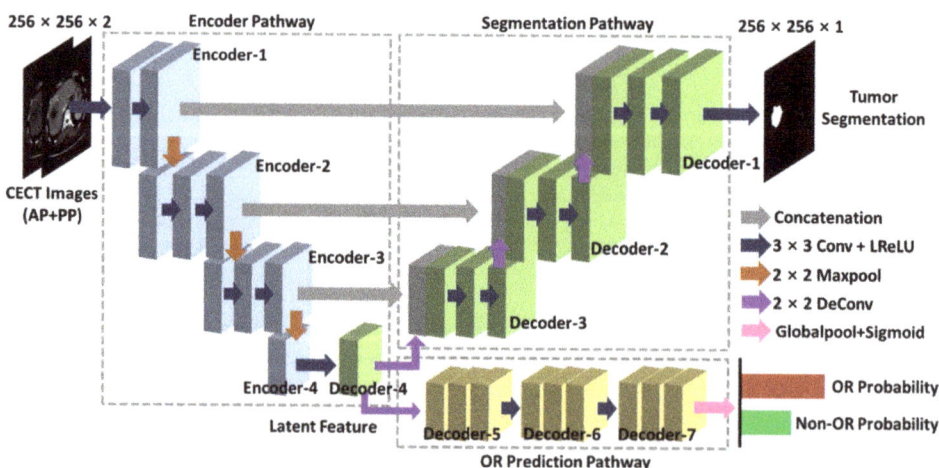

Figure 2. The structure of the proposed multi-DL (multi-task deep learning) model.

Table 1. The detailed network structure of multi-DL (multi-task deep learning).

Block Name	Layer	Parameter
Encoder-1	2 × (Conv2D + BN + LReLU) + Max-pooling	Conv: 3 × 3 × 32 filter, stride 1, same padding; Pooling: stride 2
Encoder-2	2 × (Conv2D + BN + LReLU) + Max-pooling	Conv: 3 × 3 × 64 filter, stride 1, same padding; Pooling: stride 2
Encoder-3	2 × (Conv2D + BN + LReLU) + Max-pooling	Conv: 3 × 3 × 128 filter, stride 1, same padding; Pooling: stride 2
Encoder-4	2 × (Conv2D + BN + LReLU) + Max-pooling	Conv: 3 × 3 × 256 filter, stride 1, same padding; Pooling: stride 2
Encoder-5	Conv2D + BN + LReLU	Conv: 3 × 3 × 128 filter, stride 1, same padding;
Encoder-6	Conv2D + BN + LReLU	Conv: 3 × 3 × 64 filter, stride 1, same padding;
Encoder-7	Conv2D + BN + LReLU	Conv: 3 × 3 × 32 filter, stride 1, same padding;
Decoder-1	(Conv2D + BN + LReLU) + (DeConv2D + BN + LReLU)	Conv: 3 × 3 × 32 filter, stride 1, same padding; DeConv: 3 × 3 × 32 filter, stride 2, same padding
Decoder-2	(Conv2D + BN + LReLU) + (DeConv2D + BN + LReLU)	Conv: 3 × 3 × 64 filter, stride 1, same padding; DeConv: 3 × 3 × 64 filter, stride 2, same padding
Decoder-3	(Conv2D + BN + LReLU) + (DeConv2D + BN + LReLU)	Conv: 3 × 3 × 128 filter, stride 1, same padding; DeConv: 3 × 3 × 128 filter, stride 2, same padding
Decoder-4	(Conv2D + BN + LReLU) + (DeConv2D + BN + LReLU)	Conv: 3 × 3 × 256 filter, stride 1, same padding; DeConv: 3 × 3 × 256 filter, stride 2, same padding

To verify the effectiveness of the multi-DL model, we compared the proposed method with other deep learning methods. For OR prediction, we compared ResNet50 applied in the study [26] and the single-DL-Pre model constructed of encoder pathway and prediction pathway. For tumor segmentation, we used the CNN model applied in the study [23] and encoder–decoder network in the study [18] as the comparison methods.

The loss function of the network was the combination of the cross-entropy loss and the dice loss [40]. The former was used for OR prediction, and the latter was for tumor segmentation. Dice similarity coefficient can be defined as follows:

$$\text{Dice (pre, gt)} = 2 \times (\text{pre} \cap \text{gt}) / (\text{pre} + \text{gt})$$

where pre denotes the predicted tumor region, gt denotes the ground truth tumor region and $\cap$ denotes the intersection operation.

The model was trained for 200 epochs (the number of passes of the entire training dataset the deep-learning algorithm has completed) using the Adam optimizer (a widely used algorithm that modifies the attributes of the neural network, such as weights and learning rate) [41] with the learning rate of 1×10^3. The implementation of the network was using the PyTorch framework (version 1.3.0) and Python (version 3.6) on a server equipped with a 6-core Intel CPU I7-6850K, a GPU TitanXp, and 32 GB memory.

2.5. Clinical Model Construction

The univariate analysis using logistic regression was firstly applied on all clinical variables, and those with significant differences between OR and non-OR ($p < 0.05$) were selected. Then, these variables were included in the multivariate logistic regression analysis to identify the independent risk factors associated with objective response ($p < 0.05$). Odds ratio and 95% confidence interval (CI) were calculated for each risk factor. The clinical model was constructed using the above independent risk factors using multivariate logistic regression algorithm [42].

2.6. Efficiency of Automatic Tumor Segmentation

We evaluated the efficiency of introducing automatic tumor segmentation into the model. Twenty patients were randomly selected from the training cohort and delineated by the radiologist, network processing, and network processing plus the manual adjustment. The averaged processing time was recorded and compared.

2.7. Statistical Analysis

The clinical variable distribution of the patients in the training, internal validation, and external validation cohorts were compared using Student's *t*-test or chi-squared test. For the OR prediction, performance was evaluated using the receiver operating characteristic curve (ROC) analysis and the area under the curve (AUC). Quantitative indices including accuracy (ACC), sensitivity (SEN), specificity (SPE), positive predictive value (PPV), and negative predictive value (NPV) were also computed with the confusion matrix. Youden's J statistic [43] was applied to determine the optimal operating points in ROC analysis.

The DeLong test was used to compare AUCs between different models. Survival curves were generated using the Kaplan–Meier method, and OS was compared between low- and high-risk patients with the log-rank test. For the tumor segmentation, the Dice coefficient and tumor segmentation time were compared using paired Student's *t*-test. All statistical analyses were performed using R (version 4.0.4, Foundation for Statistical Computing, Vienna, Austria). A two-tailed *p*-value of less than 0.05 was considered as statistical significance.

3. Results

Table 2 shows the demographic of HCC patients in training ($n = 136$), internal validation ($n = 50$), and external testing cohorts ($n = 62$) with the mean age of 56.9, 57.9, and 57.7, respectively. 166 patients (66.9%) were in the BCLC stage B, and most of the patients ($n = 217$, 87.5%) were infected with hepatitis B. According to the mRECIST criteria, patients in OR and Non-OR groups were 82 and 166, respectively. The median follow up was 22.3 months (IQR: 10.9–28.5 months). There was no difference in distribution among training, internal validation, and external testing cohorts among all variables. For clinical variables, BCLC stage, tumor number, and tumor size were significantly associated with the OR status in the univariate analysis. Then, these three clinical factors were processed by the multivariate analysis to build the clinical model using the logistic regression model. Results showed that the BCLC stage, tumor number, and tumor size were independent risk factors (Table 3).

Figure 3 shows the cross-entropy loss was close to 0.5 and accuracy was close to 0.85 after training of 200 epochs. Performances of different models in differentiation OR and Non-OR are shown in Figure 4A and Table 4. In the external testing cohort, the AUC of the multi-DL model was higher than both single-DL-Pre and ResNet50 which only performed the OR prediction (0.871 vs. 0.858 for single-DL-Pre, $p = 0.073$ and 0.871 vs. 0.859 for ResNet50, $p = 0.065$). Additionally, AUC of multi-DL was higher than the clinical model (0.871 vs. 0.739) with a significant difference ($p < 0.01$). Figure 5 shows the confusion matrices and quantitative indices that multi-DL obtained the highest ACC of 0.839, SEN of 0.857, SPE of 0.829, PPV of 0.720 and NPV of 0.919 among single-DL-Pre (ACC of 0.790, SEN of 0.762, SPE of 0.805, PPV of 0.667 and NPV of 0.868), ResNet50 (ACC of 0.806, SEN of 0.810, SPE of 0.805, PPV of 0.680 and NPV of 0.892), and the clinical model (ACC of 0.710, SEN of 0.714, SPE of 0.707, PPV of 0.556 and NPV of 0.829) in the external testing cohort.

Table 2. Patient characteristics in the training, internal validation, and external testing cohorts.

	Training (n = 136)	Internal Validation (n = 50)	External Testing (n = 62)	p
Mean age (years)	56.9 ± 11.9	57.9 ± 10.9	57.7 ± 13.3	0.831
F/M ratio	14:122	1:49	4:58	0.221
Child–Pugh class				0.397
A	116 (85.3)	41 (82.0)	48 (77.4)	
B	22 (14.7)	9 (18.0)	14 (22.6)	
BCLC stage				0.129
A	50 (36.8)	18 (36.0)	14 (22.6)	
B	86 (63.2)	32 (64.0)	48 (77.4)	
HBV				0.730
Presence	117 (86.0)	45 (90.0)	55 (88.7)	
Absence	19 (14.0)	5 (10.0)	7 (11.3)	
ALB (g/L)	38.8 ± 4.1	38.2 ± 5.1	38.1 ± 5.8	0.589
ALT (U/mL)	65.7 ± 58.5	77.1 ± 93.8	68.8 ± 76.6	0.630
AST (U/mL)	111.4 ± 235.4	110.8 ± 89.2	125.0 ± 112.7	0.882
PT, seconds	12.2 ± 1.7	12.0 ± 1.0	12.5 ± 1.5	0.188
PLT × 10^9/L	195.1 ± 78.1	203.8 ± 90.3	205.5 ± 120.0	0.715
TBil (umol/L)	18.6 ± 24.3	16.9 ± 8.1	17.9 ± 13.5	0.869
AFP (ng/mL)				0.202
≤400	71 (52.2)	31 (62.0)	40 (64.5)	
>400	65 (47.8)	19 (38.0)	22 (35.5)	
Tumor maximum diameter (cm)	9.0 ± 3.6	9.3 ± 3.9	9.5 ± 4.4	0.652
Multiple tumors				0.098
Single	54 (39.7)	19 (40.0)	15 (24.2)	
Multiple	82 (60.3)	31 (60.0)	47 (75.8)	
Tumor response				0.773
OR	44 (32.4)	17 (34.0)	21 (33.9)	
Non-OR	92 (67.6)	33 (66.0)	41 (66.1)	

Abbreviations: HBV, hepatitis B virus; AFP, alpha fetoprotein; ALT, alanine aminotransferase; AST, aspartate aminotransferase; ALB, albumin; PT, pro-thrombin time; TBil, total bilirubin; PLT, platelet; OR, objection response.

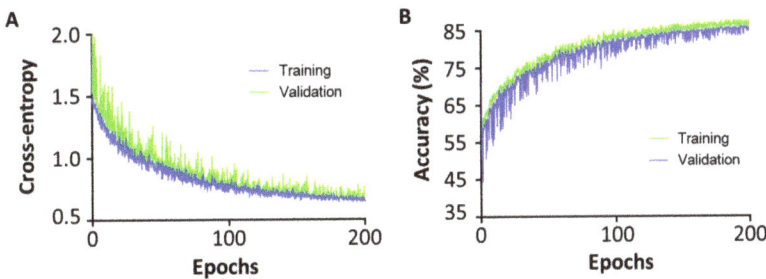

Figure 3. Training curve of multi-DL. (**A**) Cross-entropy vs. training epochs. (**B**) Accuracy vs. training epochs.

Table 3. Uni- and multivariable regression analysis of predictors of OR in the training cohort.

Clinical Variables	β	Odds Ratio (95% CI)	p Value	β	Odds Ratio (95% CI)	p Value
Mean age (years)	−0.014	0.986 (0.950–1.024)	0.470			
Sex (Female/Male)	0.142	1.152 (0.306–4.342)	0.834			
Child–Pugh class	0.139	1.150 (0.424–3.120)	0.784			
BCLC Stage (B/A)	−1.697	0.183 (0.062–0.542)	0.002 *	−1.556	0.211 (0.079–0.562)	0.002 *
HBV (Presence/Absence)	−0.587	0.556 (0.172–1.792)	0.325			
ALB (g/L)	−0.033	0.967 (0.864–1.084)	0.567			
ALT (U/mL)	−0.004	0.996 (0.987–1.004)	0.303			
AST (U/mL)	0.000	1.000 (0.996–1.003)	0.759			
PT, seconds	0.188	1.206 (0.835–1.743)	0.318			
PLT $\times 10^9$/L	0.004	1.003 (0.997–1.008)	0.371			
TBil (umol/L)	0.011	1.011 (0.981–1.041)	0.470			
AFP (>400 ng/mL/≤400 ng/mL)	−0.361	0.697 (0.297–1.634)	0.406			
Tumor maximum diameter (>5 cm/≤5 cm)	−1.399	0.247 (0.073–0.835)	0.024 *	−1.654	0.191 (0.065–0.562)	0.003 *
Multiple tumor (Single/Multiple)	1.298	3.664 (1.222–10.983)	0.020 *	1.059	2.884 (1.071–7.764)	0.036 *

* indicated $p < 0.05$.

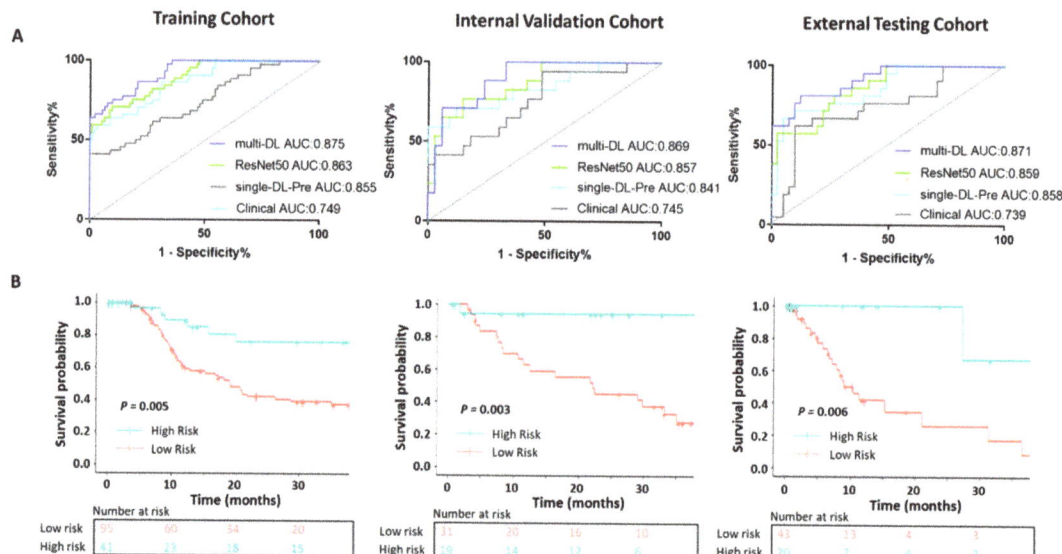

Figure 4. ROCs of OR prediction and risk stratification. (**A**) ROCs and AUCs of multi-DL, single-DL-Pre, ResNet50 and clinical model. (**B**) Survival curve of high- and low-risk patients stratified by the multi-DL model.

Table 4. Performance for multi-DL and compared methods.

Method	AUC	ACC (%)	Dice (%)
OR Prediction			
Clinical model	0.739	71.0	N/A
ResNet50 [26]	0.859	80.6	N/A
Single-DL-Pre	0.858	70.9	N/A
Tumor Segmentation			
CNN [23]	N/A	N/A	63.2
Encoder–decoder [18]	N/A	N/A	66.7
Ours			
Multi-DL	0.871	83.9	73.6

N/A: Not applicable.

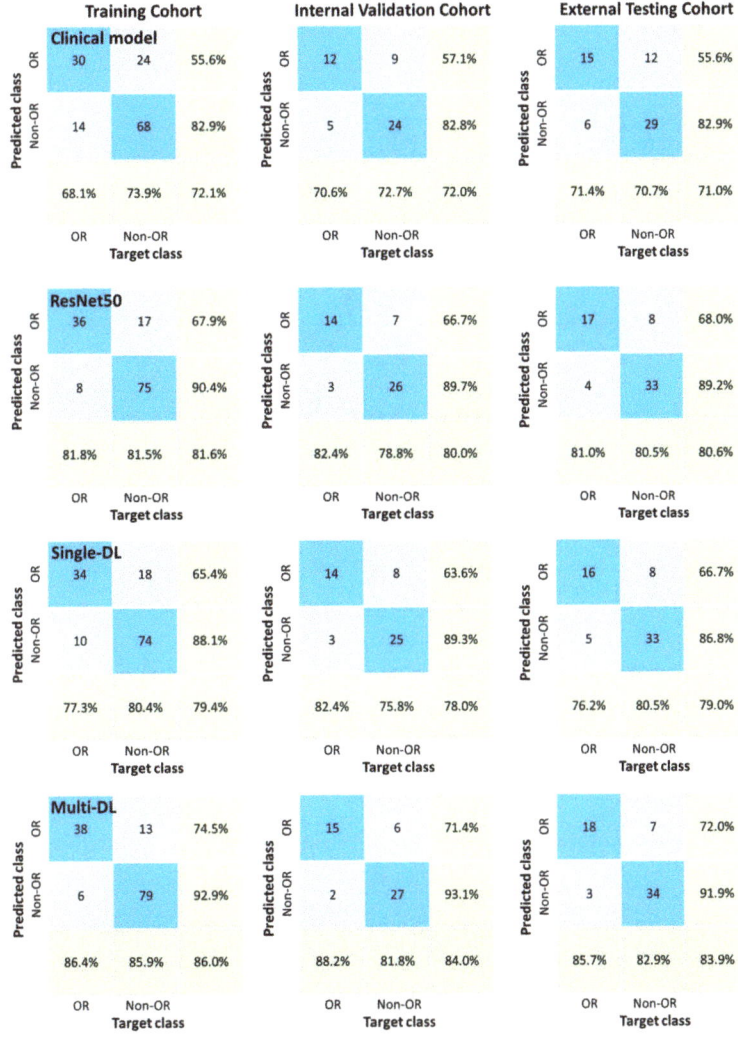

Figure 5. The confusion matrix for the clinical model, ResNet50, single-DL and multi-DL models.

The predicted OR and Non-OR patients were classified into low- and high-risk groups with the risk score threshold of 0.5. The survival curves are shown in Figure 4B. The proposed multi-DL can successfully perform the risk stratification where the low-risk and high-risk patients showed significantly different survival probability not only in training ($p = 0.005$) but also in the internal validation ($p = 0.003$) and the external testing cohort ($p = 0.006$).

Reference tumor segmentation results are shown in Figure 6. Visually, the multi-DL method can generate a more accurate lesion boundary than CNN and encoder–decoder methods. For example, in case#1, multi-DL can successfully segment the tiny hollow of the tumor while other methods failed to restore this detail. In the quantitative analysis (Table 4), the dice coefficient of the multi-DL method was significantly higher than that of encoder–decoder (73.6% vs. 66.7%, $p = 0.001$) and CNN (73.6% vs. 63.2%, $p < 0.001$), which was in accordance with the observation result. For the tumor delineation time comparison, the manual segmentation was much slower than the deep neural network processing (1.0 s/slice vs. 30.5 s/slice, $p < 0.001$) and network processing plus manual adjustment (1.0 s/slice vs. 5.2 s/slice, $p < 0.001$), which demonstrated the high efficiency of the proposed method.

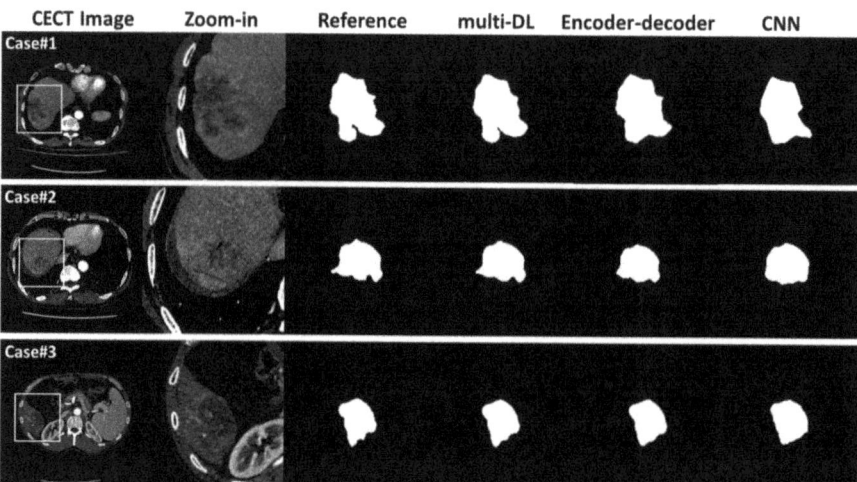

Figure 6. Tumor segmentation for three cases with reference manual segmentation, results of multi-DL, CNN, and encoder–decoder methods.

4. Discussion

In this study, a deep learning-based approach was proposed to simultaneously perform the accurate OR prediction in HCC patients with TACE treatment and automatically segment the tumor. The high performance of the proposed multi-DL method demonstrated combing two interconnected tasks (OR prediction and tumor segmentation) in a unified model could behave better than the single task.

TACE was a recommended initial treatment for HCC patients who could not receive the resection or ablation [44]. However, if patients were not appropriately selected, they could not benefit from the TACE procession, and the OS was not conferred. A previous study [45] reported that more than half of the patients had no OR to TACE. This ratio was 66.9% in our study, demonstrating the vital importance of the pre-operative prediction of OR. However, a recent study [46] reported that a restricted mean duration of response (DOR) might be a better end-point for decision-making. Still, the study only focused on two real trials with randomized phase 2 screening design, which needed further validations. Therefore, we chose OR as the end point to perform the prediction, considering the value of OR has already been demonstrated for clinical decision-making in routine practice and clinical trials [47].

Researchers have conducted relevant studies which adopted machine learning to predict OR after TACE. Abajian et al. used a supervised machine-learning method to predict the response to TACE and achieved an accuracy of 78%. Mähringer-Kunz et al. applied the CNN model to perform the survival prediction after TACE, and an accuracy of 77% was obtained. We extended the existing OR prediction framework based on previous studies by adding the tumor segmentation to form a unified model. In the proposed network, the encoder extracted and fused the inputted information to generate the latent feature, which was shared by the prediction and segmentation pathway. Therefore, the network may focus more on the tumor region and extract more cancer-related information when the network performed the OR prediction. Thus, multi-DL obtained higher accuracy in OR prediction (0.839) than ResNet50 (0.806) and the clinical model (0.710). Peng et al. recently used ResNet50 to predict OR after TACE on a large dataset including 789 patients and obtained a higher AUC of 0.97, which was higher than ResNet50 in our study (0.86). We inferred there were two reasons. Firstly, 562 patients' data were used for training in Peng's work, while only 136 patients' data were used in our study. Large-scale training data can help the neural network learn more different features, so better results were obtained. Secondly, all CT images were reconstructed using a medium sharp reconstruction algorithm with a thickness of 1 mm in Peng's study. However, in our research, CT images were collected from picture archiving and communication system (PACS) with DICOM format. They were reconstructed using different algorithms provided by different CT vendors and had different resolutions and thicknesses. Though the image pre-processing was performed in our study, CT images also had variations. Therefore, the neural network in Peng's work may learn a relatively simple task while our model had to face a more complex condition, in which the performance of the model was degraded.

The multi-task learning brought another advantage: the automatic segmentation of the tumor. The dice of tumor segmentation of the multi-DL model was higher than compared methods (73.6% vs. 63.2% for CNN and 66.7% for encoder–decoder model) and showed comparable results to those of other studies. Budak et al. adopted a cascaded convolutional encoder–decoder neural network for tumor segmentation, which achieved the dice coefficient of 64.3% [18]. Adding the attention mechanism to U-Net, AHCNet obtained the dice of 0.734 for liver tumor segmentation on CT images [48]. Chlebus et al. proposed a fully convolutional neural network with object-based postprocessing for tumor segmentation and had dice value of 0.72 [20]. In this study, the multi-DL model encoder was used to extract and fuse the inputted information to generate the latent feature, which was shared by the prediction and segmentation pathway. Then, when the segmentation pathway processed the latent feature, the OR-related tumor characteristics such as tumor size, shape, and location may also benefit tumor segmentation, thus leading to higher performance than other compared methods. However, some works were reporting higher dice values for tumor segmentation. For example, Duc et al. proposed a 3D full resolution U-Net model for liver tumor detection and segmentation, which achieved dice of 0.81 in the test set. Due to the limitation of computation resources and training data, we adopted a 2D network in our study. Therefore, the spatial context information cannot be utilized, leading to degraded performance. In the future, we will explore the 2.5D network to use the inter-slice information but with less memory assumption [49].

Another point worth discussing was the efficiency of the proposed model. Since one HCC patient may have dozens of slices containing the tumor, radiologists had to manually delineate many CT images to perform the disease evaluation or surgery planning. Therefore, $6\times$ or $30\times$ of time reduction (30 s to 5 s or 30 s to 1 s) may significantly improve the efficiency in practice. With this deep-learning algorithm or intelligent software, interventional radiotherapy procedures can be optimized to reduce the radiation exposure of patients and interventional radiologists [50]. Additionally, multi-DL had few network parameters (~1.7 M) compared with ResNet50 (~27 M). Training the neural model with many parameters was expensive, requiring more computation resources and training data. From this perspective, our method had better ease of use because it can be transferred to other medical centers where the researchers can build their own clinical solutions using data of a regular size.

There remained some limitations in this study. First, the nature of the retrospective study may bring bias into the model construction, and a large prospective study with a longer follow-up period should be conducted. Second, only 2D images were processed by the neural network, while the spatial context information was not well utilized in our study [51]. Last but not least, the doxorubicin-loaded drug-eluting beads TACE (DEB-TACE) was widely used, and it was more cost-effective than the traditional TACE treatment [52]. Though we have already applied DEB-TACE in these two medical centers, the number of patients under this treatment was relatively small. In the future, we will include more patients with DEB-TACE to validate further the robustness and effectiveness of our proposed multi-DL method.

In conclusion, we developed and validated a multi-task deep learning approach for OR prediction and tumor segmentation in HCC patients with TACE treatment, backed by internal and external testing from multiple-center datasets. The high performance of the proposed method demonstrated that combing these two interconnected tasks in a unified model could behave better than other compared methods. Furthermore, the proposed model can successfully stratify the survival risk of HCC patients and may provide a useful tool of therapeutic regime selection in clinical practice.

Supplementary Materials: The following supporting information can be downloaded at: https://www.mdpi.com/article/10.3390/jpm12020248/s1, Note S1: CECT Imaging Protocols.

Author Contributions: Conceptualization, H.C. and X.L.; Data curation, C.A.; Formal analysis, Y.L. and Z.X.; Funding acquisition, H.C.; Investigation, Y.L. and Z.X.; Methodology, Y.L. and Z.X.; Software, Y.L. and Z.X.; Supervision, H.C. and X.L.; Validation, C.A.; Writing—original draft, Y.L. and Z.X.; Writing—review and editing, C.A., H.C. and X.L. All authors have read and agreed to the published version of the manuscript.

Funding: This research was funded by Beijing Municipal Natural Science Foundation, grant number Z190024, National Natural Science Foundation of China, grant number 81930119 and 81627803.

Institutional Review Board Statement: The study was conducted in accordance with the Declaration of Helsinki and approved by the Institutional Review Board of Tsinghua University (protocol code: 20210130 and date of approval: 8 November 2021).

Informed Consent Statement: Patient consent was waived due to the retrospective nature of this study.

Data Availability Statement: The datasets used during the current study are available from the corresponding author on reasonable request.

Conflicts of Interest: The authors declare no conflict of interest.

References

1. Bray, F.; Ferlay, J.; Soerjomataram, I.; Siegel, R.L.; Torre, L.A.; Jemal, A. Global cancer statistics 2018: GLOBOCAN estimates of incidence and mortality worldwide for 36 cancers in 185 countries. *CA Cancer J. Clin.* **2018**, *68*, 394–424. [CrossRef] [PubMed]
2. Omata, M.; Cheng, A.-L.; Kokudo, N.; Kudo, M.; Lee, J.M.; Jia, J.; Tateishi, R.; Han, K.-H.; Chawla, Y.K.; Shiina, S.; et al. Asia–Pacific clinical practice guidelines on the management of hepatocellular carcinoma: A 2017 update. *Hepatol. Int.* **2017**, *11*, 317–370. [CrossRef] [PubMed]
3. Miller, K.D.; Nogueira, L.; Mariotto, A.B.; Rowland, J.H.; Yabroff, K.R.; Alfano, C.M.; Jemal, A.; Kramer, J.L.; Siegel, R.L. Cancer treatment and survivorship statistics, 2019. *CA Cancer J. Clin.* **2019**, *69*, 363–385. [CrossRef] [PubMed]
4. Miller, K.D.; Goding Sauer, A.; Ortiz, A.P.; Fedewa, S.A.; Pinheiro, P.S.; Tortolero-Luna, G.; Martinez-Tyson, D.; Jemal, A.; Siegel, R.L.J. Cancer statistics for hispanics/latinos, 2018. *CA Cancer J. Clin.* **2018**, *68*, 425–445. [CrossRef] [PubMed]
5. Kanwal, F.; Befeler, A.; Chari, R.S.; Marrero, J.; Kahn, J.; Afdhal, N.; Morgan, T.; Roberts, L.; Mohanty, S.R.; Schwartz, J.; et al. Potentially curative treatment in patients with hepatocellular cancer-results from the liver cancer research network. *Aliment. Pharmacol. Ther.* **2012**, *36*, 257–265. [CrossRef] [PubMed]
6. Cai, X. Laparoscopic liver resection: The current status and the future. *Hepatobiliary Surg. Nutr.* **2018**, *7*, 98–104. [CrossRef] [PubMed]

7. Kohles, N.; Nagel, D.; Jüngst, D.; Durner, J.; Stieber, P.; Holdenrieder, S. Prognostic relevance of oncological serum biomarkers in liver cancer patients undergoing transarterial chemoembolization therapy. *Tumor Biol.* **2012**, *33*, 33–40. [CrossRef] [PubMed]
8. Llovet, J.M.; Real, M.I.; Montaña, X.; Planas, R.; Coll, S.; Aponte, J.; Ayuso, C.; Sala, M.; Muchart, J.; Solà, R.; et al. Arterial embolisation or chemoembolisation versus symptomatic treatment in patients with unresectable hepatocellular carcinoma: A randomised controlled trial. *Lancet* **2002**, *359*, 1734–1739. [CrossRef]
9. Schulz, M.; Boix, A.S.; Niesel, K.; Alekseeva, T.; Sevenich, L. Microenvironmental Regulation of Tumor Progression and Therapeutic Response in Brain Metastasis. *Front. Immunol.* **2019**, *10*, 1713. [CrossRef]
10. Wei, X.; Zhao, L.; Ren, R.; Ji, F.; Xue, S.; Zhang, J.; Liu, Z.; Ma, Z.; Wang, X.W.; Wong, L.; et al. MiR-125b Loss Activated HIF1α/pAKT Loop, Leading to Transarterial Chemoembolization Resistance in Hepatocellular Carcinoma. *Hepatology* **2021**, *73*, 1381–1398. [CrossRef]
11. Sieghart, W.; Hucke, F.; Pinter, M.; Graziadei, I.; Vogel, W.; Müller, C.; Heinzl, H.; Trauner, M.; Peck-Radosavljevic, M. The ART of decision making: Retreatment with transarterial chemoembolization in patients with hepatocellular carcinoma. *Hepatology* **2013**, *57*, 2261–2273. [CrossRef] [PubMed]
12. Hucke, F.; Pinter, M.; Graziadei, I.; Bota, S.; Vogel, W.; Müller, C.; Heinzl, H.; Waneck, F.; Trauner, M.; Peck-Radosavljevic, M.; et al. How to STATE suitability and START transarterial chemoembolization in patients with intermediate stage hepatocellular carcinoma. *J. Hepatol.* **2014**, *61*, 1287–1296. [CrossRef] [PubMed]
13. Granito, A.; Facciorusso, A.; Sacco, R.; Bartalena, L.; Mosconi, C.; Cea, U.V.; Cappelli, A.; Antonino, M.; Modestino, F.; Brandi, N. TRANS-TACE: Prognostic role of the transient hypertransaminasemia after conventional chemoembolization for hepato-cellular carcinoma. *J. Pers. Med.* **2021**, *11*, 1041. [CrossRef] [PubMed]
14. Guo, Z.; Zhong, N.; Xu, X.; Zhang, Y.; Luo, X.; Zhu, H.; Zhang, X.; Wu, D.; Qiu, Y.; Tu, F. Prediction of Hepatocellular Carcinoma Response to Transcatheter Arterial Chemoembolization: A Real-World Study Based on Non-Contrast Computed Tomography Radiomics and General Image Features. *J. Hepatocell. Carcinoma* **2021**, *8*, 773. [CrossRef] [PubMed]
15. Kong, C.; Zhao, Z.; Chen, W.; Lv, X.; Shu, G.; Ye, M.; Song, J.; Ying, X.; Weng, Q.; Weng, W.; et al. Prediction of tumor response via a pretreatment MRI radiomics-based nomogram in HCC treated with TACE. *Eur. Radiol.* **2021**, *31*, 7500–7511. [CrossRef] [PubMed]
16. Niu, X.-K.; He, X.-F. Development of a computed tomography-based radiomics nomogram for prediction of transarterial chemoembolization refractoriness in hepatocellular carcinoma. *World J. Gastroenterol.* **2021**, *27*, 189–207. [CrossRef]
17. Topol, E.J. High-performance medicine: The convergence of human and artificial intelligence. *Nat. Med.* **2019**, *25*, 44–56. [CrossRef]
18. Budak, U.; Guo, Y.; Tanyildizi, E.; Şengür, A. Cascaded deep convolutional encoder-decoder neural networks for efficient liver tumor segmentation. *Med. Hypotheses* **2020**, *134*, 109431. [CrossRef]
19. AlMotairi, S.; Kareem, G.; Aouf, M.; Almutairi, B.; Salem, M.A.-M. Liver Tumor Segmentation in CT Scans Using Modified SegNet. *Sensors* **2020**, *20*, 1516. [CrossRef]
20. Chlebus, G.; Schenk, A.; Moltz, J.H.; Van Ginneken, B.; Hahn, H.K.; Meine, H. Automatic liver tumor segmentation in CT with fully convolutional neural networks and object-based postprocessing. *Sci. Rep.* **2018**, *8*, 15497. [CrossRef]
21. Yuan, Y. Hierarchical convolutional-deconvolutional neural networks for automatic liver and tumor segmentation. *arXiv* **2017**, arXiv:171004540.
22. Tummala, B.M.; Barpanda, S.S. Liver tumor segmentation from computed tomography images using multiscale residual dilated encoder-decoder network. *Int. J. Imaging Syst. Technol.* **2021**. [CrossRef]
23. Li, W. Automatic segmentation of liver tumor in CT images with deep convolutional neural networks. *J. Comput. Commun.* **2015**, *3*, 146. [CrossRef]
24. Liu, D.; Liu, F.; Xie, X.; Su, L.; Liu, M.; Xie, X.; Kuang, M.; Huang, G.; Wang, Y.; Zhou, H. Accurate prediction of responses to transarterial chemoembolization for patients with hepatocellular carcinoma by using artificial intelligence in contrast-enhanced ultra-sound. *Eur. Radiol.* **2020**, *30*, 2365–2376. [CrossRef] [PubMed]
25. Zhang, L.; Xia, W.; Yan, Z.-P.; Sun, J.-H.; Zhong, B.-Y.; Hou, Z.-H.; Yang, M.-J.; Zhou, G.-H.; Wang, W.-S.; Zhao, X.-Y.; et al. Deep Learning Predicts Overall Survival of Patients with Unresectable Hepatocellular Carcinoma Treated by Transarterial Chemoembolization Plus Sorafenib. *Front. Oncol.* **2020**, *10*, 2128. [CrossRef]
26. Peng, J.; Kang, S.; Ning, Z.; Deng, H.; Shen, J.; Xu, Y.; Zhang, J.; Zhao, W.; Li, X.; Gong, W.; et al. Residual convolutional neural network for predicting response of transarterial chemoembolization in hepatocellular carcinoma from CT imaging. *Eur. Radiol.* **2020**, *30*, 413–424. [CrossRef]
27. Morshid, A.; Elsayes, K.M.; Khalaf, A.M.; Elmohr, M.M.; Yu, J.; Kaseb, A.O.; Hassan, M.; Mahvash, A.; Wang, Z.; Hazle, J.D.; et al. A Machine Learning Model to Predict Hepatocellular Carcinoma Response to Transcatheter Arterial Chemoembolization. *Radiol. Artif. Intell.* **2019**, *1*, e180021. [CrossRef]
28. Abajian, A.; Murali, N.; Savic, L.J.; Laage-Gaupp, F.M.; Nezami, N.; Duncan, J.S.; Schlachter, T.; Lin, M.; Geschwind, J.-F.; Chapiro, J. Predicting treatment response to image-guided therapies using machine learning: An example for trans-arterial treatment of hepatocellular carcinoma. *JoVE* **2018**, *140*, e58382. [CrossRef]
29. Mähringer-Kunz, A.; Wagner, F.; Hahn, F.; Weinmann, A.; Brodehl, S.; Schotten, S.; Hinrichs, J.B.; Düber, C.; Galle, P.R.; Dos Santos, D.P.; et al. Predicting survival after transarterial chemoembolization for hepatocellular carcinoma using a neural network: A Pilot Study. *Liver Int.* **2020**, *40*, 694–703. [CrossRef] [PubMed]

30. Golfieri, R.; Garzillo, G.; Ascanio, S.; Renzulli, M. Focal Lesions in the Cirrhotic Liver: Their Pivotal Role in Gadoxetic Acid Enhanced MRI and Recognition by the Western Guidelines. *Dig. Dis.* **2014**, *32*, 696–704. [CrossRef] [PubMed]
31. An, C.; Zuo, M.; Li, W.; Chen, Q.; Wu, P. Infiltrative Hepatocellular Carcinoma: Transcatheter Arterial Chemoembolization Versus Hepatic Arterial Infusion Chemotherapy. *Front. Oncol.* **2021**, *11*, 747496. [CrossRef] [PubMed]
32. Huang, Z.M.; Zuo, M.X.; Gu, Y.K.; Gu, H.F.; Lai, C.X.; Zhang, T.Q.; Wang, X.C.; An, C.; Huang, J.H. Computed tomography-guided radiofrequency ablation combined with transarterial embolization assisted by a three-dimensional visualization ablation planning system for hepatocellular carcinoma in challenging locations: A preliminary study. *Abdom. Radiol.* **2020**, *45*, 1181–1192 [CrossRef] [PubMed]
33. Tovoli, F.; Renzulli, M.; Negrini, G.; Brocchi, S.; Ferrarini, A.; Andreone, A.; Benevento, F.; Golfieri, R.; Morselli-Labate, A.M.; Mastroroberto, M.; et al. Inter-operator variability and source of errors in tumour response assessment for hepatocellular carcinoma treated with sorafenib. *Eur. Radiol.* **2018**, *28*, 3611–3620. [CrossRef] [PubMed]
34. Lencioni, R.; Llovet, J.M. *Modified RECIST (mRECIST) Assessment for Hepatocellular Carcinoma*; Thieme Medical Publishers: New York, NY, USA, 2010; Volume 30, pp. 52–60. [CrossRef]
35. Kim, B.K.; Kim, S.U.; Kim, K.A.; Chung, Y.E.; Kim, M.-J.; Park, M.-S.; Park, J.Y.; Kim, D.Y.; Ahn, S.H.; Kim, M.D.; et al. Complete response at first chemoembolization is still the most robust predictor for favorable outcome in hepatocellular carcinoma. *J. Hepatol.* **2015**, *62*, 1304–1310. [CrossRef] [PubMed]
36. Olivier, R.; Cao, H. Nearest neighbor value interpolation. *Int. J. Adv. Comput. Sci. Appl.* **2012**, *3*, 25–30. [CrossRef]
37. Isensee, F.; Jaeger, P.F.; Kohl, S.A.A.; Petersen, J.; Maier-Hein, K.H. nnU-Net: A self-configuring method for deep learning-based biomedical image segmentation. *Nat. Methods* **2021**, *18*, 203–211. [CrossRef]
38. Yasrab, R.; Gu, N.; Zhang, X. An Encoder-Decoder Based Convolution Neural Network (CNN) for Future Advanced Driver Assistance System (ADAS). *Appl. Sci.* **2017**, *7*, 312. [CrossRef]
39. Ronneberger, O.; Fischer, P.; Brox, T. U-net: Convolutional Networks for Biomedical Image Segmentation. In *International Conference on Medical Image Computing and Computer-Assisted Intervention*; Springer: Cham, Switzerland, 2015; pp. 234–241.
40. Milletari, F.; Navab, N.; Ahmadi, S.-A. V-net: Fully convolutional neural networks for volumetric medical image segmentation. In Proceedings of the 2016 Fourth International Conference on 3D Vision (3DV), Stanford, CA, USA, 25–28 October 2016; pp. 565–571.
41. Kingma, D.P.; Ba, J. Adam: A method for stochastic optimization. *arXiv* **2014**, arXiv:14126980.
42. Zhao, Y.; Wang, N.; Wu, J.; Zhang, Q.; Lin, T.; Yao, Y.; Chen, Z.; Wang, M.; Sheng, L.; Liu, J.; et al. Radiomics Analysis Based on Contrast-Enhanced MRI for Prediction of Therapeutic Response to Transarterial Chemoembolization in Hepatocellular Carcinoma. *Front. Oncol.* **2021**. [CrossRef]
43. Ruopp, M.D.; Perkins, N.J.; Whitcomb, B.W.; Schisterman, E.F. Youden Index and Optimal Cut-Point Estimated from Observations Affected by a Lower Limit of Detection. *J. Math. Methods Biosci.* **2008**, *50*, 419–430. [CrossRef]
44. Park, J.; Chen, M.; Colombo, M.; Roberts, L.; Schwartz, M.; Chen, P.-J.; Kudo, M.; Johnson, P.; Wagner, S.; Orsini, L.S.; et al. Global patterns of hepatocellular carcinoma management from diagnosis to death: The BRIDGE Study. *Liver Int.* **2015**, *35*, 2155–2166. [CrossRef] [PubMed]
45. Bruix, J.; Sala, M.; Llovet, J.M. Chemoembolization for hepatocellular carcinoma. *Gastroenterology* **2004**, *127*, S179–S188. [CrossRef] [PubMed]
46. Hu, C.; Wang, M.; Wu, C.; Zhou, H.; Chen, C.; Diede, S. Comparison of Duration of Response vs Conventional Response Rates and Progression-Free Survival as Efficacy End Points in Simulated Immuno-oncology Clinical Trials. *JAMA Netw. Open* **2021**, *4*, e218175. [CrossRef] [PubMed]
47. Aykan, N.F.; Özatlı, T. Objective response rate assessment in oncology: Current situation and future expectations. *World J. Clin. Oncol.* **2020**, *11*, 53–73. [CrossRef] [PubMed]
48. Jiang, H.; Shi, T.; Bai, Z.; Huang, L. Ahcnet: An application of attention mechanism and hybrid connection for liver tumor seg-mentation in ct volumes. *IEEE Access* **2019**, *7*, 24898–24909. [CrossRef]
49. Yun, J.; Park, J.; Yu, D.; Yi, J.; Lee, M.; Park, H.J.; Lee, J.-G.; Seo, J.B.; Kim, N. Improvement of fully automated airway segmentation on volumetric computed tomographic images using a 2.5 dimensional convolutional neural net. *Med. Image Anal.* **2019**, *51*, 13–20. [CrossRef] [PubMed]
50. Compagnone, G.; Giampalma, E.; Domenichelli, S.; Renzulli, M.; Golfieri, R. Calculation of conversion factors for effective dose for various interventional radiology procedures. *Med. Phys.* **2012**, *39*, 2491–2498. [CrossRef]
51. Chang, P.; Kuoy, E.; Grinband, J.; Weinberg, B.; Thompson, M.; Homo, R.; Chen, J.; Abcede, H.; Shafie, M.; Sugrue, L.; et al. Hybrid 3D/2D Convolutional Neural Network for Hemorrhage Evaluation on Head CT. *Am. J. Neuroradiol.* **2018**, *39*, 1609–1616. [CrossRef]
52. Cucchetti, A.; Trevisani, F.; Cappelli, A.; Mosconi, C.; Renzulli, M.; Pinna, A.D.; Golfieri, R. Cost-effectiveness of doxorubicin-eluting beads versus conventional trans-arterial chemo-embolization for hepatocellular carcinoma. *Dig. Liver Dis.* **2016**, *48*, 798–805. [CrossRef]

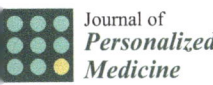

Article

Machine Learning Prediction of Visual Outcome after Surgical Decompression of Sellar Region Tumors

Nidan Qiao [1,2,3,†], Yichen Ma [4,†], Xiaochen Chen [5,†], Zhao Ye [1,2,3,6,7], Hongying Ye [8], Zhaoyun Zhang [8], Yongfei Wang [1,2,3,6,7], Zhaozeng Lu [9], Zhiliang Wang [9], Yiqin Xiao [9,*] and Yao Zhao [1,2,3,6,7,*]

1. Department of Neurosurgery, Huashan Hospital, Shanghai 200040, China; norikaisa@gmail.com (N.Q.); yezhaozj663812@126.com (Z.Y.); eamns@hotmail.com (Y.W.)
2. Neurosurgical Institute, Fudan University, Shanghai 200040, China
3. National Center for Neurological Disorders, 985 Jinguang Road, Shanghai 201107, China
4. Fudan University Graduate School, Fudan University, Shanghai 200043, China; yichenma@126.com
5. Surgical Theatre, Huashan Hospital Hongqiao Campus, Shanghai 201107, China; wonderful1211@163.com
6. Shanghai Clinical Medical Center of Neurosurgery, Shanghai 200040, China
7. Shanghai Key Laboratory of Medical Brain Function and Restoration and Neural Regeneration, Fudan University, Shanghai 200040, China
8. Department of Endocrinology, Huashan Hospital, Shanghai 200040, China; janeyhy@163.com (H.Y.); zhaoyunzhang@fudan.edu.cn (Z.Z.)
9. Department of Ophthalmology, Huashan Hospital, 12 Wulumuqi Zhong Road, Shanghai 200040, China; zzlu@fudan.edu.cn (Z.L.); zhlwang@fudan.edu.cn (Z.W.)
* Correspondence: xiaoyiqin@huashan.org.cn (Y.X.); zhaoyaohs@vip.sina.com (Y.Z.)
† These authors contributed equally to the manuscript.

Abstract: Introduction: This study aims to develop a machine learning-based model integrating clinical and ophthalmic features to predict visual outcomes after transsphenoidal resection of sellar region tumors. Methods: Adult patients with optic chiasm compression by a sellar region tumor were examined to develop a model, and an independent retrospective cohort and a prospective cohort were used to validate our model. Predictors included demographic information, and ophthalmic and laboratory test results. We defined "recovery" as more than 5% for a *p*-value in mean deviation compared with the general population in the follow-up. Seven machine learning classifiers were employed, and the best-performing algorithm was selected. A decision curve analysis was used to assess the clinical usefulness of our model by estimating net benefit. We developed a nomogram based on essential features ranked by the SHAP score. Results: We included 159 patients (57.2% male), and the mean age was 42.3 years old. Among them, 96 patients were craniopharyngiomas and 63 patients were pituitary adenomas. Larger tumors (3.3 cm vs. 2.8 cm in tumor height) and craniopharyngiomas (73.6%) were associated with a worse prognosis ($p < 0.001$). Eyes with better outcomes were those with better visual field and thicker ganglion cell layer before operation. The ensemble model yielded the highest AUC of 0.911 [95% CI, 0.885–0.938], and the corresponding accuracy was 84.3%, with 0.863 in sensitivity and 0.820 in specificity. The model yielded AUCs of 0.861 and 0.843 in the two validation cohorts. Our model provided greater net benefit than the competing extremes of intervening in all or no patients in the decision curve analysis. A model explanation using SHAP score demonstrated that visual field, ganglion cell layer, tumor height, total thyroxine, and diagnosis were the most important features in predicting visual outcome. Conclusion: SHAP score can be a valuable resource for healthcare professionals in identifying patients with a higher risk of persistent visual deficit. The large-scale and prospective application of the proposed model would strengthen its clinical utility and universal applicability in practice.

Keywords: pituitary adenoma; craniopharyngioma; optic chiasm; multicenter

1. Introduction

Pituitary adenomas (PAs) and craniopharyngiomas (CPs) are the most common brain tumors in the sellar region [1,2]. Patients complain of blurred vision when the tumor grows beyond the sella and compresses the optic chiasm. Optic nerve decompression by surgical removal of the lesion may result in visual function normalization in some patients but not in others [3–6].

The risks associated with persistent visual dysfunction include severe visual field defects, thin retinal nerve fiber layers, and pituitary macroadenomas. Careful evaluation of these risks plays a fundamental role in the clinical management of these patients. The identification of patients at high risk for persistent visual loss may be helpful as patients could be referred to further visual rehabilitation [7,8] as soon as possible after surgery. Moreover, it might serve as a cost-effective and straightforward means for preoperative patient–doctor communication.

Small sample sizes, unquantified outcomes, and partial predictors constitute the limitations of previous attempts to search for risk factors that predict for visual recovery after surgery [9–19]. However, the overall accuracy of these scores, along with their generalizability to external cohorts, remains modest, representing an unmet need for individualized patient management strategies.

From a clinical standpoint, the poor performance of existing risk scores might be related to insufficient predictive factors. Machine learning methods might overcome some of the limitations of current analytical approaches to risk prediction by applying computer algorithms to large datasets with numerous, multidimensional variables, capturing high-dimensional, non-linear relationships among clinical features to make data-driven outcome predictions. The effectiveness of this approach has been shown in several applications of sellar region tumors, where machine learning was superior in validating traditional risk stratification tools, including prediction endocrine remission after surgical or radio surgical treatment of acromegaly [20,21]. Thus, we sought to develop a machine learning-based model (Prediction of Visual Outcome in Sellar Tumors, PREVOST) integrating clinical and ophthalmic features to predict visual outcomes after transsphenoidal resection of sellar region tumors.

2. Methods

2.1. Data Sources

To develop our machine learning models, we used a derivation cohort of 159 adult patients ($\geq$18 years) with optic chiasm compression by a sellar region tumor with at least one year of follow-up. All of the patients suffered a visual field defect before surgery and were treated by transsphenoidal tumor resection and optic decompression in the Gold Pituitary Joint Unit (GPJU) between January 2019 to January 2021. The GPJU is a newly established unit that started in 2019 where patients with sellar region tumors are co-managed by a multidisciplinary team, including neurosurgeons, endocrinologists, and ophthalmologists. We excluded patients who were subtotally resected or patients who suffered a post-operation hemorrhage and needed an early emergent surgery. To test the generatability of our model, we used another retrospective cohort from Neurosurgical Institute of Fudan University (FNI), where surgeries and ophthalmic assessments were performed by different groups, to independently validate our model. We further validated our model in a prospective cohort admitted to GPJU from January 2021 to June 2021. Informed consent was obtained from patients at the time the data were collected. Predictors were assessed before surgery, and the outcome was assessed at follow-up. Institutional Review Board from both centers provided ethical approval. The overall study design is depicted in Figure 1.

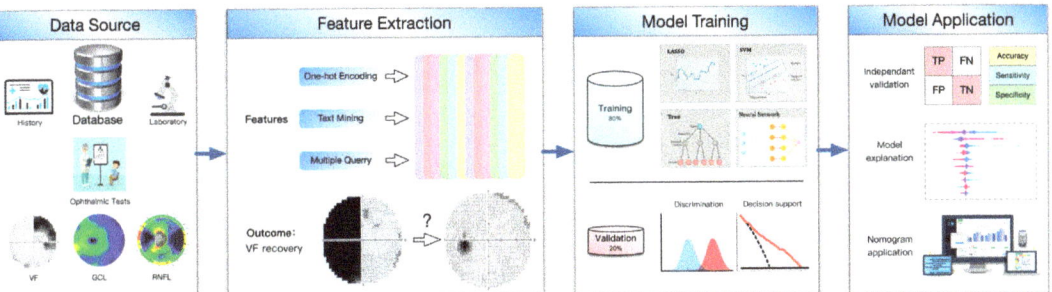

Figure 1. Overall study design.

2.2. Ophthalmic Examinations

Patients underwent a thorough ophthalmic examination by experienced ophthalmologists, including pupil, anterior, and posterior segment examination. Patients with other ocular diseases were excluded. Static automated perimetry was performed using the Humphrey 750 Visual Field Analyzer (Zeiss-Humphrey Systems, Dublin, CA, USA) and a central 30-2 threshold protocol. Fixation loss less than 20%, false-positive error less than 20%, and false-negative error less than 20% were ensured for a validated visual field. We documented the mean deviation (MD), pattern standard deviation (PSD), visual field index (VFI) on the report. The retinal nerve fiber layer (RNFL) thickness and ganglion cell layer (GCL) thickness were assessed by RTVue (Optovue, Fremont, CA, USA) using three-dimensional disc and optic nerve head (ONH) protocols.

2.3. Predictor Variables

Predictors were included based on a balance of clinical knowledge, past research, and likely clinical usefulness. The baseline model comprised visual acuity, MD (decibel, db), PSD (db), VFI (%), RNFL (μm), and GCL (μm). The full model comprised age (years), gender (female or male), BMI (kg/m^2), hypertension (yes or no), diabetes mellitus (yes or no), tumor height on MRI (cm), diagnosis (pituitary adenoma or craniopharyngioma), hemoglobin (g/L), red blood cell (1012/L), white blood cell (109/L), sodium (mmol/L), albumin (g/L), creatinine (μmol/L), ACTH (pg/mL), cortisol (μg/dL), prolactin (ng/mL), free thyroxine (pmol/L), and total thyroxine (nmol/L).

2.4. Outcome

Ophthalmic recovery after surgical decompression was categorized as a binary outcome according to the 3 to 6 month follow-up (static automated perimetry). Mean deviation in the follow-up visual field was compared with data from the general population (built-in data in the Humphrey 750 Visual Field Analyzer), and a *p*-value was calculated automatically. If the *p*-value was more than 0.05, we defined the outcome as "recovery"; otherwise, we defined the outcome as "not recovery".

2.5. Model Training

We used multiple imputations using chained equations for missing data. Seven machine learning classifiers—linear absolute shrinkage and selection operator, support vector machine, linear discriminant analysis, random forest, gradient boosting, neural network, and ensemble model—were employed to generate seven models for the prediction. The internal performance was assessed by fivefold cross-validation, by which the dataset was randomly divided into five even groups and evaluation was performed on one group at a time using the model built on the remaining 80% of the data. Model performance was assessed by the mean area under the receiver operating characteristic curve (AUC), and the best-performing algorithm was selected. The final algorithm was validated on the two validation cohorts.

2.6. Calibration

The calibration of the model was assessed graphically with calibration plots. We also recorded the Brier score, an overall measure of algorithm calibration (scores > 0.25 generally indicating a poor model).

2.7. Decision Curve Analysis

A decision curve analysis was used to assess the clinical usefulness of our model by estimating net benefit [22]. The net benefit is a metric of true positives minus false positives at a given risk threshold. The risk threshold is the amount of tolerable risk before an intervention is deemed necessary (0.5 in our case). In clinical practice, patients at high risk of not recovering were likely refered to visual rehabilitation as soon as possible after surgery. We drew a decision curve plot to visualize the net benefit of our model over varying risk thresholds compared with intervening in all patients or intervening in no patients. Classical decision theory proposes that the choice with the greatest net benefit at a chosen risk threshold should be preferred.

2.8. Feature Importance

To determine the major predictors of outcome, the importance of each feature was measured from the final model. We used the SHAP (Shapley additive explanations) score, a game-theoretic approach to explain the output of any machine learning model [23]. It measures features contributing to pushing the model output from the base value (the average model output over the training dataset we passed) to the model output.

2.9. Visual Representation

We developed a nomogram, which allows for an interactive exploration of the effect of risk factors and their combinations on the visual outcome according to their PREVOST score. The choice of variables for nomograms was based on essential features ranked by the SHAP score.

2.10. Statistical Analysis

Continuous variables with normal distribution were described as mean and standard deviation. Continuous variables with non-normal distribution were described as a median and a range. Categorical variables were described as counts and proportions. We used the linear mixed-effect models for the comparison with the control to account for intra-eye correlation. All statistical analyses were completed with R software version 3.4.2 (R Foundation for Statistical Computing, Vienna, Austria).

3. Results

The training cohort included 159 patients (91 male, 57.2%, Table 1). The mean age was 42.3 years old, and tumor volume was 9.4 (5.0–15.3) cm^3. We included 96 patients with craniopharyngioma and 63 patients with pituitary adenoma in the analysis. Among the patients with pituitary adenoma, their pathologies [24] consisted of 33 gonadotroph adenomas, 13 corticotroph adenomas, 8 somatotroph adenomas, 6 lactotroph adenomas, 2 null cell adenomas, and 1 plurihormonal PIT-1 positive adenoma. High-risk adenomas included 13 silent corticotroph adenomas, 4 lactotroph adenomas in men, 3 sparsely granulated somatotroph adenomas, and 1 plurihormonal PIT-1-positive adenoma. In total, 318 eyes were included, 172 (54.1%) eyes out of 318 eyes recovered during early follow-up. The median change in mean deviation after surgery was 40.6% compared with pre-operation. Larger tumors (3.3 cm vs. 2.8 cm in tumor height, $p < 0.001$) were associated with worse prognosis than smaller tumors, and 73.6% of the eyes unrecovered were from patients with craniopharyngiomas compared with only 26.4% of the eyes unrecovered being from patients with PAs ($p < 0.001$). The laboratory test results were similar between recovered and unrecovered eyes. Eyes with better outcomes were those with shorter disease duration (6.0 months vs. 12.0 months, $p = 0.002$), better MD (-5.0 db vs. -14.6 db, $p < 0.001$), better PSD (4.3 db vs. 11.2 db, $p < 0.001$), and thicker GCL (60.5 μm vs. 56.6 μm, $p < 0.001$) before operation. Figure 2 shows the correlation between visual severity, duration of symptoms, and size of the tumor.

Table 1. Overall characteristics of the cohort.

	Overall N = 159	Unrecovered Eyes N = 146	Recovered Eyes N = 172	p
Gender (male)	91 (57.2%)	93 (63.7%)	89 (51.7%)	0.103
Age (years old)	42.3 (16.2)	45.2 (16.5)	39.8 (15.4)	0.023
Body mass index (kg/m^2)	24.1 (3.6)	24.3 (3.2)	24.2 (4.3)	0.850
Comorbidities				
Hypertension	12 (7.5%)	9 (6.2%)	15 (8.7%)	0.518
Diabetes Mellitus	7 (4.4%)	12 (8.2%)	2 (1.2%)	0.020
Disease duration (months)	8.0 [1.0, 100.0]	12.0 [1.0, 100.0]	6.0 [1.0, 72.0]	0.002
Tumor height (cm)	3.0 (1.0)	3.3 (1.0)	2.8 (0.9)	<0.001
Diagnosis				<0.001
Pituitary adenomas	63 (39.6%)	40 (27.4%)	86 (50.0%)	
Craniopharyngiomas	96 (60.4%)	126 (73.6%)	86 (50.0%)	
Laboratory test				
Hemoglobin (g/L)	129.4 (15.9)	128.2 (17.3)	130.4 (14.5)	0.349
Red Blood Cell (10^{12}/L)	4.3 (0.5)	4.3 (0.5)	4.3 (0.5)	0.185
White Blood Cell (10^9/L)	6.6 (2.1)	6.9 (2.2)	6.4 (2.1)	0.117
Sodium (mmol/L)	140.5 (4.7)	140.4 (4.7)	140.7 (4.7)	0.670
Albumin (g/L)	43.2 (5.15)	42.8 (5.9)	43.7 (4.4)	0.239
Creatinine (μmol/L)	68.1 (15.3)	68.9 (16.7)	67.4 (14.1)	0.386
ACTH (pg/mL)	25.1 [1.1, 197.8]	23.9 [1.1, 197.8]	28.1 [3.5, 92.5]	0.936
Cortisol (μg/dL)	7.6 [0.05, 21.4]	6.6 [0.05, 48.8]	8.4 [0.1, 104.6]	0.099
Prolactin (ng/mL)	24.7 [0.4, 470.0]	21.7 [0.5, 470.0]	26.6 [0.4, 470.0]	0.052
Free Thyroxine (pmol/L)	13.8 (4.5)	13.4 (4.8)	14.2 (4.2)	0.252
Total Thyroxine (nmol/L)	80.3 (22.1)	78.9 (23.8)	81.5 (20.6)	0.429
Ophthalmology				
Visual acuity	0.6 [0.1, 1.0]	0.6 [0.1, 1.0]	0.8 [0.1, 1.0]	0.784
Visual field				
Mean deviation (db)	-8.0 [-34.2, 1.3]	-14.6 [-34.2, -0.1]	-5.0 [-32.5, 1.3]	<0.001
Pattern standard deviation (db)	7.4 [1.1, 17.7]	11.2 [1.1, 17.7]	4.3 [1.1, 17.3]	<0.001
Visual field index	70.8 (28.3)	58.7 (29.6)	81.0 (22.5)	<0.001
Retinal Nerve Fiber Layer (μm)	96.2 (33.2)	91.9 (44.5)	99.8 (18.2)	0.163
Ganglion Cell Layer (μm)	58.7 (7.1)	56.6 (7.6)	60.5 (6.1)	<0.001

Furthermore, we looked at the difference between craniopharyngiomas and pituitary adenomas (Table 2). For the ophthalmological tests, the baseline mean deviation was -8.8 [-17.2–-4.0] db in the left eye and -7.8 [-15.9–-3.3] db in the right eye. Overall, though baseline ophthalmic examinations were similar for patients with CPs and PAs, PAs were associated with better prognoses.

Among all of the algorithms trained (Table 3), the ensemble model integrating all algorithms yielded the highest AUC: 0.911 [95%CI, 0.885–0.938]. The corresponding accuracy was 84.3%, with 0.863 in sensitivity and 0.820 in specificity. The random forest model and gradient boost model ranked second and third best regarding model performance.

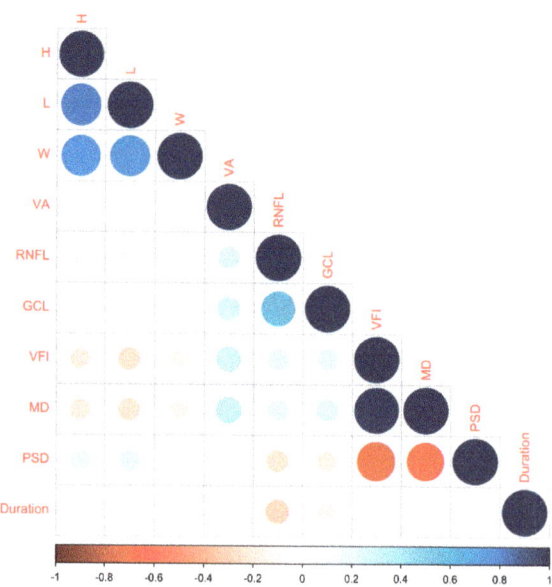

Figure 2. The correlation between visual severity, duration of symptoms, and size of the tumor. H: tumor height; L: tumor length; W: tumor width; VA: visual acuity; GCL: ganglion cell layer; VFI: visual field index; MD: mean deviation; PSD: pattern standard deviation.

Table 2. Ophthalmic examinations in patients with different diagnoses and different eyes.

	Overall N = 159	Craniopharyngioma N = 96	Pituitary Adenoma N = 63	p
Visual acuity				
Left	0.6 [0.1, 1.0]	0.7 [0.1, 1.0]	0.2 [0.1, 1.0]	0.017
Right	0.6 [0.1, 1.0]	0.8 [0.1, 1.0]	0.5 [0.1, 1.0]	0.189
Visual field				
Left				
Mean Deviation (db)	−8.8 [−34.2, 1.1]	−9.1 [−32.5, 0.1]	−7.8 [−34.2, 1.1]	0.503
Pattern Standard Deviation (db)	7.4 [1.1, 17.3]	6.0 [1.2, 16.9]	9.1 [1.1, 17.3]	0.477
Visual Field Index	69.5 (29.0)	67.5 (31.2)	72.5 (25.3)	0.288
Right				
Mean Deviation (db)	−7.8 [−32.0, 1.3]	−8.6 [−32.0, 0.0]	−6.7 [−29.7, 1.3]	0.129
Pattern Standard Deviation (db)	7.5 [1.1, 17.7]	7.6 [1.1, 16.8]	6.5 [1.1, 17.7]	0.586
Visual Field Index	72.1 (27.6)	69.9 (28.8)	75.4 (25.6)	0.222
Ganglion cell layer (μm)				
Left	58.5 (7.0)	58.9 (7.5)	57.7 (6.3)	0.290
Right	58.9 (7.1)	58.9 (7.5)	59.1 (6.4)	0.874
Retinal nerve fiber layer (μm)				
Left	99.4 (33.2)	98.3 (40.9)	101.1 (15.6)	0.609
Right	93.0 (33.0)	96.1 (38.1)	88.2 (22.5)	0.139
Recovered eyes				
Left	84 (52.8%)	42 (43.8%)	42 (66.7%)	0.008
Right	88 (55.3%)	44 (45.8%)	44 (69.8%)	0.005

We tested the model performance in two independent cohorts (Table 4). The cohorts include retrospectively collected data from FNI and prospectively collected data from GPJU. Patients in the FNI cohort had larger tumor and worse visual function than those in our training cohort. However, patients in the prospective GPJU cohort had smaller tumors and better visual function than those in our training cohort. The trained ensemble model yielded

AUCs of 0.861 and 0.843 in the retrospective FNI and prospective GPJU validation cohorts, respectively. The corresponding accuracies, sensitivities, and specificities were 86.4%, 0.842, and 0.880 and 85.0%, 0.875, and 0.833 for the two validation cohorts, respectively (Table 3). The true-positive, true-negative, false-positive, and false-negative predictions in the training and independent validation cohorts are listed in Figure 3. Most cases can be correctly classified.

Table 3. Model performance using different algorithms.

	AUC	Accuracy	Sensitivity	Specificity
Training cohort (fivefold cross validation) GPJU retrospective cohort				
LASSO	0.854 [95% CI, 0.807–0.901]	0.777	0.759	0.792
Support Vector Machine	0.875 [95% CI, 0.824–0.927]	0.786	0.764	0.806
Linear Discriminant Analysis	0.846 [95% CI, 0.794–0.897]	0.774	0.761	0.784
Random Forest	0.901 [95% CI, 0.880–0.921]	0.837	0.809	0.861
Gradient Boosting	0.889 [95% CI, 0.862–0.901]	0.799	0.789	0.807
Neural Network	0.858 [95% CI, 0.816–0.900]	0.780	0.757	0.800
Ensemble Model	0.911 [95% CI, 0.885–0.938]	0.843	0.863	0.820
Independent cohort				
FNI retrospective cohort	0.861	0.864	0.842	0.880
GPJU prospective cohort	0.843	0.850	0.875	0.833

FNI: Fudan Neurosurgical Institute. GPJU: Gold Pituitary Joint Unit.

Table 4. Comparison among three cohorts.

	Retrospective GPJU N = 159	Retrospective FNI N = 22	Prospective GPJU N = 20
Gender (male)	91 (57.2%)	17 (%)	8 (51.7%)
Age (years old)	42.3 (16.2)	41.4 (16.5)	39.0 (14.5)
Tumor height (cm)	3.0 [1.0–6.0]	3.5 [1.0–5.5]	2.4 [1.0–5.8]
Diagnosis			
Pituitary adenomas	63 (39.6%)	22 (100.0%)	15 (75.0%)
Craniopharyngiomas	96 (60.4%)	0 (0.0%)	5 (25.0%)
Ophthalmology			
Visual acuity	0.6 [0.1, 1.0]	0.4 [0.1, 1.0]	0.6 [0.1, 1.0]
Visual field			
Mean deviation (db)	−8.0 [−34.2, 1.3]	−14.3 [−29.0, 0.0]	−5.4 [−30.7, 0.4]
Pattern standard deviation (db)	7.4 [1.1, 17.7]	12.0 [1.0, 18.8]	3.8 [1.4, 16.6]
Visual field index (%)	70.8 (28.3)	56.0 (27.0)	90.0 (27.0)
Retinal Nerve Fiber Layer (μm)	96.2 (33.2)	95.8 (16.3)	103.5 (53.0)
Ganglion Cell Layer (μm)	58.7 (7.1)	87.7 (10.3)	60.2 (8.5)
Outcome: recovered	54.1%	56.8%	60.0%

FNI: Fudan Neurosurgical Institute. GPJU: Gold Pituitary Joint Unit.

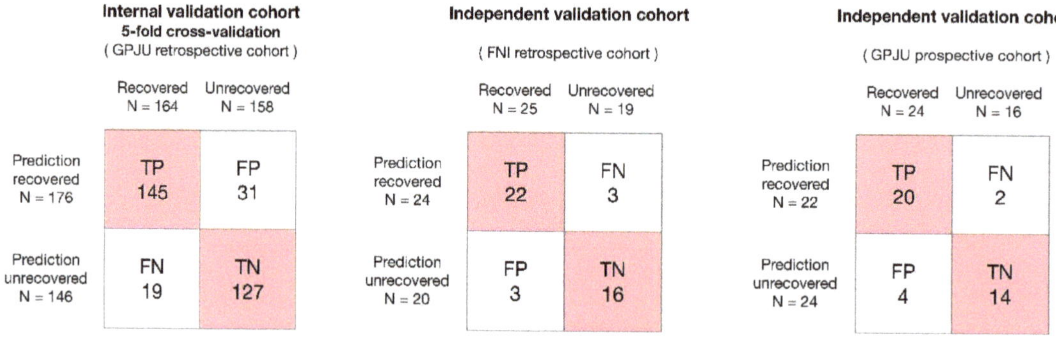

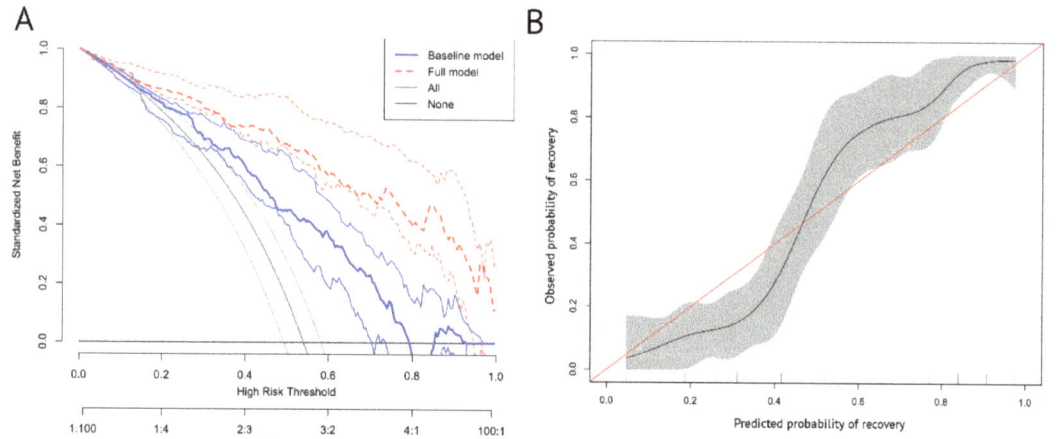

	Internal validation cohort 5-fold cross-validation (GPJU retrospective cohort)		Independent validation cohort (FNI retrospective cohort)		Independent validation cohort (GPJU prospective cohort)	
	Recovered N = 164	Unrecovered N = 158	Recovered N = 25	Unrecovered N = 19	Recovered N = 24	Unrecovered N = 16
Prediction recovered	TP 145	FP 31	TP 22	FN 3	TP 20	FN 2
Prediction unrecovered	FN 19	TN 127	FP 3	TN 16	FP 4	TN 14

Figure 3. Confusion matrix in the training and validation cohorts.

We investigated the utility of our model by plotting a decision support curve. The curve presented that the net benefit of our full model was higher than the non-model or model only using the visual field as the predictor (baseline model). PREVOST provided greater net benefit than the competing extremes of intervening in all patients or none (Figure 4A). At most risk thresholds greater than 0.1, the full model provided significant improvement in net benefit compared with the baseline model. Moreover, the model showed good calibration with low Brier scores (0.055; Figure 4B).

Figure 4. Decision support curve and calibration plot. (**A**) The curve presented that the net benefit of our full model was higher than the non-model or model only using the visual field as the predictor (baseline model). Standardized net benefit is a measure of utility that calculates a weighted sum of true positives and false positives, weighted according to the threshold. (**B**) The model showed good calibration with an intercept close to 0 and a slope close to 1. The width of the grey area represents the number of patients at each level of "predicted probability of recovery".

A model explanation using the SHAP score demonstrated that visual field, GCL, tumor height, total thyroxine, and diagnosis were the most important features in predicting visual outcome. We illustrate two cases in Figure 5, one recovered and the other unrecovered.

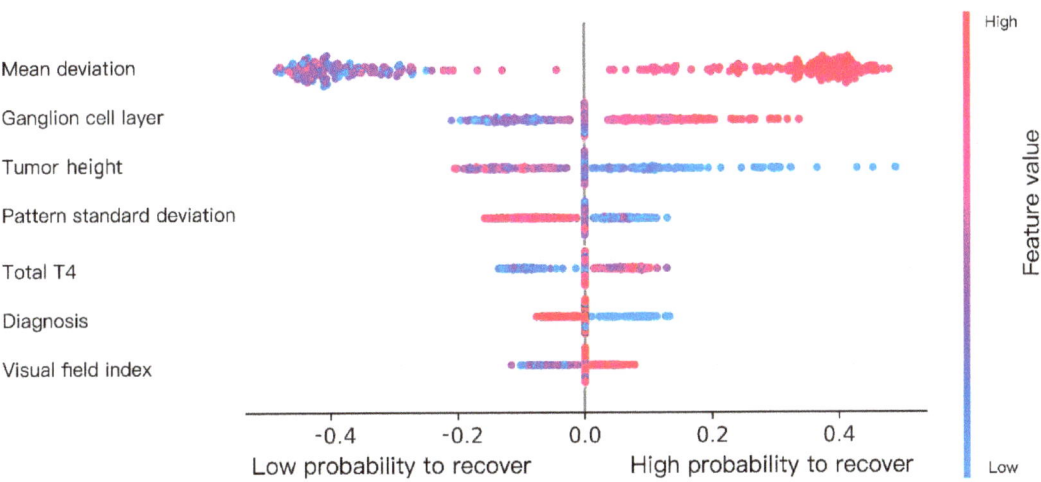

Case 1

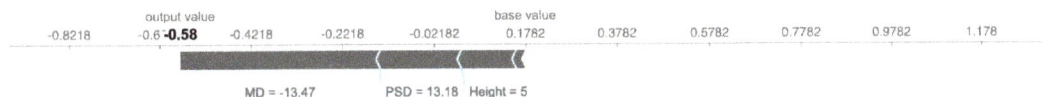

Case 2

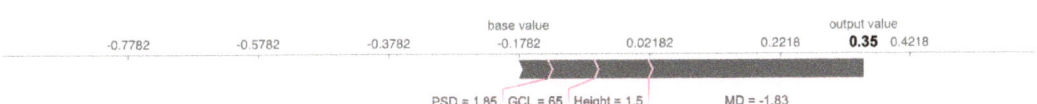

Figure 5. SHAP score-based model explanation. Every dot in the figure represents a patient. The X-axis represents the contribution to prediction (SHAP score). The variables were ordered by importance (width). Red (high) and blue (low) represent the values of the variables, e.g., for Ganglion cell layer, red means high and blue means low. Two representative cases: a severe visual field and pituitary macroadenoma contribute to the low probability of recovery (negative output) in Case 1, while a mild visual field defect, normal ganglion cell layer, and small tumor contribute to the high probability of recovery (positive output) in Case 2.

We simplified the model using these important features to construct a simple version during clinical usage. The AUC of the simple model was 0.874 [95%CI, 0.838–0.910], which was not significantly inferior to that of the original model. We constructed a nomogram based on the simple model (Figure 6). Physicians can add up corresponding scores using the graph and can obtain the recovery probability.

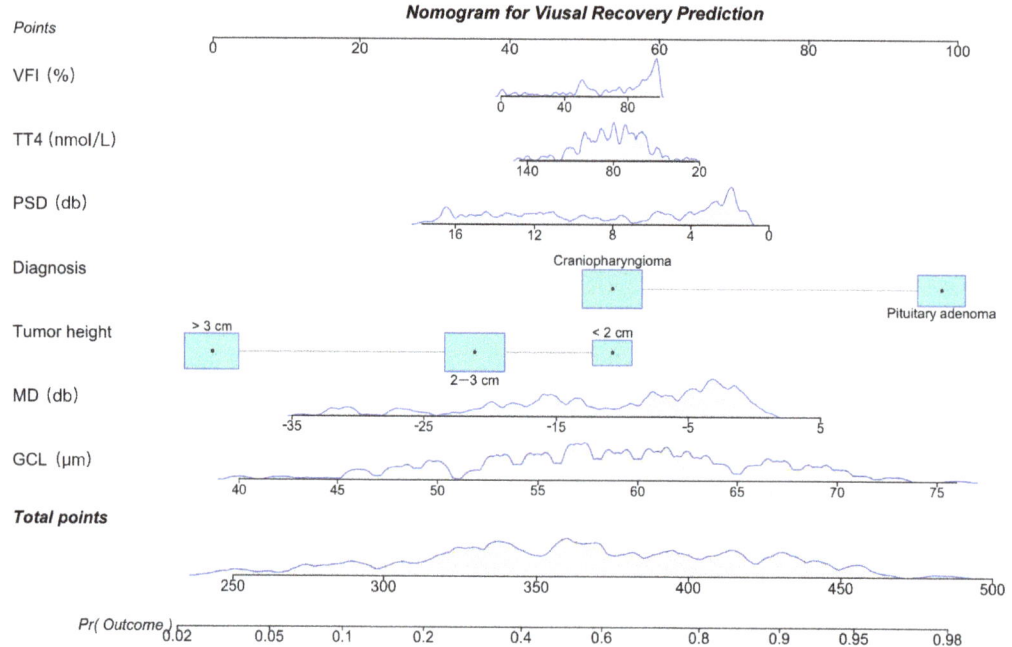

Figure 6. Nomogram for predicting visual outcome after transsphenoidal optic decompression. Physicians can add up corresponding scores using the graph and can obtain the recovery probability.

4. Discussion

We developed and independently validated PREVOST, which is, to our knowledge, the first risk-prediction algorithm specifically for visual outcomes in patients with sellar tumors. PREVOST can predict the risk of persistent visual deterioration from commonly recorded clinical information and available ophthalmic testing. The internal and external validations of PREVOST were good, with C statistics greater than 0.80. PREVOST displayed greater net benefit than alternative strategies across a range of feasible risk thresholds, although our results show that the full model should be used preferentially at most risk thresholds.

Previous studies have discussed various prognostic factors [9–19] about visual defects caused by compressive sellar region tumors. Age [5,14,25], duration of visual symptoms prior to surgery [9,12], whether the adenoma is secreting or non-secreting [25,26], tumor volume [10,27–29], pre-operative visual field deficit [9,15,19,25,27], retinal nerve fiber layer thickness [11,17–19,30], optic disc pallor [31–33], and functional MRI [13,16] were possible predictors discussed in one or several studies. However, these studies used small sample sizes, unquantified outcomes, or only a few possible predictors. In this study, however, the predictive model was developed by analyzing risk factors based on multiple factors.

Visual fields are among the most commonly included predictors in existing algorithms and are well-known contributors to visual risk, so we included them in PREVOST. Gnanalingham et al. [9] studied 41 patients with visual disturbance caused by pituitary adenomas and found that the extent of the visual recovery was mainly dependent on the preoperative visual field deficit. Yu et al. concluded that low preoperative mean deviation was one of the independent influencing factors for improving the visual field after pituitary adenomas resection [25]. Tuomas et al. also concluded that severe preoperative visual impairment resulted in poorer postoperative visual outcomes [27]. In accordance with past results, our study also established the prognostic value of preoperative visual fields. The duration of visual symptoms was another risk factor in previous studies [9,12], but it was not correlated with pre-operative visual function and was also excluded in the simplified model due to possible recall bias.

The prognostic value of GCL has been previously assessed by several researchers [11,17–19,30]. Maud Jacob et al. [11] evaluated 37 eyes of 19 patients suffering from pituitary adenomas and found that a lower RNFL thickness was a potent prognostic factor. The findings on RNFL thickness in our study were similar to the recently published research by Danesh-Meyer et al. [18], who studied 205 eyes from 107 patients and found that patients with normal preoperative RNFL thickness showed an increased propensity for visual recovery.

Tumor height was associated with visual recovery in several studies [10,27–29], and we included it in PREVOST. Blood-based predictors, such as cortisol and ACTH, were relatively infrequently included in visual risk-prediction algorithms. We found that the inclusion of blood-based predictors improved all predictive performance metrics. However, blood-based monitoring might not always be possible, and we found that the simple model still provided reliable performance estimates.

Patients and clinicians might prefer to tolerate a slightly higher risk threshold when the proposed intervention could be deemed more burdensome or might increase the risk of other adverse effects. The risk threshold for our PREVOST model was set to be 0.5. However, trials of treatments such as visual rehabilitation are scarce in these patients, but evidence suggests that such treatments might benefit visual outcomes [7,8].

The limitations of the study include non-universal representation and a lack of external prospective validation. We only included patients with craniopharyngiomas and pituitary adenomas in our study because these were the two major lesions that produce visual disturbance. Other cases, such as meningioma, could potentially be added to update the algorithm in future studies. Though the model was validated in an external cohort, with the two centers being similar in surgical volume and experience, the generalization of our model in other institutions is unknown. An external validation of PREVOST on prospective samples is required since simulation studies have suggested a minimum of 100 outcome events for an accurate validation analysis.

5. Conclusions

A new prognostic model for visual recovery after trans-sphenoidal sellar region tumor resection was developed based on an ensemble machine learning analytical approach. The score can become a valuable resource for healthcare professionals by identifying patients with a higher risk of persistent visual deficit. The large-scale and prospective application of the proposed model would strengthen its clinical utility and universal applicability in practice.

Author Contributions: Conceptualization, Y.Z. and Y.X.; methodology, N.Q. and Y.M.; software, N.Q.; validation, Y.M. and X.C.; formal analysis, N.Q.; investigation, Z.L. and Z.W.; data curation, Y.M. and Z.Y.; writing—original draft preparation, N.Q.; writing—review and editing, Y.X. and Y.Z.; visualization, H.Y. and Z.Z.; supervision, Y.W. All authors have read and agreed to the published version of the manuscript.

Funding: This study is supported by grant No.17YF1426700 from the Shanghai Committee of Science and Technology of China and the National Natural Science Foundation No. 82073640.

Institutional Review Board Statement: The study was conducted in accordance with the Declaration of Helsinki, and approved by the Institutional Review Board (or Ethics Committee) of Huashan Hospitan (KY2010-259).

Informed Consent Statement: Informed consent was obtained from all subjects involved in the study.

Data Availability Statement: De-identified data will be available upon request.

Conflicts of Interest: The authors declare no conflict of interest.

Consent to Participate: Patients consented before their clinical data were logged into the database.

Consent for Publication: All authors agreed to this publication.

Availability of Data and Material: De-identified data are available upon request.

Code Availability: All statistical analyses were completed in R software version 3.4.2, and code is available upon request.

References

1. Chen, Y.; De Wang, C.; Su, Z.P.; Chen, Y.X.; Cai, L.; Zhuge, Q.C.; Wu, Z.B. Natural history of postoperative nonfunctioning pituitary adenomas: A systematic review and meta-analysis. *Neuroendocrinology* **2012**, *96*, 333–342. [CrossRef] [PubMed]
2. Fernandez-Balsells, M.; Murad, M.H.; Barwise, A.; Gallegos-Orozco, J.F.; Paul, A.; Lane, M.A.; Lampropulos, J.F.; Natividad, I.; Perestelo-Pérez, L.; De León-Lovatón, P.G.P.; et al. Natural history of nonfunctioning pituitary adenomas and incidentalomas: A systematic review and metaanalysis. *J. Clin. Endocrinol. Metab.* **2011**, *96*, 905–912. [CrossRef] [PubMed]
3. Barker, F.G.; Klibanski, A.; Swearingen, B. Transsphenoidal surgery for pituitary tumors in the United States, 1996–2000: Mortality, morbidity, and the effects of hospital and surgeon volume. *J. Clin. Endocrinol. Metab.* **2003**, *88*, 4709–4719. [CrossRef] [PubMed]
4. Moon, C.H.; Hwang, S.-C.; Ohn, Y.-H.; Park, T.K. The time course of visual field recovery and changes of retinal ganglion cells after optic chiasmal decompression. *Investig. Opthalmol. Vis. Sci.* **2011**, *52*, 7966–7973. [CrossRef] [PubMed]
5. Dekkers, O.M.; de Keizer, R.J.W.; Roelfsema, F.; Klaauw, A.A.V.; Honkoop, P.J.; van Dulken, H.; Smit, J.W.A.; Romijn, J.A.; Pereira, A.M. Progressive improvement of impaired visual acuity during the first year after transsphenoidal surgery for non-functioning pituitary macroadenoma. *Pituitary* **2007**, *10*, 61–65. [CrossRef]
6. Sullivan, L.J.; O'Day, J.; McNeill, P. Visual outcomes of pituitary adenoma surgery. St. Vincent's Hospital 1968–1987. *J. Clin. Neuro-Ophthalmol.* **1991**, *11*, 262–267.
7. Romano, J.G.; Schulz, P.; Kenkel, S.; Todd, D.P. Visual field changes after a rehabilitation intervention: Vision restoration therapy. *J. Neurol. Sci.* **2008**, *273*, 70–74. [CrossRef]
8. Oeverhaus, M.; Dekowski, D.; Hirche, H.; Esser, J.; Schaperdoth-Gerlings, B.; Eckstein, A. Visual rehabilitation of patients with corneal diseases. *BMC Ophthalmol.* **2020**, *20*, 184. [CrossRef]
9. Gnanalingham, K.K.; Bhattacharjee, S.; Pennington, R.; Ng, J.; Mendoza, N. The time course of visual field recovery following transsphenoidal surgery for pituitary adenomas: Predictive factors for a good outcome. *J. Neurol. Neurosurg. Psychiatry* **2005**, *76*, 415–419. [CrossRef]
10. Hudson, H.; Rissell, C.; Gauderman, W.J.; Feldon, S. Pituitary tumor volume as a predictor of postoperative visual field recovery. Quantitative analysis using automated static perimetry and computed tomography morphometry. *J. Clin. Neuro-Ophthalmol.* **1991**, *11*, 280–283.
11. Jacob, M.; Raverot, G.; Jouanneau, E.; Borson-Chazot, F.; Perrin, G.; Rabilloud, M.; Tilikete, C.; Bernard, M.; Vighetto, A. Predicting visual outcome after treatment of pituitary adenomas with optical coherence tomography. *Am. J. Ophthalmol.* **2009**, *147*, 64–70.e2. [CrossRef] [PubMed]
12. Bulters, D.O.; Shenouda, E.; Evans, B.T.; Mathad, N.; Lang, D.A. Visual recovery following optic nerve decompression for chronic compressive neuropathy. *Acta Neurochir.* **2009**, *151*, 325–334. [CrossRef] [PubMed]
13. Anik, I.; Anik, Y.; Koc, K.; Ceylan, S.; Genc, H.; Altintas, O.; Ozdamar, D.; Ceylan, D.B. Evaluation of early visual recovery in pituitary macroadenomas after endoscopic endonasal ranssphenoidal surgery: Quantitative assessment with diffusion tensor imaging (DTI). *Acta Neurochir.* **2011**, *153*, 831–842. [CrossRef] [PubMed]
14. Barzaghi, L.R.; Medone, M.; Losa, M.; Bianchi, S.; Giovanelli, M.; Mortini, P. Prognostic factors of visual field improvement after trans-sphenoidal approach for pituitary macroadenomas: Review of the literature and analysis by quantitative method. *Neurosurg. Rev.* **2011**, *35*, 369–379. [CrossRef] [PubMed]
15. Lee, S.; Kim, S.-J.; Yu, Y.S.; Kim, Y.H.; Paek, S.H.; Kim, D.G.; Jung, H.-W. Prognostic factors for visual recovery after transsphenoidal pituitary adenectomy. *Br. J. Neurosurg.* **2013**, *27*, 425–429. [CrossRef]
16. Paul, D.A.; Gaffin-Cahn, E.; Hintz, E.B.; Adeclat, G.J.; Zhu, T.; Williams, Z.R.; Vates, G.E.; Mahon, B.Z. White matter changes linked to visual recovery after nerve decompression. *Sci. Transl. Med.* **2014**, *6*, 266ra173. [CrossRef]
17. Yoneoka, Y.; Hatase, T.; Watanabe, N.; Jinguji, S.; Okada, M.; Takagi, M.; Fujii, Y. Early morphological recovery of the optic chiasm is associated with excellent visual outcome in patients with compressive chiasmal syndrome caused by pituitary tu-mors. *Neurol. Res.* **2015**, *37*, 1–8. [CrossRef]
18. Danesh-Meyer, H.V.; Wong, A.; Papchenko, T.; Matheos, K.; Stylli, S.; Nichols, A.; Frampton, C.; Daniell, M.; Savino, P.J.; Kaye, A.H. Optical coherence tomography predicts visual outcome for pituitary tumors. *J. Clin. Neurosci.* **2015**, *22*, 1098–1104. [CrossRef]
19. Lee, J.; Kim, S.W.; Kim, D.W.; Shin, J.Y.; Choi, M.; Oh, M.C.; Kim, E.H.; Kim, S.H.; Byeon, S.H. Predictive model for recovery of visual field after surgery of pituitary adenoma. *J. Neuro-Oncol.* **2016**, *130*, 155–164. [CrossRef]
20. Fan, Y.; Jiang, S.; Hua, M.; Feng, S.; Feng, M.; Wang, R. Machine learning-based radiomics predicts radiotherapeutic response in patients with acromegaly. *Front. Endocrinol.* **2019**, *10*, 588. [CrossRef]
21. Qiao, N.; Shen, M.; He, W.; He, M.; Zhang, Z.; Ye, H.; Li, Y.; Shou, X.; Li, S.; Jiang, C.; et al. Machine learning in predicting early remission in patients after surgical treatment of acromegaly: A multicenter study. *Pituitary* **2021**, *24*, 53–61. [CrossRef] [PubMed]
22. Van Calster, B.; Wynants, L.; Verbeek, J.F.; Verbakel, J.; Christodoulou, E.; Vickers, A.J.; Roobol, M.J.; Steyerberg, E.W. Reporting and interpreting decision curve analysis: A guide for investigators. *Eur. Urol.* **2018**, *74*, 796–804. [CrossRef] [PubMed]

23. Lundberg, S.M.; Nair, B.; Vavilala, M.S.; Horibe, M.; Eisses, M.J.; Adams, T.; Liston, D.E.; Low, D.K.-W.; Newman, S.-F.; Kim, J.; et al. Explainable machine-learning predictions for the prevention of hypoxaemia during surgery. *Nat. Biomed. Eng.* **2018**, *2*, 749–760. [CrossRef] [PubMed]
24. Lloyd, R.V.; Osamura, R.Y.; Klöppel, G.; Rosai, J. Tumours of the pituitary gland. Introduction. In *WHO Classification of Tumours of Endocrine Organs*, 4th ed.; Lloyd, R.V., Osamura, R.Y., Klöppel, G., Rosai, J., Eds.; IARC: Lyon, France, 2017; Volume 10, p. 13.
25. Yu, F.-F.; Chen, L.-L.; Su, Y.-H.; Huo, L.-H.; Lin, X.-X.; Liao, R.-D. Factors influencing improvement of visual field after transsphenoidal resection of pituitary macroadenomas: A retrospective cohort study. *Int. J. Ophthalmol.* **2015**, *8*, 1224–1228. [CrossRef] [PubMed]
26. Trautmann, J.C.; Laws, E.R. Visual status after transsphenoidal surgery at the mayo clinic, 1971–1982. *Am. J. Ophthalmol.* **1983**, *96*, 200–208. [CrossRef]
27. Luomaranta, T.; Raappana, A.; Saarela, V.; Liinamaa, M.J. Factors affecting the visual outcome of pituitary adenoma patients treated with endoscopic transsphenoidal surgery. *World Neurosurg.* **2017**, *105*, 422–431. [CrossRef]
28. Ryu, W.H.A.; Starreveld, Y.; Burton, J.M.; Liu, J.; Costello, F.; the PITNET Study Group. The utility of magnetic resonance imaging in assessing patients with pituitary tumors compressing the anterior visual pathway. *J. Neuro-Ophthalmol.* **2017**, *37*, 230–238. [CrossRef]
29. Grkovic, D.; Bedov, T. Outcome of visual acuity after surgical removal of pituitary adenomas. *Srp. Arh. Za Celok. Lek.* **2013**, *141*, 296–303. [CrossRef]
30. Danesh-Meyer, H.V.; Papchenko, T.; Savino, P.J.; Law, A.; Evans, J.; Gamble, G. In Vivo retinal nerve fiber layer thickness measured by optical coherence tomography predicts visual recovery after surgery for parachiasmal tumors. *Investig. Opthalmol. Vis. Sci.* **2008**, *49*, 1879–1885. [CrossRef]
31. Johansson, C.; Lindblom, B. The role of optical coherence tomography in the detection of pituitary adenoma. *Acta Ophthalmol.* **2009**, *87*, 776–779. [CrossRef]
32. Tanito, M.; Itai, N.; Goto, T.; Ohira, A.; Chihara, E. Abnormalities of scanning laser polarimetry associated with pituitary adenoma. *Am. J. Ophthalmol.* **2003**, *135*, 565–567. [CrossRef]
33. Marcus, M.; Vitale, S.; Calvert, P.C.; Miller, N.R. Visual parameters in patients with pituitary adenoma before and after transsphenoidal surgery. *Aust. N. Z. J. Ophthalmol.* **1991**, *19*, 111–118. [CrossRef] [PubMed]

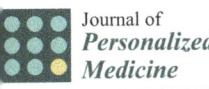

Journal of Personalized Medicine

Article

Predicting Venous Thrombosis in Osteoarthritis Using a Machine Learning Algorithm: A Population-Based Cohort Study

Chao Lu [1,†], Jiayin Song [1,†], Hui Li [1,2,†], Wenxing Yu [1], Yangquan Hao [1], Ke Xu [1,*] and Peng Xu [1,*]

[1] Department of Joint Surgery, Xi'an Hong Hui Hospital, Xi'an Jiaotong University Health Science Center, Xi'an 710054, China; luchao0925@163.com (C.L.); jean_songdm@sina.com (J.S.); lihui1326148739@163.com (H.L.); yuwenxing110@163.com (W.Y.); haoyq2008@126.com (Y.H.)

[2] Department of Traditional Chinese and Western Medicine, The First Clinical College of Shaanxi University of Chinese Medicine, Shaanxi University of Chinese Medicine, Xi'an 712046, China

* Correspondence: santxuke1986@126.com (K.X.); sousou369@163.com (P.X.)

† These authors contributed equally to this work.

Abstract: Osteoarthritis (OA) is the most common joint disease associated with pain and disability. OA patients are at a high risk for venous thrombosis (VTE). Here, we developed an interpretable machine learning (ML)-based model to predict VTE risk in patients with OA. To establish a prediction model, we used six ML algorithms, of which 35 variables were employed. Recursive feature elimination (RFE) was used to screen the most related clinical variables associated with VTE. SHapley additive exPlanations (SHAP) were applied to interpret the ML mode and determine the importance of the selected features. Overall, 3169 patients with OA (average age: 66.52 ± 7.28 years) were recruited from Xi'an Honghui Hospital. Of these, 352 and 2817 patients were diagnosed with and without VTE, respectively. The XGBoost algorithm showed the best performance. According to the RFE algorithms, 15 variables were retained for further modeling with the XGBoost algorithm. The top three predictors were Kellgren–Lawrence grade, age, and hypertension. Our study showed that the XGBoost model with 15 variables has a high potential to predict VTE risk in patients with OA.

Keywords: osteoarthritis; venous thrombosis; VTE risk prediction; machine learning algorithm; population-based cohort study

1. Introduction

Osteoarthritis (OA) is the most common joint disease worldwide, with an age-associated increase in both incidence and prevalence [1,2]. It is estimated that approximately 302 million people globally suffer from this disease, and the associated healthcare resources and financial burden can be substantial [3,4]. OA, a primary cause of pain, disability, and joint replacement, is characterized by disease affecting the whole joint, including articular cartilage degradation, synovium and ligament inflammation, and changes to the subchondral bone [5–7]. Despite the symptomatic treatment of pain, stiffness, and swelling, there are no FDA-approved disease-modifying drugs [8]. As a complex disease, a multitude of possible etiologies contribute to the development of OA, including obesity, sedentary lifestyle, trauma, and aging [9–11]. Early prevention and elimination of risk factors are critical in delaying disease progression [12]. Nevertheless, despite these identifiable underlying causes, OA still cannot be effectively prevented.

Venous thrombosis is a relatively common and potentially fatal condition in patients, and an increased risk of VTE has been reported in arthritis, particularly in rheumatic arthritis (RA) [13–16]. Li et al. reported that RA patients have an increased risk of VTE, pulmonary embolism, and deep vein thrombosis after diagnosis in comparison with the general population [17]. This suggests that VTE may play a vital role in chronic and systemic inflammatory autoimmune disease. However, the relationship between OA and VTE has not been elucidated. A recent study in a large population-based cohort revealed that knee or hip osteoarthritis might increase incident VTE risk to 40% and 80%, respectively, when compared to those without OA, which may be partly mediated through joint replacement [18].

Thus, predicting the VTE risk among OA patients is critical to reduce morbidity and mortality from VTE in OA patients. Machine learning (ML) is a computer-based method of data analysis that is often used to construct predictive models based on large datasets [19]. In this study, we aimed to develop a model using the ML algorithm to identify those at high risk of VTE in OA patients

2. Materials and Methods

We performed a single-center cross-sectional study of OA patients in Xi'an Honghui Hospital between January 2018 and December 2020. Patients were consecutively recruited from joint surgery department and were examined by venous ultrasound of the legs to assess VTE risk. The inclusion criteria were as follows: (1) diagnosed with knee osteoarthritis (guidelines for the diagnosis and treatment of osteoarthritis (2018 edition)) [20]; (2) radiographically evaluated by X-ray at Kellgren–Lawrence grade stages 3–4. Those with heart stent, ischemic stroke, cancers, or incomplete laboratory data were excluded from the study. The study was approved by the Ethics Committee of Xi'an Honghui Hospital and conducted in accordance with the Declaration of Helsinki. Written informed consent was waived owing to the retrospective nature of the study. All confidential patient information was deleted from the entire dataset prior to the analysis.

All patient demographics and laboratory data at admission were extracted manually from electronic medical records using a standardized case report form.

2.1. Machine Learning Algorithms

To develop machine learning models, 35 parameters were used for the analysis. Before developing the ML models, laboratory indices, which were continuous variables, were converted into categorical variables based on their normal range values. In addition, the patient's age was treated as a continuous variable, with missing values replaced by median values. All patients were randomly divided into a training set and test set at a ratio of 8:2.

Six ML algorithms, namely logistic regression (LR), random forest (RF), extreme gradient boosting (XGBoost), adaptive boosting (AdaBoost), gradient boosting decision tree (GBDT), and light gradient boosting machine (LGBM), were used to predict the VTE risk. We used the receiver operating characteristic (ROC) curve as the evaluation metric to compare the performance of the ML algorithm between the training and testing sets. The best performance model was chosen, and recursive feature elimination (RFE) was employed to screen the optimized variable combinations. For model interpretation, the Shapley additive exPlanations (SHAP) algorithm was used to calculate the Shapley value of each variable based on game theory to further explain the best performance model.

2.2. Statistical Analysis

All statistical analyses were conducted using Python software (version 3.8). A Fisher's exact test or an x^2 test was conducted for binary variables, and Student's t-test was used for continuous variables. Owing to the imbalance of the dataset, the synthetic minority oversampling technique (SMOTE) was used to deal with the training set. Six ML algorithms were used to screen for the best performance prediction model. Using the RFE algorithm, all variables were filtered one by one to obtain the best combination, which was then established in a selected ML prediction model. We also used the SHAP algorithm to interpret and evaluate the optimized model. Statistical significance was set at $p \leq 0.05$.

3. Results

We excluded subjects with missing data and subsequently enrolled 3169 patients with an average age of 66.52 ± 7.28 years in the study (Figure 1). Of them, 2400 patients were male and 769 patients were female, accounting for 75.73% and 24.27% of all patients, respectively. All patients were divided into the VTE and non-VTE groups. There were 352 patients with VTE, with an average age of 68.05 ± 6.84 and 2817 patients without VTE, with an average age of 66.33 ± 7.31. In the VTE group, 281 patients were male (79.83%) and 71 patients were female (20.17%). In the non-VTE group, 2119 patients were male (75.22%) and 698 were female (24.78%). The baseline characteristics of patients stratified by VTE are summarized in Table 1.

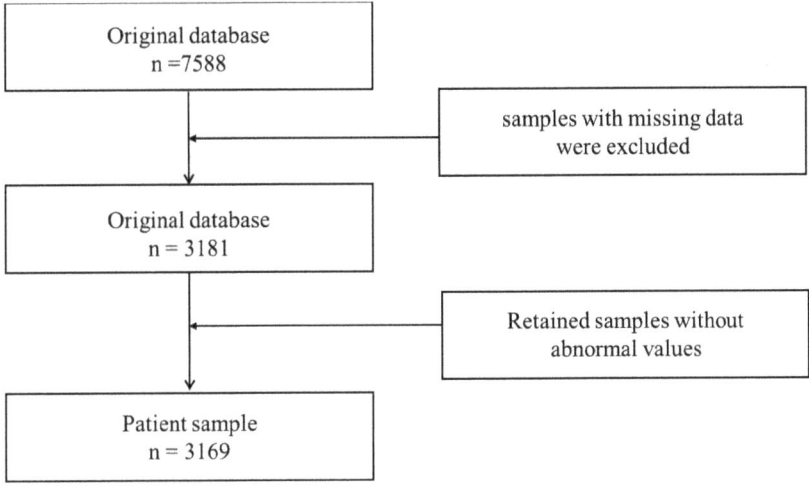

Figure 1. Flow chart of patients for enrollment.

Table 1. Characteristics of the patients stratified by VTE or not.

	Class [a]	Total	None-Venous Thrombosis	Venous Thrombosis	p [b]
N		3169	2817	352	
Age (year) [b]		66.52 ± 7.28	66.33 ± 7.31	68.05 ± 6.84	<0.001
Gender					
	Male	2400 (75.73%)	2119 (75.22%)	281 (79.83%)	0.066
	Female	769 (24.27%)	698 (24.78%)	71 (20.17%)	
Hypertension					
	No	1730 (54.59%)	1543 (54.77%)	187 (53.12%)	0.597
	Yes	1439 (45.41%)	1274 (45.23%)	165 (46.88%)	
Diabetes					
	No	2751 (86.81%)	2437 (86.51%)	314 (89.20%)	0.185
	Yes	418 (13.19%)	380 (13.49%)	38 (10.80%)	
Coronary heart disease					
	No	2207 (69.64%)	1974 (70.07%)	233 (66.19%)	0.152
	Yes	962 (30.36%)	843 (29.93%)	119 (33.81%)	

Table 1. Cont.

	Class [a]	Total	None-Venous Thrombosis	Venous Thrombosis	p [b]
Kellgren–Lawrence grade					
	0	2269 (71.60%)	1943 (68.97%)	326 (92.61%)	<0.001
	III	181 (5.71%)	178 (6.32%)	3 (0.85%)	
	IV	719 (22.69%)	696 (24.71%)	23 (6.54%)	
Eosinophil ratio					
	Normal Range	2746 (86.65%)	2431 (86.30%)	315 (89.49%)	0.115
	Abnormal	423 (13.35%)	386 (13.70%)	37 (10.51%)	
Hematocrit					
	Normal Range	2535 (79.99%)	2254 (80.01%)	281 (79.83%)	0.991
	Abnormal	634 (20.01%)	563 (19.99%)	71 (20.17%)	
Mean platelet volume					
	Normal Range	2782 (87.79%)	2462 (87.40%)	320 (90.91%)	0.070
	Abnormal	387 (12.21%)	355 (12.60%)	32 (9.09%)	
Thrombocytocrit					
	Normal Range	2858 (90.19%)	2527 (89.71%)	331 (94.03%)	0.013
	Abnormal	311 (9.81%)	290 (10.29%)	21 (5.97%)	
platelet-larger cell ratio					
	Normal Range	2390 (75.42%)	2112 (74.97%)	278 (78.98%)	0.114
	Abnormal	779 (24.58%)	705 (25.03%)	74 (21.02%)	
Uric acid					
	Normal Range	2554 (80.59%)	2261 (80.26%)	293 (83.24%)	0.208
	Abnormal	615 (19.41%)	556 (19.74%)	59 (16.76%)	
Glucose					
	Normal Range	2665 (84.10%)	2369 (84.10%)	296 (84.09%)	0.941
	Abnormal	504 (15.90%)	448 (15.90%)	56 (15.91%)	
Antistreptococcal hemolysin "O"					
	Normal Range	3074 (97.00%)	2726 (96.77%)	348 (98.86%)	0.045
	Abnormal	95 (3.00%)	91 (3.23%)	4 (1.14%)	
Anti-CCP antibody					
	Normal Range	2549 (80.44%)	2255 (80.05%)	294 (83.52%)	0.140
	Abnormal	620 (19.56%)	562 (19.95%)	58 (16.48%)	
Rheumatoid factors					
	Normal Range	2902 (91.57%)	2577 (91.48%)	325 (92.33%)	0.661
	Abnormal	267 (8.43%)	240 (8.52%)	27 (7.67%)	

[a] Continuous variable are transformed to dichotomous variables according to their normal range. [b] Values are presented as mean ± SD.

The patients were randomly stratified (8:2) into training and testing sets to evaluate the model performance. Finally, a total of 35 characteristics were enrolled in the six ML algorithms, including LR, RF, XGBoost, AdaBoost, GBDT, and LGBM, to identify the model with the best predictive performance. Our results showed that the XGBoost model demonstrated the best performance, with an area under the curve (AUC) of 0.741 (95% CI: 0.676, 0.806) (Figure 2A,B). The AUC values of the other models are shown in Table 2.

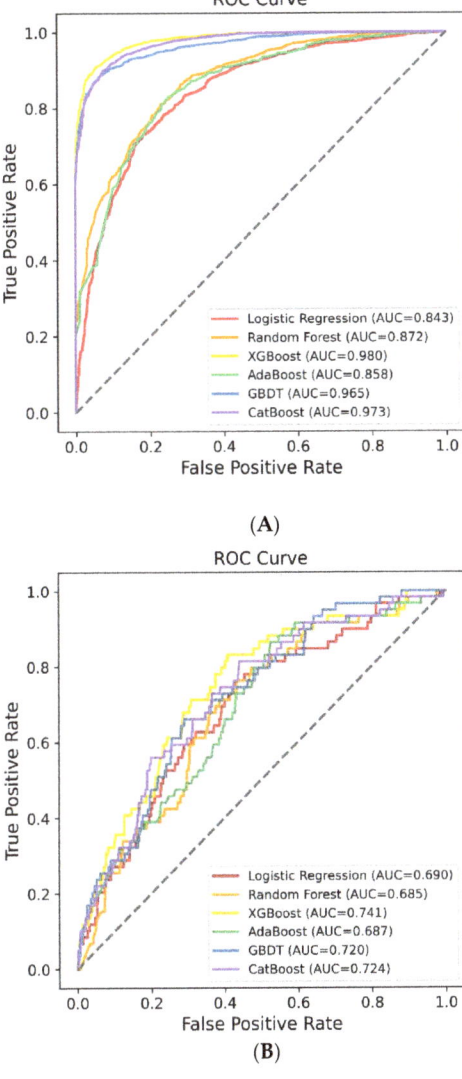

Figure 2. The receiver operating characteristic (ROC) curves of the machine learning models on the training set (**A**) and testing set (**B**).

Table 2. The area under the curve (AUC) of training set and testing set.

	Training Set (AUC, 95% CI)	Testing Set (AUC, 95% CI)
LR	0.843 (0.832, 0.855)	0.690 (0.620, 0.760)
RF	0.872 (0.862, 0.882)	0.685 (0.618, 0.753)
XGBoost	0.980 (0.977, 0.983)	0.741 (0.676, 0.806)
AdaBoost	0.858 (0.847, 0.868)	0.687 (0.619, 0.755)
GBDT	0.965 (0.960, 0.970)	0.720 (0.656, 0.784)
CatBoost	0.973 (0.969, 0.977)	0.724 (0.657, 0.790)

To further optimize the XGBoost model, the RFE method was used to screen the most important variables that can predict the VTE risk. Finally, 15 variables were employed to establish the final prediction model, and the new XGBoost model showed that the AUC of the testing dataset was 0.727 (95% CI = 0.662, 0.792) (Figure 3A,B).

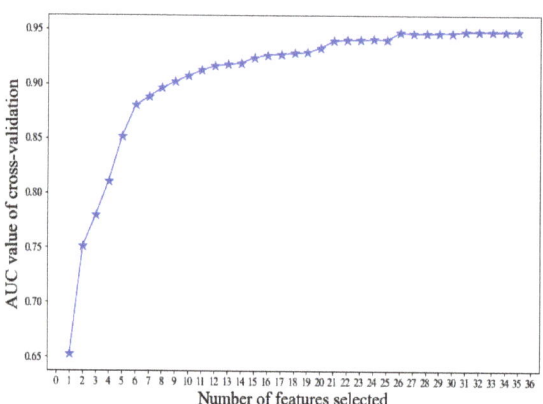

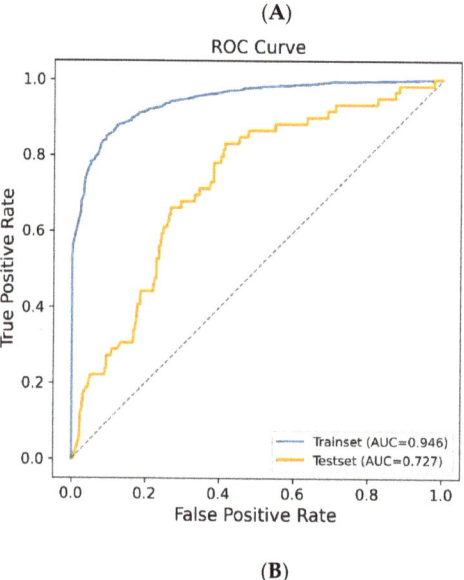

Figure 3. Using the RFE method to screen the optimal variables. (**A**) The most import variables, screened by the RFE method; (**B**) The receiver operating characteristic (ROC) curves of XGBoost model on the training set and testing set.

Interpretation and Evaluation of Machine Learning Model

The SHAP method was also used to interpret the relative importance of each variable in the XGBoost model. Our results showed that age, eosinophil ratio (EOSR), hematocrit (HCT), mean platelet volume (MPV), thrombocytocrit (PCT), platelet-larger cell ratio (P-LCR), uric acid (UA), glucose, antistreptococcal hemolysin "O" (ASO), anti-cyclic citrullinated peptide antibody (ACPA), rheumatoid factor (RF), Kellgren–Lawrence grade (K–L grade), history of hypertension, diabetes, and coronary artery disease (CAD) were associated with the risk of VTE in OA patients. Particularly, K–L grade, age, and hypertension were the three vital variables (Figure 4A,B).

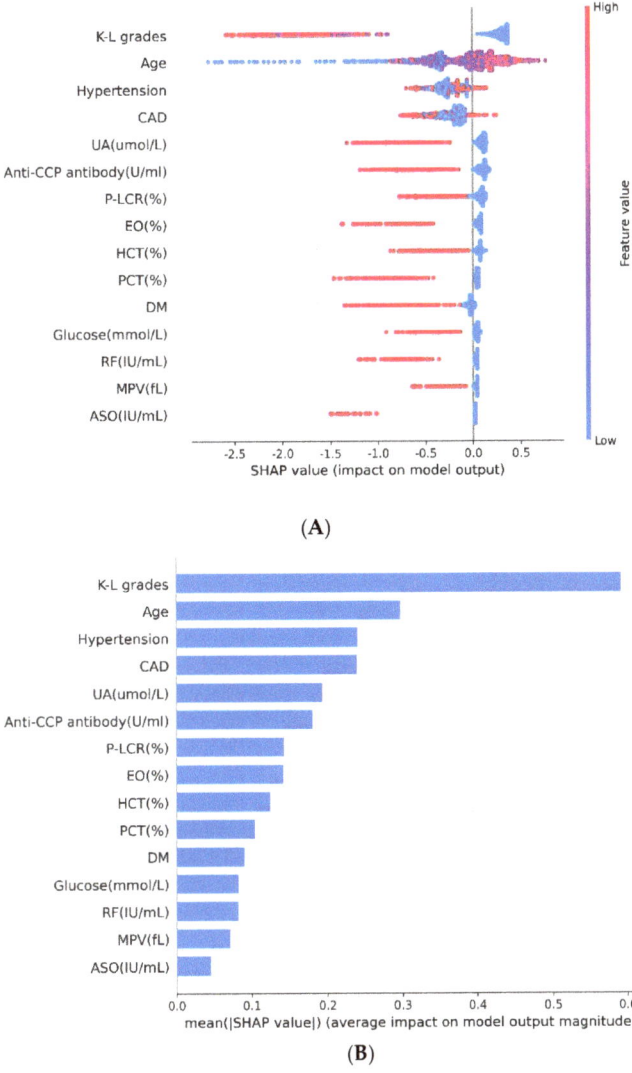

Figure 4. Interpretation and Evaluation of Machine Learning Model. (**A**) SHAP analysis on the dataset, which shows the 15 most important features and their impact on the model output. Each dot represents one patient, with blue color meaning the lowest range and red color meaning the highest range of the feature; (**B**) Ranking of the features' importance indicated by SHAP analysis.

4. Discussion

Extensive efforts have been made to delay OA patients progress to the end stage. In this hospital-based cross-sectional study, we used the ML algorithm to predict VTE risk in patients with OA. We found that using the XGBoost model with 15 variables can predict VTE risk in OA patients, and this may have a growing prevalence due to the global ageing population.

OA is not simply a matter of mechanical damage to the joint but involves several additional risk factors [21]. Nevertheless, some patients still inevitably rapidly progress to the end stages [22]. The 11th leading cause of disability worldwide has resulted in a rapid increase in orthopedic surgeries over the last few decades [4]. Rather than medication, lifestyle modification is the most promising avenue for the prevention of OA [3,23]. Many risk factors, including VTE, have been identified, and these may be partly mediated through knee or hip replacement. In a large population-based cohort study, Zeng et al. reported that VTE increased by approximately 40% among individuals with knee OA and by 80% among individuals with hip OA compared to those without OA [18].

Machine learning is a crucial branch of artificial intelligence that utilizes historical data to predict the likelihood of a future outcome [24,25]. As a multidisciplinary approach, ML algorithms are increasingly being utilized to predict outcomes in lower-extremity total joint arthroplasty [26]. Lu et al. used ML to establish a model to predict surgical outcomes after non-compartmental knee arthroplasty [27]. Kunze et al. developed machine learning algorithms based on partially modifiable risk factors for predicting dissatisfaction after arthroplasty [28]. In this study, we found that the XGBoost algorithm was the best performing algorithm. In this prediction model, 15 variables were found to be associated with VTE risk. In addition to the conventional risk factors such as age, hypertension, and diabetes, our study found that CAD, EOSR, HCT, MPV, PCT, P-LCR, UA, ASO, ACPA, RF, and Kellgren–Lawrence grade were also correlated with VTE. These have not been reported elsewhere.

The present study has certain limitations. First, although ML algorithms are widely used in medical practice, the predictive value is limited due to the "black box" characteristic. Thus, rather than being used as a clinical judgment tool, an ML algorithm model should be used as a reference for physicians. Second, all the data analyzed in the present study were from a single institution, and the imbalance of gender ratio has limited the generalization of our results. Additionally, because of the nature of an observational study, some unmeasured confounding effects may persist; thus, additional validation and assessment of the relationship between the variables and VTE in OA patients should be performed in a large population. Nevertheless, despite such limitations, to our knowledge, this is the first study to use a machine learning method to predict VTE risk in OA patients.

5. Conclusions

In conclusion, we developed a XGBoost model with a high accuracy in the prediction of VTE risk in patients with OA, which might supply a complementary tool for the screening of populations at high risk of VTE.

Author Contributions: Conceptualization, P.X.; methodology, C.L. and J.S.; formal analysis, C.L. and J.S.; investigation, H.L. and W.Y.; resources, Y.H.; writing—original draft preparation, C.L.; supervision, P.X. and K.X. All authors have read and agreed to the published version of the manuscript.

Funding: This research was funded by National Natural Science Foundation of China, grant number 82072432.

Institutional Review Board Statement: The study was approved by the Ethics Committee of Xi'an Honghui Hospital and conducted in accordance with the Declaration of Helsinki.

Informed Consent Statement: Written informed consent was waived owing to the retrospective nature of the study. All confidential patient information was deleted from the entire dataset prior to the analysis.

Data Availability Statement: The authors confirm that all data underlying the findings are fully available and can be obtained after submitting a request to the corresponding author.

Conflicts of Interest: The authors declare no conflict of interest.

References

1. Barnett, R. Osteoarthritis. *Lancet* **2018**, *391*, 1985. [CrossRef]
2. Villafane, J.H.; Valdes, K.; Pedersini, P.; Berjano, P. Osteoarthritis: A call for research on central pain mechanism and personalized prevention strategies. *Clin. Rheumatol.* **2019**, *38*, 583–584. [CrossRef]

3. Kolasinski, S.L.; Neogi, T.; Hochberg, M.C.; Oatis, C.; Guyatt, G.; Block, J.; Callahan, L.; Copenhaver, C.; Dodge, C.; Felson, D.; et al. 2019 American college of rheumatology/arthritis foundation guideline for the management of osteoarthritis of the hand, hip, and knee. *Arthritis Rheumatol.* **2020**, *72*, 220–233. [CrossRef]
4. Palazzo, C.; Nguyen, C.; Lefevre-Colau, M.M.; Rannou, F.; Poiraudeau, S. Risk factors and burden of osteoarthritis. *Ann. Phys. Rehabil. Med.* **2016**, *59*, 134–138. [CrossRef]
5. Abramoff, B.; Caldera, F.E. Osteoarthritis: Pathology, diagnosis, and treatment options. *Med. Clin. N. Am.* **2020**, *104*, 293–311. [CrossRef] [PubMed]
6. Goldring, S.R.; Goldring, M.B. Changes in the osteochondral unit during osteoarthritis: Structure, function and cartilage-bone crosstalk. *Nat. Rev. Rheumatol.* **2016**, *12*, 632–644. [CrossRef] [PubMed]
7. Sanchez-Romero, E.A.; Pecos-Martin, D.; Calvo-Lobo, C.; Garcia-Jimenez, D.; Ochoa-Saez, V.; Burgos-Caballero, V.; Fernandez-Carnero, J. Clinical features and myofascial pain syndrome in older adults with knee osteoarthritis by sex and age distribution: A cross-sectional study. *Knee* **2019**, *26*, 165–173. [CrossRef] [PubMed]
8. Trouvin, A.P.; Perrot, S. Pain in osteoarthritis. Implications for optimal management. *Joint Bone Spine* **2018**, *85*, 429–434. [CrossRef] [PubMed]
9. O'Neill, T.W.; Mccabe, P.S.; Mcbeth, J. Update on the epidemiology, risk factors and disease outcomes of osteoarthritis. *Best Pract. Res. Clin. Rheumatol.* **2018**, *32*, 312–326. [CrossRef]
10. Prieto-Alhambra, D.; Judge, A.; Javaid, M.K.; Cooper, C.; Diez-Perez, A.; Arden, N.K. Incidence and risk factors for clinically diagnosed knee, hip and hand osteoarthritis: Influences of age, gender and osteoarthritis affecting other joints. *Ann. Rheum. Dis.* **2014**, *73*, 1659–1664. [CrossRef]
11. Sanchez, R.E.; Melendez, O.E.; Alonso, P.J.; Martin, P.S.; Turroni, S.; Marchese, L.; Villafane, J.H. Relationship between the gut microbiome and osteoarthritis pain: Review of the literature. *Nutrients* **2021**, *13*, 716. [CrossRef]
12. Vina, E.R.; Kwoh, C.K. Epidemiology of osteoarthritis: Literature update. *Curr. Opin. Rheumatol.* **2018**, *30*, 160–167. [CrossRef] [PubMed]
13. Holmqvist, M.E.; Neovius, M.; Eriksson, J.; Mantel, A.; Wallberg-Jonsson, S.; Jacobsson, L.T.; Askling, J. Risk of venous thromboembolism in patients with rheumatoid arthritis and association with disease duration and hospitalization. *JAMA* **2012**, *308*, 1350–1356. [CrossRef] [PubMed]
14. Bacani, A.K.; Gabriel, S.E.; Crowson, C.S.; Heit, J.A.; Matteson, E.L. Noncardiac vascular disease in rheumatoid arthritis: Increase in venous thromboembolic events? *Arthritis Rheum.* **2012**, *64*, 53–61. [CrossRef]
15. Ketfi, C.; Boutigny, A.; Mohamedi, N.; Bouajil, S.; Magnan, B.; Amah, G.; Dillinger, J.G. Risk of venous thromboembolism in rheumatoid arthritis. *Jt. Bone Spine* **2021**, *88*, 105122. [CrossRef] [PubMed]
16. Chung, W.S.; Peng, C.L.; Lin, C.L.; Chang, Y.J.; Chen, Y.F.; Chiang, J.Y.; Sung, F.C.; Kao, C.H. Rheumatoid arthritis increases the risk of deep vein thrombosis and pulmonary thromboembolism: A nationwide cohort study. *Ann. Rheum. Dis.* **2014**, *73*, 1774–1780. [CrossRef]
17. Li, L.; Lu, N.; Avina-Galindo, A.M.; Zheng, Y.; Lacaille, D.; Esdaile, J.M.; Choi, H.K.; Avina-Zubieta, J.A. The risk and trend of pulmonary embolism and deep vein thrombosis in rheumatoid arthritis: A general population-based study. *Rheumatology* **2021**, *60*, 188–195. [CrossRef]
18. Zeng, C.; Bennell, K.; Yang, Z.; Nguyen, U.; Lu, N.; Wei, J.; Lei, G.; Zhang, Y. Risk of venous thromboembolism in knee, hip and hand osteoarthritis: A general population-based cohort study. *Ann. Rheum. Dis.* **2020**, *79*, 1616–1624. [CrossRef]
19. Deo, R.C. Machine learning in medicine. *Circulation* **2015**, *132*, 1920–1930. [CrossRef]
20. Association, T.J.S.B.; Wang, K. Guidelines for the diagnosis and treatment of osteoarthritis (2018 edition). *Chin. J. Orthop.* **2018**, *38*, 705–715.
21. Jiang, T.; Yao, Y.; Xu, X.; Song, K.; Pan, P.; Chen, D.; Xu, Z.; Dai, J.; Qin, J.; Shi, D.; et al. Prevalence and risk factors of preoperative deep vein thrombosis in patients with end-stage knee osteoarthritis. *Ann. Vasc. Surg.* **2020**, *64*, 175–180. [CrossRef] [PubMed]
22. O'Brien, M.S.; Mcdougall, J.J. Age and frailty as risk factors for the development of osteoarthritis. *Mech. Ageing Dev.* **2019**, *180*, 21–28. [CrossRef]
23. Chen, W.H.; Tsai, W.C.; Wang, H.T.; Wang, C.H.; Tseng, Y.T. Can early rehabilitation after osteoarthritis reduce knee and hip arthroplasty risk?: A national representative cohort study. *Medicine* **2019**, *98*, e15723. [CrossRef] [PubMed]
24. Badillo, S.; Banfai, B.; Birzele, F.; Davydov, I.I.; Hutchinson, L.; Kam-Thong, T.; Siebourg-Polster, J.; Steiert, B.; Zhang, J.D. An introduction to machine learning. *Clin. Pharmacol. Ther.* **2020**, *107*, 871–885. [CrossRef]
25. Helm, J.M.; Swiergosz, A.M.; Haeberle, H.S.; Karnuta, J.M.; Schaffer, J.L.; Krebs, V.E.; Spitzer, A.I.; Ramkumar, P.N. Machine learning and artificial intelligence: Definitions, applications, and future directions. *Curr. Rev. Musculoskelet. Med.* **2020**, *13*, 69–76. [CrossRef] [PubMed]
26. Haeberle, H.S.; Helm, J.M.; Navarro, S.M.; Karnuta, J.M.; Schaffer, J.L.; Callaghan, J.J.; Mont, M.A.; Kamath, A.F.; Krebs, V.E.; Ramkumar, P.N. Artificial intelligence and machine learning in lower extremity arthroplasty: A review. *J. Arthroplast.* **2019**, *34*, 2201–2203. [CrossRef]
27. Lu, Y.; Khazi, Z.M.; Agarwalla, A.; Forsythe, B.; Taunton, M.J. Development of a machine learning algorithm to predict nonroutine discharge following unicompartmental knee arthroplasty. *J. Arthroplast.* **2021**, *36*, 1568–1576. [CrossRef]
28. Kunze, K.N.; Polce, E.M.; Sadauskas, A.J.; Levine, B.R. Development of machine learning algorithms to predict patient dissatisfaction after primary total knee arthroplasty. *J. Arthroplast.* **2020**, *35*, 3117–3122. [CrossRef]

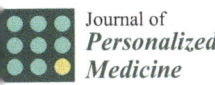

Article

Machine Learning-Based Approaches for Prediction of Patients' Functional Outcome and Mortality after Spontaneous Intracerebral Hemorrhage

Rui Guo [1,†], Renjie Zhang [1,2,†], Ran Liu [3], Yi Liu [1], Hao Li [1], Lu Ma [1], Min He [1], Chao You [1,4] and Rui Tian [1,*]

1. Department of Neurosurgery, West China Hospital, Sichuan University, Chengdu 610041, China; 13980774725@163.com (R.G.); zrjwch@163.com (R.Z.); liuyi@wchscu.cn (Y.L.); coscolh@126.com (H.L.); alex80350305@163.com (L.M.); heminhx@aliyun.com (M.H.); youchao@vip.126.com (C.Y.)
2. Department of Clinical Medicine, West China Medical College, Sichuan University, Chengdu 610041, China
3. Engineering Research Center of Medical Information Technology, Ministry of Education, West China Hospital, Sichuan University, Chengdu 610041, China; 283897787@163.com
4. West China Brain Research Centre, West China Hospital, Sichuan University, Chengdu 610041, China
* Correspondence: tianrui17419@wchscu.cn
† Rui Guo and Renjie Zhang have contributed equally to this work and share first authorship.

Abstract: Spontaneous intracerebral hemorrhage (SICH) has been common in China with high morbidity and mortality rates. This study aims to develop a machine learning (ML)-based predictive model for the 90-day evaluation after SICH. We retrospectively reviewed 751 patients with SICH diagnosis and analyzed clinical, radiographic, and laboratory data. A modified Rankin scale (mRS) of 0–2 was defined as a favorable functional outcome, while an mRS of 3–6 was defined as an unfavorable functional outcome. We evaluated 90-day functional outcome and mortality to develop six ML-based predictive models and compared their efficacy with a traditional risk stratification scale, the intracerebral hemorrhage (ICH) score. The predictive performance was evaluated by the areas under the receiver operating characteristic curves (AUC). A total of 553 patients (73.6%) reached the functional outcome at the 3rd month, with the 90-day mortality rate of 10.2%. Logistic regression (LR) and logistic regression CV (LRCV) showed the best predictive performance for functional outcome (AUC = 0.890 and 0.887, respectively), and category boosting presented the best predictive performance for the mortality (AUC = 0.841). Therefore, ML might be of potential assistance in the prediction of the prognosis of SICH.

Keywords: spontaneous intracerebral hemorrhage (SICH); machine learning; 90-day function outcome; mortality

Citation: Guo, R.; Zhang, R.; Liu, R.; Liu, Y.; Li, H.; Ma, L.; He, M.; You, C.; Tian, R. Machine Learning-Based Approaches for Prediction of Patients' Functional Outcome and Mortality after Spontaneous Intracerebral Hemorrhage. *J. Pers. Med.* **2022**, *12*, 112. https://doi.org/10.3390/jpm12010112

Academic Editor: Youxin Wang

Received: 26 October 2021
Accepted: 23 December 2021
Published: 14 January 2022

Publisher's Note: MDPI stays neutral with regard to jurisdictional claims in published maps and institutional affiliations.

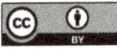

Copyright: © 2022 by the authors. Licensee MDPI, Basel, Switzerland. This article is an open access article distributed under the terms and conditions of the Creative Commons Attribution (CC BY) license (https://creativecommons.org/licenses/by/4.0/).

1. Introduction

Spontaneous intracerebral hemorrhage (SICH), which accounts for 10–30% of all strokes, is the most fatal and disabling type of hemorrhage [1–3]. China has one of the highest disease burdens of SICH in the world [1,4]. Because of the high disability and mortality rates of SICH, outcome-prediction models combining clinical presentations, laboratory data and imaging findings are of great significance and can ensure the optimal care [5]. Several prognostic tools have been proposed for outcome prediction in intracerebral hemorrhage (ICH) such as ICH score [6]. These tools are potentially useful for predicting prognosis, facilitating communication between clinicians, and selecting patients for interventions [7–9]. However, the predictive performance of the 90-day functional outcome and mortality of these tools remains unknown. Besides, the ICH score only consists of the Glasgow Coma Scale (GCS), ICH volume, age, location, and intraventricular extension of the hematoma [6]. Recent studies showed that some laboratory results, such as levels of monocytes and lymphocytes [10–14], offered potential predictive benefits to the outcome of SICH, suggesting that a more accurate model could be made including more variables. Moreover, there is still no widely recognized tool for predicting the prognosis of Chinese SICH patients [15].

As a type of artificial intelligence, machine learning (ML) has several advantages in detecting the possible interactions among attributes and may be useful in the identification of prognostic markers. The key feature of ML is to allow computers to detect underlying patterns by iteratively learning from data, based on which a new model can be created, which prevents the influence from the researchers' intervention. In recent years, ML have been widely applied to the outcome prediction models for cerebrovascular diseases such as ischemic stroke [16,17], aneurysmal subarachnoid hemorrhage [18], and arteriovenous malformations [19]. However, ML-based outcome-prediction models for the SICH in Chinese patients are still rare. The aim of this study was to develop a prognostic model with ML methods to predict the functional outcome and mortality in Chinese patients with SICH according to the initial information on admission to hospital and to compare them with ICH score, the traditional risk stratification scale.

2. Materials and Methods

2.1. Study Population

We retrospectively reviewed SICH patients admitted to West China Hospital during a 2-year period, from 1 January 2018, to 31 December 2019. The diagnosis of SICH was confirmed by head computed tomography (CT) within the first 24 h after admission.

All continuous patients who were diagnosed with SICH during this period and were followed up for more than 3 months were included for further analysis. Extremely severe cases whose families refused any therapy after diagnosis were excluded in this study.

2.2. Data Collection

The study was conducted according to the guidelines of the Declaration of Helsinki and was approved by the Ethics Committee of West China Hospital (protocol code 1.1; 1 July 2017). The data used to develop the ML models were collected from the electronic medical records, including clinical, radiographic, and laboratory variables at the first evaluation. The demographic information, vital signs, radiographic findings, laboratory results, previous medical history, and treatments were collected. The first vital signs (body temperature [BT], heart rate [HR], and blood pressure) after hospital arrival were used. Length of time in the emergency room (ER) meant the period from when the patient first arrived ER to when the patients were transferred to the neurosurgery department or the operating room. The level of consciousness was assessed with GCS. Location of the hematoma (supratentorial, infratentorial, and both supra- and infratentorial), intraventricular hemorrhage (IVH), and the initial hematoma volume were evaluated by CT scan independently by two experienced doctors. The hematoma volume was measured using the ABC/2 method [20], in which A is the greatest diameter on the largest hemorrhage slice, B is the diameter perpendicular to A, and C is the approximate number of axial slices with hemorrhage multiplied by the slice thickness. Levels of complete blood count, blood glucose (BG), triglyceride, total cholesterol, high density lipoprotein cholesterol, low density lipoprotein cholesterol, creatinine, uric acid, sodium, chlorine, fibrinogen, and D-dimer were evaluated in the laboratory of our hospital. Estimated glomerular filtration rate (eGFR) was calculated based on the Chronic Kidney Disease Epidemiology Collaboration (CKD-EPI) equation. The previous medical history, including hypertension, diabetes mellitus (DM), coronary heart disease, kidney diseases, and pulmonary diseases, was obtained by the patients' self-reports or the medical treatment they received.

2.3. In-Hospital Treatments and Outcomes

In-hospital treatments included conservative treatment or surgery (surgical hematoma evacuation). Generally, patients who had a supratentorial hematoma of ≥30 mL or infratentorial hematoma of ≥10 mL were recommended for surgery.

All patients were followed up for at least 3 months. The primary outcome was the functional disability at the 3rd month evaluated by the modified Rankin Scale ([mRS] from 0, no functional deficit, to 6, death). An mRS of 0–2 was defined as a favorable functional outcome, while an mRS of 3–6 was defined as an unfavorable functional outcome in this study. Survival at the 3rd month was evaluated as the secondary outcome.

2.4. Machine Learning ML Algorithms

Firstly, all candidate variables were tested with univariate analysis.

Subsequently, recursive feature elimination with cross-validation (RFECV) was used to obtain the best feature combination for each model. RFECV included two parts: recursive features elimination (RFE) and cross-validation. Given an external estimator, RFE was used to select features by recursively considering increasingly small sets of features. For each ML algorithm, firstly, the estimator was trained on the initial set of features which contained all 41 variables, and the importance of each feature was obtained. Then, the least important feature was pruned from the current set of features. This procedure was recursively repeated on the pruned set until the optimal combination of features was got.

Six ML algorithms, which are efficient and widely used methods for the binary classification, were used in this study. Logistic regression (LR) and LRCV are most wildly used statistical models which in their basic form use a logistic function to model a binary dependent variable [21]. LR and LRCV are of high efficiency, especially for analogously linear datasets, and they are much faster in training models than other ML-based algorithms like support vector machine (SVM) and random forest (RF). SVM is one of the most robust prediction methods, being based on statistical learning frameworks or the Vapnik–Chervonenkis theory. It can efficiently perform not only a linear classification but also a non-linear classification using the kernel trick [22]. RF operates by constructing a multitude of decision trees at training time. For classification tasks, the output of the RF is the class selected by most trees [23]. RF is usually flexible and easy to use in various conditions. Extreme gradient boosting (XGBoost) and category boosting (CatBoost) are typical and widely used ensemble learning algorithms. Ensemble methods use multiple learning algorithms to obtain a better predictive performance than that which could be obtained from any of the constituent learning algorithms alone [24].

In the current study, a five-fold cross-validation was used to build and assess the LR, LRCV, SVM, RF, XGBoost, and CatBoost models. All samples were divided into five approximately equally sized subsamples. Four subsamples were used as training data and the remaining one subsample was retained as the validation set for testing the models. The process was then repeated five times, with each of the five sub-samples used exactly once for validation. The five results from the repetition were then averaged to produce a final estimation. The area under the receiver operator characteristic curve (AUC) was used to evaluate the predictive performance of each model.

2.5. Comparison to the Intracerebral Hemorrhage (ICH) Score

The ICH score was calculated as described previously [6] based on GCS, ICH volume, IVH, location of the hematoma, and age. Its performance (AUC) was compared with the developed ML-based models using a pairwise *t*-test which was commonly used in the previous studies to assess the performance [25–27].

2.6. Statistical Analysis

All statistical analyses were performed in Python programming language, version 3.7 (Python Software Foundation). Qualitative data are described as the frequency and percentage. Fisher's exact test or Chi-square test were used to compare the categorical variables in subgroups. Quantitative data were first tested for normality by the D'Agostino–Pearson test. Normal data are expressed as the mean ± standard deviation (SD), while non-normal data are displayed as the median and interquartile range (IQR). Student's *t*-test was used for the comparison of normal variables, while the Wilcoxon test was used for the comparison of non-normal variables. The performance (AUC) of the different models was compared using the pairwise *t*-test. For all the statistical hypothesis, *p* values < 0.05 were considered significant.

3. Results

3.1. Patient Characteristics

As shown in Figure 1, a total of 829 patients admitted with the diagnosis of SICH in our hospital during the 2-year period (from 1 January 2018, to 31 December 2019) were retrospectively reviewed. Seventy-eight patients were excluded because their family refused any further therapy after the diagnosis. The remaining 751 patients were further analyzed. The overall 90-day mortality was 10.2% ($n = 76$), while 553 patients (73.6%) presented favorable functional outcome at 90-day follow up. The cohort characteristics were presented in Table 1. The raw data supporting the conclusions of this article will be made available by the authors through contacting the corresponding author, without undue reservation.

Table 1. Clinical characteristics of the patients with spontaneous intracerebral hemorrhage (SICH).

Variables	Functional Outcome			Mortality		
	Favorable ($n = 553$)	Unfavorable ($n = 198$)	*p*-Value	Survival ($n = 675$)	Death ($n = 76$)	*p*-Value
Demographics						
Age, years	54.0 (46.0–66.0)	58.9 (43.7–74.0)	0.004 **	54.0 (46.0–66.0)	65.5 (52.5–77.0)	<0.001 ***
Gender, n (%)			0.70			0.20
Female	189 (74.70%)	64 (25.30%)		232 (92.06%)	20 (7.94%)	
Male	364 (73.09%)	134 (26.91%)		443 (88.78%)	56 (11.22%)	
Clinical features						
Location, n (%)			<0.001 ***			<0.001 ***
Supratentorial	475 (78.51%)	130 (21.49%)		556 (91.90%)	49 (8.10%)	
Infratentorial	72 (58.06%)	52 (41.94%)		106 (85.48%)	18 (14.52%)	
Supra and Infra	6 (27.27%)	16 (72.73%)		13 (59.09%)	9 (40.91%)	
Initial volume, mL	25.0 (15.0–35.0)	34.9 (19.3–50.5)	<0.001 ***	25.0 (15.0–35.0)	35.0 (20.0–46.2)	<0.001 ***
IVH, n (%)			<0.001 ***			0.001 **
Yes	253 (63.73%)	144 (36.27%)		342 (86.15%)	55 (13.85%)	
No	300 (84.75%)	54 (15.25%)		333 (94.07%)	21 (5.93%)	
GCS	13 (9–15)	8 (6–8)	<0.001 ***	13 (9–15)	7 (4–10)	<0.001 ***
Length of time in ER, h	1.08 (0.57–2.35)	1.13 (0.65–2.35)	0.48	1.03 (0.57–2.35)	1.47 (0.85–2.35)	0.02 *
BT, °C	36.6 (36.5–36.8)	36.8 (36.5–37.0)	<0.001 ***	36.6 (36.5–36.9)	36.8 (36.5–37.0)	0.02 *
HR, bpm	82 (72–92)	86 (75 -102)	0.001 **	82 (72–93)	94 (80–112)	<0.001 ***
Systolic BP, mmHg	165 (144–183)	164 (130–199)	0.48	165 (144–182)	168 (128 -208)	0.18
Diastolic BP, mmHg	96 (82–107)	92 (81–109)	0.10	96 (82–108)	93.5 (78–107)	0.12
Medical history						
Hypertension, n (%)			0.48			0.24
Yes	429 (72.96%)	159 (27.04%)		524 (77.63%)	64 (82.89%)	
No	124 (76.07%)	39 (23.93%)		151 (22.37%)	12 (15.79%)	
DM, n (%)			0.09			0.007 **
Yes	50 (64.94%)	27 (35.06%)		62 (80.52%)	15 (19.48%)	
No	503 (74.63%)	171 (25.37%)		613 (90.95%)	61 (9.05%)	
Coronary heart disease, n (%)			0.21			0.29
Yes	34 (65.38%)	18 (34.62%)		44 (84.62%)	8 (15.38%)	
No	519 (74.25%)	180 (25.75%)		631 (90.27%)	68 (9.73%)	
Kidney diseases, n (%)			0.16			0.15
Yes	30 (63.83%)	167 (36.17%)		38 (82.61%)	8 (17.39%)	
No	523 (74.29%)	181 (25.71%)		637 (90.35%)	68 (9.65%)	

Table 1. Cont.

Variables	Functional Outcome			Mortality		
	Favorable (n = 553)	Unfavorable (n = 198)	p-Value	Survival (n = 675)	Death (n = 76)	p-Value
Pulmonary diseases, n (%)			0.07			0.15
Yes	68 (66.02%)	35 (33.98%)		88 (85.44%)	15 (14.56%)	
No	485 (74.85%)	163 (25.15%)		587 (90.59%)	61 (9.41%)	
Cigarette smoking, n (%)			0.43			0.31
Yes	175 (75.76%)	56 (24.24%)		212 (91.77%)	19 (8.23%)	
No	378 (75.76%)	142 (27.31%)		463 (89.04%)	57 (10.96%)	
Alcohol consumption, n (%)			0.41			0.76
Yes	170 (75.89%)	54 (24.11%)		203 (90.62%)	21 (9.38%)	
No	383 (72.68%)	144 (27.32%)		472 (89.56%)	54 (10.44%)	
Family history of stroke, n (%)			0.19			0.74
Yes	11 (57.89%)	8 (42.11%)		18 (94.74%)	1 (5.26%)	
No	542 (74.04%)	190 (25.96%)		657 (89.75%)	75 (10.25%)	
Coagulative disorders, n (%)			0.05			0.86
Yes	6 (46.15%)	7 (53.85%)		11 (84.62%)	2 (15.38%)	
No	547 (74.12%)	191 (25.88%)		664 (89.97%)	74 (10.03%)	
Anticoagulation therapy, n (%)			0.19			0.66
Yes	11 (57.89%)	8 (42.11%)		16 (84.21%)	3 (15.79%)	
No	542 (74.04%)	190 (25.96%)		659 (90.03%)	73 (9.97%)	
Antiplatelet therapy, n (%)			0.61			0.07
Yes	2 (50.00%)	2 (50.00%)		2 (50.00%)	2 (50.00%)	
No	551 (73.76%)	196 (26.24%)		673 (90.09%)	74 (9.91%)	
Laboratory studies						
BG, mmol/L	7.16 (6.07–8.85)	9.25 (7.35–11.64)	<0.001 ***	7.38 (6.24–9.41)	9.37 (7.35–12.45)	<0.001 ***
Creatinine, μmol/L	69 (56–84)	72 (60–96)	0.004 **	69 (56–85)	79 (64–116)	<0.001 ***
Uric acid, μmol/L	324 (250–407)	338 (257–419)	0.26	321 (250–407)	348 (288–439)	0.03 *
TG, mmol/L	1.14 (0.80–1.72)	1.21 (0.87–1.73)	0.09	1.13 (0.81–1.69)	1.38 (0.88–1.99)	0.03 *
Cholesterol, mmol/L	4.42 (3.78–5.06)	4.34 (3.68–5.06)	0.36	4.40 (3.76–5.06)	4.36 (3.66–5.12)	0.50
HDLC, mmol/L	1.29 (1.03–1.61)	1.33 (1.03–1.66)	0.19	1.30 (1.04–1.63)	1.31 (1.02–1.61)	0.33
LDLC, mmol/L	2.60 (2.08–3.21)	2.51 (1.91–3.24)	0.11	2.60 (2.05–3.21)	2.40 (1.83–3.3)	0.07
Sodium, mmol/L	138.4 (136.1–140.3)	138.3 (134.0–142.6)	0.29	138.4 (136.1–140.4)	137.9 (133.6–142.3)	0.45
Chlorine, mmol/L	101.4 (98.8–104.3)	100.5 (95.5–105.4)	0.002 **	101.3 (98.6–104.3)	99.6 (94.8–104.4)	0.001 **
eGFR, mL/min	91.0 (87.7–103.5)	91.0 (77.2–100.9)	<0.001 ***	91.0 (87.0–103.6)	86.0 (63.6–91.0)	<0.001 ***
Platelet, 10^9 cells/L	170 (129–217)	184 (136–222)	0.12	175 (131–218)	175 (98–252)	0.35
WBC, 10^9 cells/L	10.11 (7.58–12.99)	11.91 (9.22–15.43)	<0.001 ***	10.54 (7.76–13.22)	11.62 (8.24–16.45)	0.006 **
ANC, 10^9 cells/L	8.43 (5.67–11.25)	10.33 (7.09–13.26)	<0.001 ***	8.81 (5.91–11.51)	9.64 (6.17–13.57)	0.03 *
ALC, 10^9 cells/L	1.09 (0.76–1.48)	1.17 (0.72–1.82)	0.08	1.09 (0.75–1.51)	1.19 (0.73–1.99)	0.06
AMC, 10^9 cells/L	0.39 (0.26–0.53)	0.42 (0.28–0.62)	0.006 **	0.4 (0.26–0.54)	0.47 (0.30–0.62)	0.02 *
Hematocrit	0.41 (0.38–0.44)	0.41 (0.37–0.44)	0.29	0.41 (0.38–0.44)	0.42 (0.37–0.44)	0.23
Fibrinogen, g/L	2.77 (2.26–3.41)	2.74 (2.16–3.57)	0.44	2.75 (2.24–3.42)	2.77 (2.28–3.61)	0.27
D-dimer, mg/L FEU	0.64 (0.31–1.94)	1.43 (0.63–2.84)	<0.001 ***	0.72 (0.32–2.16)	2.37 (0.80–5.24)	<0.001 ***
Treatment, n (%)			0.92			0.74
Surgery	172 (73.19%)	63 (26.81%)		213 (90.64%)	22 (9.36%)	
Conservative	381 (73.84%)	135 (26.16%)		462 (89.53%)	54 (10.47%)	

* $p < 0.05$; ** $p < 0.01$; *** $p < 0.001$. ANC, absolute neutrophil count; ALC, absolute lymphocyte count; AMC, absolute monocyte count; BG, blood glucose; BT, body temperature; DM, diabetes mellitus; eGFR, estimated glomerular filtration rate; ER, emergency room; GCS, Glasgow Coma Scale; HR, heart rate; IVH, intraventricular hemorrhage; TG, triglyceride; WBC, white blood cell; HDLC, high-density lipoprotein cholesterol; LDLC, low-density lipoprotein cholesterol.

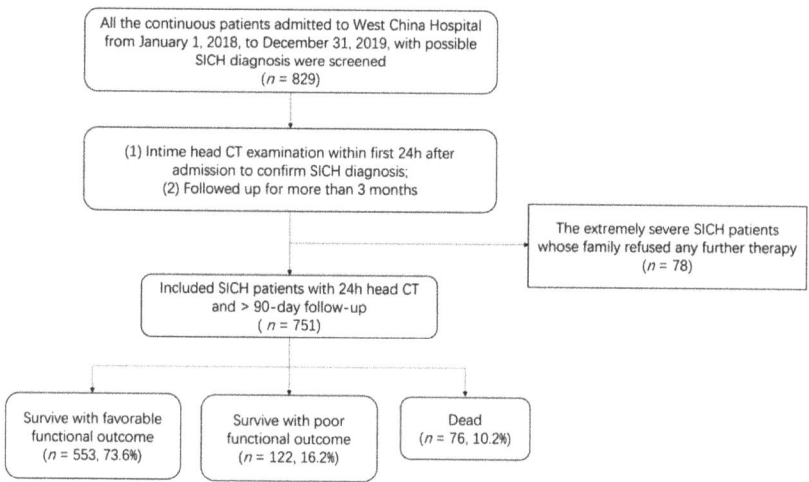

Figure 1. Flowchart of SICH patient inclusion and exclusion.

3.2. Predictive Performance of the ML-Based Models

The intact algorithms for all the models with the optimal parameters were shown in the Supplementary Materials.

Among all the ML-based models, LR and LRCV showed the best predictive performance for the functional outcome at the 3rd month (AUC = 0.890 and 0.887, respectively, Table 2 and Figure 2), followed by CatBoost, XGBoost, RF, and SVM (AUC = 0.871, 0.864, 0.862, 0.849, respectively). In both LR and LRCV models, location of the hematoma, coagulation disorders, AMC, GCS, and intraventricular hemorrhage contributed materially to the models (Table 3).

The predictive performance for the 90-day mortality was assessed by the similar method. As shown in Table 2 and Figure 3, CatBoost and LRCV provided the best predictive performance for the mortality outcome (AUC = 0.841 and 0.844, respectively). The AUCs of the other four models were as follows: LR, 0.837; XGBoost, 0.820; RF, 0.818; SVM, 0.777. As shown in Table 3, GCS, Age, D-dimer, and HR contributed largely to CatBoost, while AMC, location of the hematoma, and history of diabetes mellitus contributed significantly to LRCV.

Table 2. Predictive performance for the 90-day functional outcome and mortality after spontaneous intracerebral hemorrhage.

Algorithm	Functional Outcome		Mortality	
	AUC, Mean	AUC, 95%CI	AUC, Mean	AUC, 95% CI
ICH score	0.856	0.827–0.884	0.790	0.712–0.867
LR	0.890	0.858–0.922	0.837	0.780–0.894
LRCV	0.887	0.855–0.920	0.844	0.807–0.881
SVM	0.849	0.804–0.894	0.777	0.720–0.833
RF	0.862	0.813–0.912	0.818	0.718–0.917
XGBoost	0.863	0.815–0.911	0.820	0.741–0.899
CatBoost	0.871	0.829–0.913	0.841	0.774–0.907

AUC, area under the receiver operator characteristic curve; CatBoost, Category Boosting; CI, confidence interval; ICH, intracerebral hemorrhage; LR, logistic regression; SD, standard deviation; SVM; support vector machine; RF, random forest; XGBoost, extreme gradient boosting.

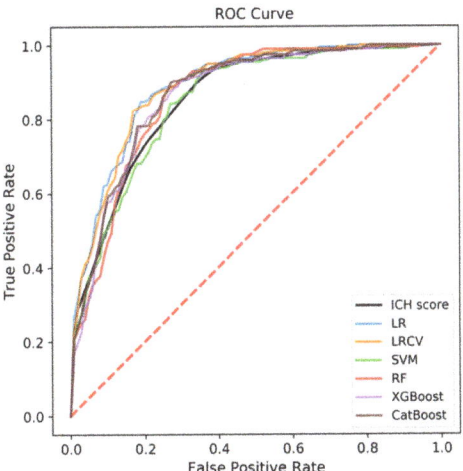

Figure 2. The receiver operating characteristic (ROC) curve of all the six machine learning (ML)-based models compared with the traditional ICH Score, with respect to predictive performance for the functional outcome at the third month.

Table 3. List of variables used in the final model.

Algorithm	Variables for Functional Outcome [a]	Variables for Mortality [a]
LR	Coagulation disorders, Location of the hematoma, GCS, IVH, AMC, BG, BT, D-dimer, Age, ANC, Chlorine	Location of the hematoma, AMC, GCS, DM, WBC, D-Dimer, ANC, BG, Age, Chlorine, IVH, HR, Time in ER, BT
LRCV	Coagulation disorders, Location of the hematoma, AMC, GCS, IVH, BG, ANC, WBC, D-dimer, Age, BT	AMC, Location of the hematoma, DM, GCS, WBC, ANC, IVH, D-Dimer, Age, Chlorine, BG, TG, HR, Hematoma volume, BT
SVM [b]	-	-
RF	GCS, BG, Hematoma volume, Location of the hematoma, D-Dimer, IVH	GCS, D-dimer, Age, BG, HR, eGFR, Time in ER, Hematoma volume, Chlorine, ANC, WBC, Location of the hematoma, Creatine, Uric acid, TG, BT, IVH, DM
XGBoost	GCS, BG, D-dimer, Location of the hematoma, eGFR, Hematoma volume, Age, WBC, Creatine, Chlorine	GCS, D-dimer, Age, WBC, Location of the hematoma, Hematoma volume, eGFR, HR, Chlorine, Time in ER, Creatine, ANC, TG
CatBoost	GCS, BG, D-dimer	GCS, Age, D-dimer, HR, Time in ER, Chlorine, eGFR, Location of the hematoma, Hematoma volume

[a] Variables are listed according to the importance. [b] Because of the mechanism of SVM, the importance of variables cannot be accessed. AMC, absolute monocyte count; ANC, absolute neutrophil count; BG, blood glucose; BT, body temperature; CatBoost, Category Boosting; DM, diabetes mellitus; eGFR, estimated glomerular filtration rate; ER, emergency room; GCS, Glasgow Coma Scale; HR, heart rate; IVH, intraventricular hemorrhage; LR, logistic regression; RF, random forest; SVM; support vector machine; TG, triglyceride; WBC, white blood cell; XGBoost, extreme gradient boosting.

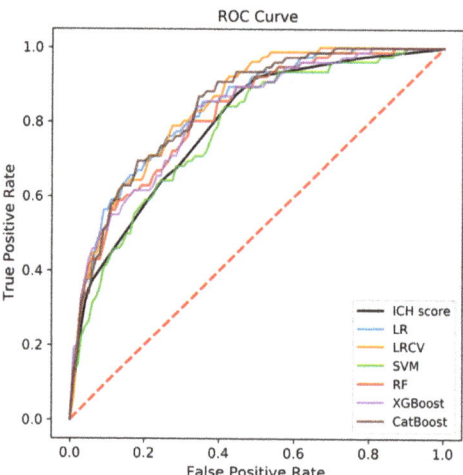

Figure 3. The ROC curve of all the six ML-based models compared with the traditional ICH Score, with respect to predictive performance for the 90-day mortality at the third month.

3.3. Comparison to ICH Score

As shown in Supplementary Table S1, predictive performance for the functional outcome of LR (AUC = 0.890, $p < 0.001$) and LRCV (AUC = 0.887, $p = 0.001$) were significantly better than that of ICH score (AUC = 0.856). Besides, CatBoost (AUC = 0.841, $p = 0.03$) and XGBoost (AUC = 0.820, $p = 0.05$) showed significantly better performance to predict the 90-day mortality than ICH score (AUC = 0.790).

4. Discussion

The prognosis prediction of SICH has long been dependent on the ICH score. Recent studies revealed the promising role of some laboratory results (such as levels of monocytes and lymphocytes) in the SICH outcome prediction. However, the ICH score, a traditional and widely-used prognostic predictive method, consists of the GCS, ICH volume, age, location, and intraventricular extension of the hematoma [6], without involvement of any laboratory results. In this study, we built distinctive ML-based models to develop a more accurate model involving multiple variables, in order to predict the 90-day functional outcome and mortality with better efficacy.

In this study, we developed 6 ML-based models for predicting the outcome of SICH. We analyzed the clinical characteristics, radiographic results, laboratory results, and previous medical history of 751 consecutive SICH patients by reviewing their medical records. The results showed that LR and LRCV were the most accurate models to predict the functional outcome with an AUC of 0.890 and 0.887, respectively, both of which were significantly better than that of ICH score. Besides, CatBoost and LRCV showed the best performance in the prediction of the 90-day mortality (AUC = 0.841 and 0.844, respectively), and they were also significantly more accurate than ICH score.

Patients with the favorable functional outcome were significantly different from those with the unfavorable functional outcome in 15 variables, including age (younger), location of the hematoma (supratentorial), initial hematoma volume (smaller), IVH (without), GCS (greater), BT (lower), HR (lower), BG (lower), creatinine (lower), chlorine (higher), eGFR (higher), WBC (lower), absolute neutrophil count (ANC, lower), absolute monocyte count (AMC, lower), and D-dimer (lower, $p = 0.004$, <0.001, <0.001, <0.001, <0.001, <0.001, 0.001, <0.001, 0.004, 0.002, <0.001, <0.001, <0.001, 0.006, <0.001, respectively).

Similar results were shown when considering 90-day mortality (Table 1). Patients who survived 90 days after SICH were significantly different from the others in age (younger), location of the hematoma (supratentorial), hematoma volume (smaller), GCS (higher), time in ER (shorter), BT (lower), HR (lower), DM (without), BG (lower), creatine (lower), uric acid (lower), triglyceride (lower), chlorine (higher), eGFR (higher), WBC (lower), ANC (lower), AMC (lower), and D-dimer (lower).

Both the univariate analysis and the feature importance analysis of the ML-based models illuminated that the level of the absolute monocyte cells provided a significant contribution to the prediction of both 90-day mortality and functional outcome. Higher levels of monocytes indicated a poor outcome of SICH. The recruitment of monocytes is a key feature of inflammation [28]. In 2016, Morotti et al. [10] illuminated that a higher level of monocyte on admission was directly associated with a higher risk of hematoma expansion, which might suggest a more unfavorable outcome. Indeed, many previous studies concluded that an elevated level of the monocyte was an independent risk factor for 30-day mortality in SICH patients, suggesting that monocyte level on admission might help predict the outcome of SICH [11–14], which was consistent with our study. Using ML technology, the monocyte level was proved to have significant predictive benefit of the 90-day outcome of SICH, which also suggested that additional knowledge could be obtained, benefiting from ML algorithms.

In clinical practice, the most widely used risk stratification scale for ICH, the ICH score, consists of GCS, ICH volume, age, location, and intraventricular extension of the hematoma [6]. The ICH score predicts the 30-day mortality after ICH. As our results displayed, some ML-based models performed significantly better than the ICH score in predicting both 90-day functional outcome and 90-day mortality. Overall, our results demonstrate how the data mining approach can be used as an alternative to the conventional approach, achieving comparable performance to well accepted prognostic models.

In this study, RFE was used to select the optimal combination of features by recursively considering smaller and smaller sets of features according to the importance, which enumerated almost all the combinations. Although this method is not so efficient, it is the best way to improve the performance of the model. Besides RFE, minimum redundancy maximum relevance (MrMr) and the Boruta algorithm are also efficient and widely-used methods for feature selection. According to Peng et al., MrMr can use either mutual information, correlation, or distance/similarity scores to select features. However, this algorithm may underestimate the importance of each of the seemingly insignificant variables with poor performance, which may turn significant when organized into ML-based models. Thus, MrMr is mostly used when variables are categorical. However, there are many quantitative variables in our datasets. Similar to MrMr, the Boruta algorithm optimizes the combination of variables by reducing the relevancy between the selected variables and increasing the relevancy between the variables and outcomes. Although these methods are more efficient in feature selection, RFE can provide a better performing model by enumeration.

This study has several clinical and methodological implications. Firstly, the factors which were previously neglected could be discovered. Together with these factors, the predictive performance could be improved using machine learning approaches. Secondly, the best model in the present study only contained a small number of variables. Thus, these models can be used easily in clinical practice to provide an accessible prediction of the outcome in SICH patients, which helps both the doctors and patients' families to choose the optimal management. Based on our studies, online websites were developed [http://114.251.235.51:1226/ich_recover_predict (accessed on 2 January 2022) for 90-day functional outcome; http://114.251.235.51:1226/ich_death_predict (accessed on 2 January 2022) for 90-day mortality]. Furthermore, our results eliminated that the predictive performance of the ML-based models remained high even when plenty of variables were input. Nowadays, since the electronic medical records are widely used, much larger datasets are needed to be manipulated in the future. ML algorithms are much more suitable to deal with the increasing number of variables than the traditional statistical methods.

However, our study had several limitations. First, some patients in critical conditions were not included in the study because of early withdrawal of care. Second, the sample size of our retrospective study may limit the improvement of the model performance. Third, the primary aim of this study was to predict the 90-day outcome of ICH patients based on the initial information on admission to hospital, thus serial changes of variables after admission were not considered. Moreover, external validation is lacking in the present study, which may restrict the generalizability of our results. Future studies with larger samples may help provide a higher predictive power.

5. Conclusions

In conclusion, the prediction of functional outcome and mortality after SICH is a challenge. Our findings suggested that the ML-based model is of high potential. The CatBoost and LRCV models are of good predictive performance for 90-day mortality with considerable accuracy, while the LRCV and LR models are of reliable predictive performance for 90-day functional outcome, all of which were better than ICH score, the traditional and widely-used risk stratification scale. These models might provide additional assistance in the prediction of functional outcome or mortality for SICH patients.

Supplementary Materials: The following are available online at https://www.mdpi.com/article/10.3390/jpm12010112/s1. Supplementary Table S1: The comparison between the ML models and the ICH score. Supplementary Code: The intact algorithms.

Author Contributions: Conceptualization, R.T. and R.G.; methodology, R.G. and R.Z.; software, R.Z. and R.L.; validation, R.G., R.Z. and R.T.; formal analysis, R.Z.; data curation, R.Z. and R.L.; writing—original draft preparation, R.G.; writing—review and editing, R.Z. and R.T.; visualization, R.T. and R.L.; supervision, H.L., L.M., M.H. and C.Y.; project administration, C.Y. and R.T.; funding acquisition, R.T., Y.L., L.M. and M.H. All authors have read and agreed to the published version of the manuscript.

Funding: This research was funded by (1) National Key R&D Program of China, grant number 2018YFA0108603; (2) 1·3·5 Project for Disciplines of Excellence, West China Hospital, Sichuan University, grant number 2021HXFH014; (3) Clinical Research Innovation Project, West China Hospital, Sichuan University, grant number 2019HXCX07.

Institutional Review Board Statement: The study was conducted according to the guidelines of the Declaration of Helsinki and was approved by the Ethics Committee of West China Hospital (protocol code 1.1; 1 July 2017).

Informed Consent Statement: Informed consent was obtained from all subjects involved in the study.

Data Availability Statement: The data presented in this study are available on request from the corresponding author. The data are not publicly available due to data-safety restrictions.

Acknowledgments: The authors thank the patients who were involved in this study.

Conflicts of Interest: The authors declare no conflict of interest. The funders had no role in the design of the study; in the collection, analyses, or interpretation of data; in the writing of the manuscript, or in the decision to publish the results.

References

1. Feigin, V.L.; Stark, B.A.; Johnson, C.O.; Roth, G.A.; Bisignano, C.; Abady, G.G.; Abbasifard, M.; Abbasi-Kangevari, M.; Abd-Allah, F.; Abedi, V.; et al. Global, regional, and national burden of stroke and its risk factors, 1990–2019: A systematic analysis for the Global Burden of Disease Study 2019. *Lancet Neurol.* **2021**, *20*, 795–820. [CrossRef]
2. Shoamanesh, A.; Patrice Lindsay, M.; Castellucci, L.A.; Cayley, A.; Crowther, M.; de Wit, K.; English, S.W.; Hoosein, S.; Huynh, T.; Kelly, M.; et al. Canadian stroke best practice recommendations: Management of Spontaneous Intracerebral Hemorrhage, 7th Edition Update 2020. *Int. J. Stroke Off. J. Int. Stroke Soc.* **2021**, *16*, 321–341. [CrossRef]
3. Steiner, T.; Salman, R.A.-S.; Beer, R.; Christensen, H.; Cordonnier, C.; Csiba, L.; Forsting, M.; Harnof, S.; Klijn, C.; Krieger, D.; et al. European Stroke Organisation (ESO) Guidelines for the Management of Spontaneous Intracerebral Hemorrhage. *Int. J. Stroke* **2014**, *9*, 840–855. [CrossRef] [PubMed]
4. Flaherty, M.L.; Woo, D.; Haverbusch, M.; Sekar, P.; Khoury, J.; Sauerbeck, L.; Moomaw, C.J.; Schneider, A.; Kissela, B.; Kleindorfer, D.; et al. Racial Variations in Location and Risk of Intracerebral Hemorrhage. *Stroke* **2005**, *36*, 934–937. [CrossRef]

5. Gregório, T.; Pipa, S.; Cavaleiro, P.; Atanásio, G.; Albuquerque, I.; Chaves, P.C.; Azevedo, L. Prognostic models for intracerebral hemorrhage: Systematic review and meta-analysis. *BMC Med. Res. Methodol.* **2018**, *18*, 145. [CrossRef]
6. Hemphill, J.C., 3rd; Bonovich, D.C.; Besmertis, L.; Manley, G.T.; Johnston, S.C. The ICH score: A simple, reliable grading scale for intracerebral hemorrhage. *Stroke* **2001**, *32*, 891–897. [CrossRef]
7. Gupta, V.P.; Garton, A.L.; Sisti, J.A.; Christophe, B.R.; Lord, A.; Lewis, A.; Frey, H.-P.; Claassen, J.; Connolly, E.S. Prognosticating Functional Outcome After Intracerebral Hemorrhage: The ICHOP Score. *World Neurosurg.* **2017**, *101*, 577–583. [CrossRef]
8. Hall, A.N.; Weaver, B.; Liotta, E.; Maas, M.B.; Faigle, R.; Mroczek, D.K.; Naidech, A.M. Identifying Modifiable Predictors of Patient Outcomes After Intracerebral Hemorrhage with Machine Learning. *Neurocritical Care* **2021**, *34*, 73–84. [CrossRef]
9. Wang, H.-L.; Hsu, W.-Y.; Lee, M.-H.; Weng, H.-H.; Chang, S.-W.; Yang, J.-T.; Tsai, Y.-H. Automatic Machine-Learning-Based Outcome Prediction in Patients With Primary Intracerebral Hemorrhage. *Front. Neurol.* **2019**, *10*, 910. [CrossRef] [PubMed]
10. Morotti, A.; Phuah, C.-L.; Anderson, C.D.; Jessel, M.J.; Schwab, K.; Ayres, A.M.; Pezzini, A.; Padovani, A.; Gurol, E.; Viswanathan, A.; et al. Leukocyte Count and Intracerebral Hemorrhage Expansion. *Stroke* **2016**, *47*, 1473–1478. [CrossRef] [PubMed]
11. Adeoye, O.; Walsh, K.; Woo, J.G.; Haverbusch, M.; Moomaw, C.J.; Broderick, J.P.; Kissela, B.M.; Kleindorfer, D.; Flaherty, M.L.; Woo, D. Peripheral Monocyte Count Is Associated with Case Fatality after Intracerebral Hemorrhage. *J. Stroke Cerebrovasc. Dis. Off. J. Natl. Stroke Assoc.* **2014**, *23*, e107–e111. [CrossRef]
12. Mackey, J.; Blatsioris, A.D.; Saha, C.; Moser, E.A.S.; Carter, R.J.L.; Cohen-Gadol, A.A.; Leipzig, T.J.; Williams, L.S. Higher Monocyte Count is Associated with 30-Day Case Fatality in Intracerebral Hemorrhage. *Neurocritical Care* **2021**, *34*, 456–464. [CrossRef] [PubMed]
13. Walsh, K.B.; Sekar, P.; Langefeld, C.D.; Moomaw, C.J.; Elkind, M.S.; Boehme, A.K.; James, M.; Osborne, J.; Sheth, K.N.; Woo, D.; et al. Monocyte Count and 30-Day Case Fatality in Intracerebral Hemorrhage. *Stroke* **2015**, *46*, 2302–2304. [CrossRef] [PubMed]
14. Li, J.; Yuan, Y.; Liao, X.; Yu, Z.; Li, H.; Zheng, J. Prognostic Significance of Admission Systemic Inflammation Response Index in Patients With Spontaneous Intracerebral Hemorrhage: A Propensity Score Matching Analysis. *Front. Neurol.* **2021**, *12*, 718032. [CrossRef]
15. Wu, S.; Wu, B.; Liu, M.; Chen, Z.; Wang, W.; Anderson, C.S.; Sandercock, P.; Wang, Y.; Huang, Y.; Cui, L.; et al. Stroke in China: Advances and challenges in epidemiology, prevention, and management. *Lancet Neurol.* **2019**, *18*, 394–405. [CrossRef]
16. Kuang, H.; Qiu, W.; Boers, A.M.; Brown, S.; Muir, K.; Majoie, C.B.; Dippel, D.W.; White, P.; Epstein, J.; Mitchell, P.J.; et al. Computed Tomography Perfusion–Based Machine Learning Model Better Predicts Follow-Up Infarction in Patients with Acute Ischemic Stroke. *Stroke* **2021**, *52*, 223–231. [CrossRef] [PubMed]
17. Teo, Y.H.; Lim, I.C.Z.; Tseng, F.S.; Teo, Y.N.; Kow, C.S.; Ng, Z.H.C.; Ko, N.C.K.; Sia, C.-H.; Leow, A.S.T.; Yeung, W.; et al. Predicting Clinical Outcomes in Acute Ischemic Stroke Patients Undergoing Endovascular Thrombectomy with Machine Learning: A Systematic Review and Meta-analysis. *Clin. Neuroradiol.* **2021**, *31*, 1121–1130. [CrossRef] [PubMed]
18. Rubbert, C.; Patil, K.R.; Beseoglu, K.; Mathys, C.; May, R.; Kaschner, M.G.; Sigl, B.; Teichert, N.A.; Boos, J.; Turowski, B.; et al. Prediction of outcome after aneurysmal subarachnoid haemorrhage using data from patient admission. *Eur. Radiol.* **2018**, *28*, 4949–4958. [CrossRef] [PubMed]
19. Asadi, H.; Kok, H.K.; Looby, S.; Brennan, P.; O'Hare, A.; Thornton, J. Outcomes and Complications After Endovascular Treatment of Brain Arteriovenous Malformations: A Prognostication Attempt Using Artificial Intelligence. *World Neurosurg.* **2016**, *96*, 562–569. [CrossRef] [PubMed]
20. Divani, A.A.; Majidi, S.; Luo, X.; Souslian, F.G.; Zhang, J.; Abosch, A.; Tummala, R.P. The ABCs of Accurate Volumetric Measurement of Cerebral Hematoma. *Stroke* **2011**, *42*, 1569–1574. [CrossRef]
21. Tolles, J.; Meurer, W.J. Logistic Regression: Relating Patient Characteristics to Outcomes. *JAMA* **2016**, *316*, 533–534. [CrossRef] [PubMed]
22. Cortes, C.; Vapnik, V. Support-vector networks. *Mach. Learn.* **1995**, *20*, 273–297. [CrossRef]
23. Ho, T.K. The random subspace method for constructing decision forests. *IEEE Trans. Pattern Anal. Mach. Intell.* **1998**, *20*, 832–844. [CrossRef]
24. Opitz, D.; Maclin, R. Popular Ensemble Methods: An Empirical Study. *J. Artif. Intell. Res.* **1999**, *11*, 169–198. [CrossRef]
25. Al-Mallah, M.H.; Elshawi, R.; Ahmed, A.M.; Qureshi, W.T.; Brawner, C.A.; Blaha, M.J.; Ahmed, H.M.; Ehrman, J.K.; Keteyian, S.J.; Sakr, S. Using Machine Learning to Define the Association between Cardiorespiratory Fitness and All-Cause Mortality (from the Henry Ford Exercise Testing Project). *Am. J. Cardiol.* **2017**, *120*, 2078–2084. [CrossRef] [PubMed]
26. Shouval, R.; Hadanny, A.; Shlomo, N.; Iakobishvili, Z.; Unger, R.; Zahger, D.; Alcalai, R.; Atar, S.; Gottlieb, S.; Matetzky, S.; et al. Machine learning for prediction of 30-day mortality after ST elevation myocardial infraction: An Acute Coronary Syndrome Israeli Survey data mining study. *Int. J. Cardiol.* **2017**, *246*, 7–13. [CrossRef] [PubMed]
27. Liu, Y.; Liu, X.; Hong, X.; Liu, P.; Bao, X.; Yao, Y.; Xing, B.; Li, Y.; Huang, Y.; Zhu, H.; et al. Prediction of Recurrence after Transsphenoidal Surgery for Cushing's Disease: The Use of Machine Learning Algorithms. *Neuroendocrinology* **2019**, *108*, 201–210. [CrossRef] [PubMed]
28. Kratofil, R.M.; Kubes, P.; Deniset, J.F. Monocyte Conversion During Inflammation and Injury. *Arter. Thromb. Vasc. Biol.* **2017**, *37*, 35–42. [CrossRef] [PubMed]

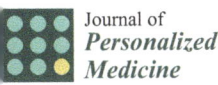

Article

Random Forest Model in the Diagnosis of Dementia Patients with Normal Mini-Mental State Examination Scores

Jie Wang [1], Zhuo Wang [2], Ning Liu [2], Caiyan Liu [1], Chenhui Mao [1], Liling Dong [1], Jie Li [1], Xinying Huang [1], Dan Lei [1], Shanshan Chu [1], Jianyong Wang [2,*] and Jing Gao [1,*]

1. Department of Neurology, State Key Laboratory of Complex Severe and Rare Diseases, Peking Union Medical College Hospital, Chinese Academy of Medical Science and Peking Union Medical College, Beijing 100730, China; wangjie_smu@163.com (J.W.); liucy-pumch@163.com (C.L.); maochenhui@pumch.cn (C.M.); sophie_d@163.com (L.D.); jielicathy@126.com (J.L.); hxypumch@163.com (X.H.); ld94616@163.com (D.L.); chuss9486@163.com (S.C.)
2. Department of Computer Science and Technology, Tsinghua University, Beijing 100084, China; wang-z18@mails.tsinghua.edu.cn (Z.W.); victorliucs@gmail.com (N.L.)
* Correspondence: jianyong@tsinghua.edu.cn (J.W.); gj107@163.com (J.G.); Tel.: +86-10-62789150 (J.W.); +86-13011809777 (J.G.)

Citation: Wang, J.; Wang, Z.; Liu, N.; Liu, C.; Mao, C.; Dong, L.; Li, J.; Huang, X.; Lei, D.; Chu, S.; et al. Random Forest Model in the Diagnosis of Dementia Patients with Normal Mini-Mental State Examination Scores. *J. Pers. Med.* **2022**, *12*, 37. https://doi.org/10.3390/jpm12010037

Academic Editor: Niels Bergsland

Received: 23 November 2021
Accepted: 31 December 2021
Published: 4 January 2022

Publisher's Note: MDPI stays neutral with regard to jurisdictional claims in published maps and institutional affiliations.

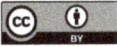

Copyright: © 2022 by the authors. Licensee MDPI, Basel, Switzerland. This article is an open access article distributed under the terms and conditions of the Creative Commons Attribution (CC BY) license (https://creativecommons.org/licenses/by/4.0/).

Abstract: Background: Mini-Mental State Examination (MMSE) is the most widely used tool in cognitive screening. Some individuals with normal MMSE scores have extensive cognitive impairment. Systematic neuropsychological assessment should be performed in these patients. This study aimed to optimize the systematic neuropsychological test battery (NTB) by machine learning and develop new classification models for distinguishing mild cognitive impairment (MCI) and dementia among individuals with MMSE $\geq$ 26. **Methods:** 375 participants with MMSE $\geq$ 26 were assigned a diagnosis of cognitively unimpaired (CU) (n = 67), MCI (n = 174), or dementia (n = 134). We compared the performance of five machine learning algorithms, including logistic regression, decision tree, SVM, XGBoost, and random forest (RF), in identifying MCI and dementia. **Results:** RF performed best in identifying MCI and dementia. Six neuropsychological subtests with high-importance features were selected to form a simplified NTB, and the test time was cut in half. The AUC of the RF model was 0.89 for distinguishing MCI from CU, and 0.84 for distinguishing dementia from nondementia. **Conclusions:** This simplified cognitive assessment model can be useful for the diagnosis of MCI and dementia in patients with normal MMSE. It not only optimizes the content of cognitive evaluation, but also improves diagnosis and reduces missed diagnosis.

Keywords: machine learning; dementia; cognitive dysfunction; neuropsychological tests; mental status and dementia tests

1. Introduction

The prevalence of dementia is rising with the aging of the population, affecting the quality of life and increasing the burden on society and the family [1]. Mild cognitive impairment (MCI) is considered a transitional stage between normal aging and dementia, with a higher risk of developing dementia. The diagnosis of MCI and dementia early has prognostic value [2,3].

The most widely used screening tool for dementia is the Mini-Mental State Examination (MMSE) [4], a 30-point instrument that assesses several domains including orientation, attention, language, memory, and executive function. MMSE has good sensitivity and specificity for detecting dementia. Creavin et al. reported that in the community, a pooled sensitivity of 0.85 and specificity of 0.90 at a cut point of 24, and sensitivity of 0.87 and specificity of 0.82 at a cut point of 25 [5]. Pooled estimates of 15 studies showed a sensitivity of 0.89 and specificity of 0.89 at a cut point of 23 or less or 24 or less [6]. However, the sensitivity (0.20–0.93) and specificity (0.48–0.93) to detect MCI vary significantly in different studies, meaning less consistent estimates for test accuracy [6]. Thus, its ability to distinguish between cognitively impaired subjects and cognitively unimpaired (CU) adults is limited [7–9], leading to the possibility that some patients with normal MMSE scores but cognitive impairment may be missed.

For these individuals with normal MMSE scores, a more comprehensive cognitive assessment is needed. The systematic neuropsychological test battery (NTB) designed by the Peking Union Medical College Hospital (PUMCH) consists of more than 20 subtests to evaluate five cognitive domains: executive function, visuospatial ability, language, memory, and abstract reasoning and calculation [10]. It takes into account Chinese culture and language and is suitable for the Chinese elderly to detect MCI and dementia. All these subtests have been used and validated in the Chinese population, and normative population data were available. However, administering such a comprehensive battery is time-consuming.

Recent studies had shown that machine learning (ML) exhibited excellent performance in identifying MCI and dementia [11–17], but these mostly used biomarker data such as neuroimaging and CSF components that were expensive technologies [12,13,16]. ML diagnostic models based on cognitive data were gradually being applied [11,15,18,19]. Random forest (RF), an ensemble ML method based on a set of decision trees, has positive significance in processing complex neuropsychological data and excellent predictive performance for the diagnosis of cognitive impairment [15]. Using the feature selection method in RF, we can determine the importance of features and delete insignificant ones, thereby reducing the complexity of the NTB.

Therefore, the purpose of this study was to use RF to simplify the NTB and shorten evaluation time. Several important neuropsychological subtests were selected, and new RF models were developed to classify CU, MCI, and dementia for people with normal MMSE scores.

2. Materials and Methods

2.1. Participants

375 (67 CU adults, 174 MCI patients and 134 dementia patients) participants were enrolled consecutively from the PUMCH dementia cohort, the Dementia Clinic of the Department of Neurology of PUMCH between May 2009 to April 2021. They received a detailed clinical evaluation that included medical history taking, physical and neurological examinations, a systemic of neuropsychological tests, laboratory testing, and neuroimaging studies (head CT or MRI). The inclusion criteria included MMSE score $\geq$ 26, with normal function in motor, sensory, balance, reflex, and ability to complete all neuropsychological tests. Patients with significant functional disabilities, a history of major psychiatric illness, or any other central nervous system disorders other than cognitive impairment were excluded.

2.2. Neuropsychological Examinations

Cognitive tests included the Chinese version of the MMSE [20] and the PUMCH version of Montreal cognitive assessment (MoCA-P) [10]. Previous studies had shown that MMSE scores were influenced by age, gender, and particularly years of education [9]. Several studies that investigated the normative data of the MMSE in the Chinese population got different optimal cut-off points ranging from 19 to 26 for dementia screening [9,21,22]. In this study, we defined $\geq$26 points as normal MMSE scores. A Chinese version of ADL was used to determine impairment in everyday functioning [23], which was revised and supplemented according to the scale of Lawton and Brody [24], consisting of eight activities focused on instrumental ADL (IADL) (including using telephone, shopping, food preparation, housekeeping, laundry, transportation, managing medications, and handling finances) and 12 activities focused on the basic ADL (BADL) (e.g., dressing, bathing, eating, getting in or out of bed, using the toilet and so on). Each item of ADL range from 1 to 4 (1 = can do it myself, 2 = have some difficulty doing but can still do it by myself, 3 = need help to do it, 4 = cannot do it at all). The lowest ADL score was 20 points, indicating that the patient's ability was completely normal, and the highest was 80 points. The Hospital Anxiety and Depression (HAD) scale was used to screen for anxiety and depression among patients [25]. Participants were administered the above assessments as the diagnostic neuropsychological measures.

All subjects underwent the systemic NTB to evaluate five cognitive domains. These were: (1) Executive function: category verbal fluency [26], the digit symbol test (DST) [27], the trail making test A (TMT A) [28], the clock drawing test [8], paired-associate learning (PAL) of The Clinical Memory Test [29], the block design test of the Aphasia Battery of Chinese [30], and modified Luria three-step task [31]; (2) Visuospatial ability: the block design test and figure copying of the Aphasia Battery of Chinese [30], the copy of a modified Rey-Osterrieth figure [32], and gestures imitation; (3) Language: several subtests of the Aphasia Battery of Chinese including spontaneous speech, auditory comprehension, repetition, and naming [30]; (4) Memory: PAL, the logical memory test (LMT) of the modified Wechsler Memory Scale [33], and the auditory verbal learning test-Huashan version (AVLT-H) [34] were used to assess verbal memory. Nonverbal memory was measured by the modified Rey-Osterreith with a 10-min free recall; and (5) Abstract reasoning and calculation: subtests of the Wechsler Adult Intelligence Scale including similarities and calculations [27]. All subtests of NTB were not used to assist in making the clinical diagnosis of MCI or dementia, but as screening tests for machine learning.

2.3. Diagnostic Criteria

A clinical diagnosis of CU, MCI, or dementia was made based on all available information including clinical history and neuropsychological measures. MCI and dementia were diagnosed based on clinical judgment and/or on cognitive test performance according to the clinical criteria of the National Institute on Aging and the Alzheimer's Association (NIA-AA) guidelines [35–37]. Dementia diagnostic criteria included the following: evidence of decline from a previous level of cognitive performance; cognitive impairment diagnosed through history-taking and/or cognitive assessment; evidence of impairment in activities in daily living (ADL score > 23, IADL score > 11). MCI diagnostic criteria included the following: evidence of decline from a previous level of cognitive performance; no evidence of impairment in activities in daily living (ADL score $\leq$ 23, IADL score $\leq$ 11); not meeting the criteria for dementia. Subjects in the CU group had no or only mild cognitive decline, and neuropsychological tests were in the normal range.

2.4. Statistical Analysis

Continuous variables were described as mean $\pm$ standard deviation (M $\pm$ SD) and categorical variables as numbers and percentages (n, %). ANOVA with Bonferroni post-hoc tests or chi-square analysis was applied to detect significant differences between the different subgroups. A p-value of <0.05 was considered statistically significant. Statistical analysis was performed by SPSS version 24.0 software (Chicago, IL, USA).

2.5. Machine Learning

We manually extracted 64 features, including basic demographic information (sex, age, education years, etc.) and neuropsychological scores of NTB. All features were listed in Supplementary Table S1. At first, we used RF to calculate the importance of all features and perform feature selection. We tested all features with five-fold cross-validation and used mean area under the curves (AUC) as the performance metric. Different features had different importance in diagnosing dementia. Selecting the top-ranked features and filtering out the bottom-ranked features can simplify the classification process.

Next, other classification models, including logistic regression, decision tree, SVM, and XGBoost were trained and compared with RF. The performance of various models was evaluated by accuracy, precision, recall, F1 score, and AUC.

After selecting the features with high importance or the features we were interested in, 5-fold cross-validation was employed to train classification models, and the corresponding receiver operating characteristic (ROC) curves were also plotted. For each model, we got three ROC curves to distinguish CU, MCI, and dementia. The performance of each model effectiveness was evaluated using the mean ROC of the 5-fold cross-validation, the mean AUC, sensitivity, and specificity. AUC takes a value between 0 and 1, where AUC = 1 represents perfect diagnostic accuracy. Sensitivity is the true positive rate and specificity is the true negative rate. Sensitivity and specificity were calculated according to the maximal Youden's Index (sensitivity + specificity−1).

Classification models were built by using Python 3.7.9 with the package scikit-learn 0.23.2.

3. Results

3.1. Participants' Characteristics

375 participants, 161 men and 214 women, aged 65.51 ± 11.46 years, were recruited. Of these, 67 (17.9%) were CU, 174 (46.4%) had MCI, and 134 (35.7%) had dementia. Table 1 shows the baseline demographic and cognitive profiles of the three groups. The dementia group was significantly older than the MCI group, and years of education were significantly higher in the CUs than in the subjects with MCI and dementia. There was no significant gender difference between the three groups. For MMSE and MoCA-P scores, CU > MCI > dementia ($p < 0.001$); for ADL, IADL and BADL, CU = MCI < dementia.

Table 1. Comparison of demographic details and cognitive data among the groups.

	Total n = 375	CU n = 67	MCI n = 174	Dementia n = 134	χ^2/F [a]	Post Hoc Tests [b,c]
Age (years)	65.51 ± 11.46	63.24 ± 12.00	64.16 ± 11.61	68.41 ± 10.44	7.05 **	1 = 2 < 3
Gender (% female)	214 (57.1%)	43 (64.2%)	99 (56.9%)	72 (53.7%)	1.99	-
Education years	12.28 ± 3.91	13.88 ± 3.34	11.93 ± 3.98	11.96 ± 3.92	6.63 **	1 > 2 = 3
MMSE	27.80 ± 1.31	28.70 ± 1.17	27.95 ± 1.22	27.15 ± 1.17	40.42 **	1 > 2 > 3
MoCA-P	24.35 ± 3.08	27.18 ± 1.65	24.64 ± 2.77	22.54 ± 2.82	71.52 **	1 > 2 > 3
ADL	24.34 ± 4.57	21.78 ± 2.05	22.26 ± 2.53	28.31 ± 4.85	136.32 **	1 = 2 < 3
IADL	11.39 ± 3.30	9.45 ± 1.82	9.82 ± 1.99	14.39 ± 3.11	160.18 **	1 = 2 < 3
BADL	12.95 ± 1.92	12.33 ± 0.73	12.45 ± 1.01	13.93 ± 2.69	31.29 **	1 = 2 < 3
HAD-anxiety	4.66 ± 3.38	4.45 ± 3.15	4.48 ± 3.52	5.01 ± 3.29	1.06	-
HAD-depression	4.88 ± 3.48	4.50 ± 3.50	4.46 ± 3.44	5.64 ± 3.41	4.86 *	1 = 2 < 3

Data were shown as mean ± standard deviation (SD) or frequency (percentage, %). [a] Test statistic: F = one-way ANOVA value; χ^2 = chi-square test value. [b] 1: CU group; 2: MCI group; and 3: Dementia group. [c] Pairwise comparisons among the three groups of subjects were conducted using the Bonferroni post hoc tests. * $p < 0.05$; ** $p < 0.001$. Abbreviations: ADL = Activities of Daily Living; BADL = Basic ADL; CU = Cognitively Unimpaired; HAD = Hospital Anxiety and Depression; IADL = Instrumental ADL; MCI = Mild Cognitive Impairment; MMSE = Mini-Mental State Examination; MoCA-P = PUMCH version of Montreal Cognitive Assessment; PUMCH = Peking Union Medical College Hospital.

3.2. Assessment of Feature Importance

We extracted all features (64 features) into the RF classification model and calculated feature importance. ROC analysis for the detection of MCI and dementia and the top 20 features were shown in Figure 1. ROC-AUC of all features for distinguishing MCI from CU was 0.90 ± 0.04, sensitivity and specificity were 0.89 and 0.77 (Figure 1A), and the most important feature was PAL-T (total score of the three learning trials of PAL) (Figure 1B). ROC-AUC of all features for distinguishing dementia from MCI was 0.81 ± 0.07, sensitivity and specificity were 0.75 and 0.74 (Figure 1C), and the most important feature was AVLT N5 (the fifth long-delayed free recall trial of AVLT-H) (Figure 1D). ROC-AUC of all features for distinguishing dementia from non-dementia was 0.87 ± 0.04, sensitivity and specificity were 0.90 and 0.73 (Figure 1E), and the most important feature was AVLT N5 (Figure 1F).

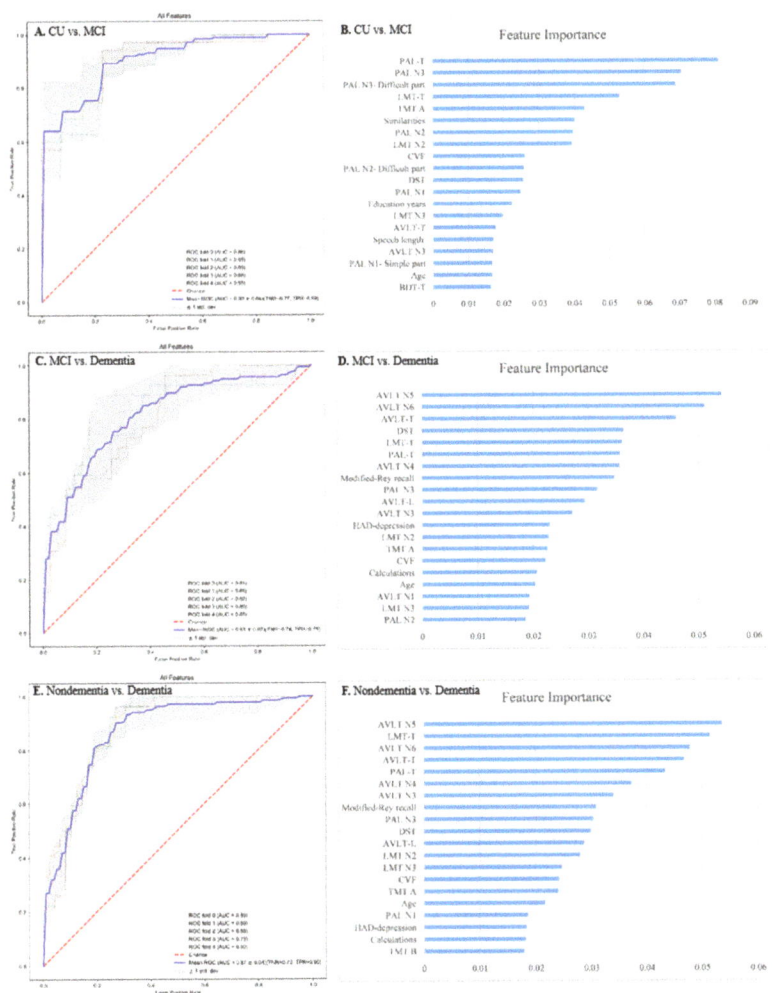

Figure 1. Receiver operating characteristic (ROC) curve analysis for the detection of MCI and dementia and the optimal 20 features. (**A**) ROC curve of all features for the detection of MCI from CU. (**B**) 20 top-ranked features for the detection of MCI from CU. (**C**) ROC curve of all features for the detection of dementia from MCI. (**D**) 20 top-ranked features for the detection of dementia from MCI. (**E**) ROC curve of all features for the detection of dementia from non-dementia. (**F**) 20 top-ranked features for the detection of dementia from non-dementia. Abbreviations: AVLT N1 = the first learning trial of AVLT-H (auditory verbal learning test-Huashan version); AVLT N3 = the third learning trial of AVLT-H; AVLT N4 = the fourth short delayed free recall trial of AVLT-H; AVLT N5 = the fifth long delayed free recall trial of AVLT-H; AVLT N6 = the sixth delayed category cue recall trial of AVLT-H; AVLT-L = total score of AVLT N1, N2,and N3; AVLT-T = total score of AVLT N1, N2, N3, N4 and N5; BDT-T = total score of the block design test; CVF = category verbal fluency; DST = Digit Symbol Test; HAD = hospital anxiety and depression; LMT N2 = the second story of logical memory test (LMT); LMT N3 = the third story of LMT; LMT-T = total score of LMT; PAL N1 = The first learning trial of PAL (paired-associate learning); PAL N1-Simple part = simple word pairs of PAL N1; PAL N2 = The second learning trial of PAL; PAL N2-Difficult part = difficult word pairs of PAL N2; PAL N3 = The third learning trial of PAL; PAL N3-Difficult part = difficult word pairs of PAL N3; PAL-T = total score of PAL N1, N2, and N3; TMT A = trail making test A; TMT B = trail making test B.

3.3. Performance of Various Classification Models

Table 2 shows the performance of various classification models. The accuracies of the logistic regression, decision tree, SVM, XGBoost, and RF models were 0.605, 0.597, 0.624, 0.664, and 0.680, while the AUCs were 0.796, 0.696, 0.809, 0.816, and 0.852. Among these methods, The RF classifier achieved the most stable performance with high accuracy compared with other classifiers.

Table 2. Performance of models trained by various methods.

	Accuracy	Precision	Recall	F1 Score	ROC-AUC
Logistic Regression	60.53	60.80	60.08	60.12	79.62
Decision Tree	59.73	60.48	60.86	60.21	69.55
SVM	62.40	65.37	59.29	61.17	80.87
XGBoost	66.40	67.78	66.15	66.70	81.61
Random Forest	68.00	71.09	66.73	68.02	85.17

3.4. Selecting the Optimal Neuropsychological Tests to Establish Diagnostic Models

Finally, we selected six interested neuropsychological subtests with 22 high importance features (including AVLT-H, PAL, modified Rey figure, LMT, DST, and TMT A). The selected features contained in each neuropsychological subtest were listed in Supplementary Table S2. These features trained four new RF diagnosis models. The Performance (ROC AUC, sensitivity, and specificity) of these four models were shown in Table 3. If we selected three selected subtests (AVLT-H, PAL, and modified Rey figure) with 19 features to establish the diagnosis model, AUC to detect CU from MCI, MCI from dementia, dementia from nondementia was 0.86, 0.77, 0.84, respectively. If we selected four subtests (AVLT-H, PAL, modified Rey figure, and LMT) with 20 features, AUC to discriminate CU from MCI, MCI from dementia, dementia from non-dementia was 0.87, 0.79, 0.83. If we selected five subtests (AVLT-H, PAL, modified Rey figure, LMT, and DST) with 21 features, AUC to detect CU from MCI, MCI from dementia, dementia from nondementia was 0.86, 0.77, 0.84, respectively. When we chose all six important subtests with 22 selected features to establish the RF classification model, AUC to detect CU from MCI was 0.89 (sensitivity = 0.87 and specificity = 0.85), AUC to detect MCI from dementia was 0.79 (sensitivity = 0.84 and specificity = 0.63), and AUC to detect dementia from nondementia was 0.84 (sensitivity = 0.72 and specificity = 0.81). RF Model based on 22 neuropsychological features was almost equivalent to the model established using all 64 features. At the same time, the cognitive tests time was reduced from more than an hour to 30 min.

Table 3. Performance of the four new RF diagnosis models on the classification of CU, MCI, and Dementia.

New Diagnosis Models	Subtests of Interest	Number of Features	ROC AUC for CU vs. MCI (Sensitivity, Specificity)	ROC AUC for MCI vs. Dementia (Sensitivity, Specificity)	ROC AUC for Dementia vs. Nondementia (Sensitivity, Specificity)
Model-1	PAL, AVLT-H, Modified-Rey	19	0.86 (0.79, 0.84)	0.77 (0.68, 0.76)	0.84 (0.72, 0.81)
Model-2	PAL, AVLT-H, Modified-Rey, LMT	20	0.87 (0.78, 0.84)	0.79 (0.76, 0.66)	0.83 (0.70, 0.83)
Model-3	PAL, AVLT-H, Modified-Rey, LMT, DST	21	0.87 (0.83, 0.84)	0.79 (0.81, 0.65)	0.84 (0.84, 0.71)
Model-4	PAL, AVLT-H, Modified-Rey, LMT, DST, TMT A	22	0.89 (0.92, 0.74)	0.79 (0.84, 0.63)	0.84 (0.85, 0.73)

Abbreviations: AVLT-H = Auditory Verbal Learning Test-Huashan version; CU = Cognitively Unimpaired; DST = Digit Symbol Test; LMT = Logical Memory Test; MCI = Mild Cognitive Impairment; Modified-Rey = Modified Rey-Osterreith figure; PAL = Paired-Associate Learning.

4. Discussion

The present study found that 35.7 percent of subjects with MMSE scores ≥ 26 had evidence of dementia. Similar results have been obtained from previous studies [38,39]. This suggests that MMSE, as the only cognitive testing tool, is not sufficient to diagnose cognitive impairment. According to the 2011 NIA-AA criteria of "dementia", when clinical history and bedside cognitive tests cannot provide evidence of cognitive impairment, neuropsychological tests should be performed [36]. In this study, we applied the RF algorithm to determine the contribution of different cognitive tests and to screen out efficient neuropsychological features for better diagnosis of cognitive impairment. Our results showed that the RF algorithm has satisfactory performance in the task of diagnosing MCI (AUC = 0.89) and dementia (AUC = 0.84). The ML method helped develop a simplified version of NTB for CU, MCI, and dementia classification in patients with MMSE scores ≥ 26. The diagnostic model finally included six neuropsychological tests with highly important features, and other low-importance tests were deleted, thus greatly shortening the evaluation time.

The NTB is suitable for the Chinese cultural background and language habits, but the normative data of its subtests have not been updated for a long time. As the education level and living conditions of the Chinese have improved significantly in recent decades, the clinical value of the norms has been limited. Reestablishing the norms for large samples is time-consuming and requires organization and resources to conduct. In addition, the norms are influenced by many factors such as age, gender, education level, and residence (rural or urban). ML has the potential to solve the above problems by allowing multi-dimensional interactions between variables [15]. It also can rank variables that are critical to assessing cognitive impairment, which can be used to optimize neuropsychological testing [40,41]. RF can handle both linear and non-linear data and offers an advanced method to deal with outliers or missing values [42]. It has been used to solve classification and regression problems and can serve as a powerful tool to distinguish MCI and dementia [43]. Studies have found that the RF algorithm has excellent efficiency in diagnosing dementia based on neuropsychological testing [15]. Kleiman et al. reported that RF two-class classification showed greater clinical utility compared to the three-class approach in classifying cognitive impairment [44]. Therefore, our two-class models for distinguishing MCI from CU, dementia from MCI, or dementia from nondementia.

One review [45] that included 59 studies indicated that MMSE, as a global cognitive screening tool, showed the highest discrimination coefficient in the ML automatic classification of cognitive impairment. However, previous studies did not focus on people with normal MMSE scores when developing diagnostic models or optimizing neuropsychological tests using ML methods [45]. In these studies, subjects with MCI and mild dementia had significantly lower baseline scores on the bedside cognitive tests than our sample [11,41,44,46,47]. For example, Quintana et al. [47] reported that the mean MMSE score of the MCI group and dementia group was 25.77 ± 2.22, 20.37 ± 3.98, respectively. In the Chiu et al. [11] study, the mean MMSE and MoCA scores in the very mild dementia group were 19.7 ± 4.7, 12.4 ± 6.0, respectively. Lower MMSE scores indicate more severe impairment of cognition, and the diagnostic accuracy of the ML model developed based on this situation will be higher, which means that it is more difficult to detect dementia in people with normal MMSE. Classification models using ML on demographical and neuropsychological data in the literature showed wide heterogeneity in performance metrics. Weakley et al. [48] reported a sensitivity and specificity of 0.84 and 0.89 for differentiating MCI from CU, and 0.95 and 0.97 for dementia and CU, and Battista et al. [41] with 0.98 and 0.81 for MCI, and 1.00 and 0.96 for dementia. In this work, the selected sample were subjects whose MMSE was higher than the cut-off value. This is the first time to address the question that classifies people with normal MMSE. Our results showed that the RF model has good sensitivity (0.87) and specificity (0.85) for differentiating MCI from CU, as well as good sensitivity (0.85) and specificity (0.73) for dementia from nondementia.

RF had also been proven to be more effective in feature selection. Previous studies that focused on ML and cognitive measures had the disadvantage of having fewer neuropsychological features [47,49], or they just focused on the comparison between MCI and CU or CU and dementia [50,51]. Our study included 20 neuropsychological tests and compared CU, MCI, and dementia groups. The most frequent optimal neuropsychological tests reported in the literature were episodic memory [41,47,49] (like AVLT, logical memory test) and semantic fluency [46,47,52]. However, these neuropsychological measures mainly focus on Alzheimer's disease and dementia and cannot examine the damage of multiple cognitive domains. In our research, the combination of six tests is sufficient to cover multiple cognitive domains including executive function, visual perception function, language, memory, and attention, which can help diagnose all-cause dementia. AVLT-H and LMT, which assess both immediate and delayed recall, are popular methods for detecting episodic memory impairment [53,54]. PAL measures the strength of memory binding of twelve word-pairs [29]. The word pairs are presented verbally, one pair at a time. Then the participant hears the first word of each word-pair and is asked to answer the last word. PAL assesses episodic memory and executive function and could successfully detect MCI and dementia [55,56]. Modified Rey includes copy and delayed recall of the complex figure, assessing visuospatial ability and nonverbal memory. Good performance of DST and TMT A requires intact motor speed, attention, and visual perception functions, which is an important executive domain involved in semantic information processing [57]. The 2011 NIA-AA staging criteria also suggests some neuropsychological tests that are considered to be predictors of conversion from MCI to dementia [33]. These tests are generally consistent with those selected in our study.

In addition, the RF algorithm could be used not only to optimize the NTB but also to simplify individual subtests. For example, AVLT-H begins with three learning trials, followed by the fourth short delayed free recall trial, the fifth long-delayed free recall trial, the sixth category cue recall trial, and the recognition trial [53]. When ranking variables' importance, we found that AVLT N5 was the most important feature. Therefore, we choose to administer the first five trials of AVLT-H in the future practical application and delete the sixth category cue recall trial and the recognition trial. The second story of LMT was the best predictor among the three stories, so only the second story needs to be completed when performing this neuropsychological test.

There were two main limitations to this study. First, this study was a retrospective, single-center, observational study with inherent selection bias. Prospective, multi-centered, large-scale studies are therefore warranted. A second limitation is that we did not subclassify dementia. Subjects in the dementia group were patients with all-cause dementia, most of which is Alzheimer's disease and vascular dementia, and other dementia subtypes such as frontotemporal dementia and dementia with Lewy body were rare. This might cause some features to become less important. For example, language-related features such as repetition and naming were removed. Future research needs to consider dementia subtypes.

5. Conclusions

The present study showed that the RF algorithm can be a useful tool to classify CU, MCI, and dementia among a population with normal MMSE. We found that the optimized NTB, consisting of six neuropsychological tests (AVLT-H, PAL, modified Rey figure, LMT, DST, and TMT A), enables detection of MCI and dementia with good sensitivity and specificity. As cognitive markers, neuropsychological assessments have the excellent performance to identify cognitive disorders. For low- and middle-income countries, this has advantages over using classifiers based on more invasive, expensive, and time-consuming methods such as cerebrospinal fluid markers.

Supplementary Materials: The following are available online at https://www.mdpi.com/article/10.3390/jpm12010037/s1, Table S1: 64 features that extracted, Table S2: Six neuropsychological subtests and they selected features.

Author Contributions: Conceptualization, J.W. (Jie Wang) and J.G.; Data curation, J.W. (Jie Wang), Z.W., N.L., C.L., C.M., L.D., J.L., X.H., D.L., S.C. and J.G.; Formal analysis, J.W. (Jie Wang), Z.W., N.L. and J.W. (Jianyong Wang); Funding acquisition, J.G.; Investigation, J.W. (Jie Wang), C.L., C.M., L.D., J.L., X.H., D.L., S.C. and J.G.; Methodology, J.W. (Jie Wang), Z.W., N.L., J.W. (Jianyong Wang) and J.G.; Project administration, J.G.; Resources, J.W. (Jianyong Wang) and J.G.; Software, Z.W., N.L. and J.W. (Jianyong Wang); Writing—original draft, J.W. (Jie Wang); Writing—review & editing, Z.W. and J.G. All authors have read and agreed to the published version of the manuscript.

Funding: This research was funded by the National Key Research and Development Program of China [2020YFA0804500, 2016YFC1306300], CAMS Innovation Fund for Medical Sciences (CIFMS) (2020-I2MC&T-B-010, 2016-I2M-1-004), National Natural Science Foundation of China [81550021, 30470618], and the strategic priority research program (Pilot study) 'biological basis of aging and therapeutic strategies' of the Chinese Academy of Sciences [grant XDPB10].

Informed Consent Statement: All subjects gave their informed consent for inclusion before they participated in the study.

Data Availability Statement: The data that support the findings of this study are available from the corresponding author upon reasonable request.

Acknowledgments: The authors are deeply grateful to the patients and clinicians who participated in this work.

Conflicts of Interest: The authors report no competing interests.

References

1. Feigin, V.L.; Nichols, E.; Alam, T.; Bannick, M.S.; Beghi, E.; Blake, N.; Culpepper, W.J.; Dorsey, E.R.; Elbaz, A.; Ellenbogen, R.G.; et al. Global, regional, and national burden of neurological disorders, 1990–2016: A systematic analysis for the Global Burden of Disease Study 2016. *Lancet Neurol.* **2019**, *18*, 459–480. [CrossRef]
2. Roberts, R.O.; Knopman, D.S.; Mielke, M.M.; Cha, R.H.; Pankratz, V.S.; Christianson, T.J.; Geda, Y.E.; Boeve, B.F.; Ivnik, R.J.; Tangalos, E.G.; et al. Higher risk of progression to dementia in mild cognitive impairment cases who revert to normal. *Neurology* **2014**, *82*, 317–325. [CrossRef] [PubMed]
3. Olazarán, J.; Reisberg, B.; Clare, L.; Cruz, I.; Peña-Casanova, J.; Del Ser, T.; Woods, B.; Beck, C.; Auer, S.; Lai, C.; et al. Nonpharmacological Therapies in Alzheimer's Disease: A Systematic Review of Efficacy. *Dement. Geriatr. Cogn. Disord.* **2010**, *30*, 161–178. [CrossRef] [PubMed]
4. Folstein, M.F.; Folstein, S.E.; McHugh, P.R. "Mini-mental state". A practical method for grading the cognitive state of patients for the clinician. *J. Psychiatr. Res.* **1975**, *12*, 189–198. [CrossRef]
5. Creavin, S.T.; Wisniewski, S.; Noel-Storr, A.H.; Trevelyan, C.M.; Hampton, T.; Rayment, D.; Thom, V.M.; Nash, K.J.; Elhamoui, H.; Milligan, R.; et al. Mini-Mental State Examination (MMSE) for the detection of dementia in clinically unevaluated people aged 65 and over in community and primary care populations. *Cochrane Database Syst. Rev.* **2016**, *1*, CD011145. [CrossRef] [PubMed]
6. Patnode, C.D.; Perdue, L.A.; Rossom, R.C.; Rushkin, M.C.; Redmond, N.; Thomas, R.G.; Lin, J.S. Screening for Cognitive Impairment in Older Adults: Updated Evidence Report and Systematic Review for the US Preventive Services Task Force. *JAMA* **2020**, *323*, 764–785. [CrossRef]
7. Breton, A.; Casey, D.; Arnaoutoglou, N.A. Cognitive tests for the detection of mild cognitive impairment (MCI), the prodromal stage of dementia: Meta-analysis of diagnostic accuracy studies. *Int. J. Geriatr. Psychiatry* **2019**, *34*, 233–242. [CrossRef]
8. Nasreddine, Z.S.; Phillips, N.A.; Bédirian, V.; Charbonneau, S.; Whitehead, V.; Collin, I.; Cummings, J.L.; Chertkow, H. The Montreal Cognitive Assessment, MoCA: A Brief Screening Tool For Mild Cognitive Impairment. *J. Am. Geriatr. Soc.* **2005**, *53*, 695–699. [CrossRef] [PubMed]
9. Li, H.; Jia, J.; Yang, Z. Mini-Mental State Examination in Elderly Chinese: A Population-Based Normative Study. *J. Alzheimer's Dis.* **2016**, *53*, 487–496. [CrossRef] [PubMed]
10. Tan, J.P.; Li, N.; Gao, J.; Wang, L.-N.; Zhao, Y.-M.; Yu, B.-C.; Du, W.; Zhang, W.-J.; Cui, L.-Q.; Wang, Q.-S.; et al. Optimal Cutoff Scores for Dementia and Mild Cognitive Impairment of the Montreal Cognitive Assessment among Elderly and Oldest-Old Chinese Population. *J. Alzheimer's Dis.* **2014**, *43*, 1403–1412. [CrossRef]
11. Chiu, P.Y.; Tang, H.; Wei, C.Y.; Zhang, C.; Hung, G.U.; Zhou, W. NMD-12: A new machine-learning derived screening instrument to detect mild cognitive impairment and dementia. *PLoS ONE* **2019**, *14*, e0213430. [CrossRef] [PubMed]
12. Davatzikos, C. Machine learning in neuroimaging: Progress and challenges. *NeuroImage* **2019**, *197*, 652–656. [CrossRef]

13. Shigemizu, D.; Akiyama, S.; Asanomi, Y.; Boroevich, K.; Sharma, A.; Tsunoda, T.; Sakurai, T.; Ozaki, K.; Ochiya, T.; Niida, S. A comparison of machine learning classifiers for dementia with Lewy bodies using miRNA expression data. *BMC Med. Genom.* **2019**, *12*, 150. [CrossRef]
14. Shehzad, A.; Rockwood, K.; Stanley, J.; Dunn, T.; Howlett, S.E. Use of Patient-Reported Symptoms from an Online Symptom Tracking Tool for Dementia Severity Staging: Development and Validation of a Machine Learning Approach. *J. Med. Internet Res.* **2020**, *22*, e20840. [CrossRef]
15. Yim, D.; Yeo, T.Y.; Park, M.H. Mild cognitive impairment, dementia, and cognitive dysfunction screening using machine learning. *J. Int. Med. Res.* **2020**, *48*, 300060520936881. [CrossRef]
16. Yilmaz, A.; Ustun, I.; Ugur, Z.; Akyol, S.; Hu, W.T.; Fiandaca, M.S.; Mapstone, M.; Federoff, H.; Maddens, M.; Graham, S.F. A Community-Based Study Identifying Metabolic Biomarkers of Mild Cognitive Impairment and Alzheimer's Disease Using Artificial Intelligence and Machine Learning. *J. Alzheimer's Dis.* **2020**, *78*, 1381–1392. [CrossRef] [PubMed]
17. Khatri, U.; Kwon, G.R. An Efficient Combination among sMRI, CSF, Cognitive Score, and APOE ε4 Biomarkers for Classification of AD and MCI Using Extreme Learning Machine. *Comput. Intell. Neurosci.* **2020**, *2020*, 8015156. [CrossRef] [PubMed]
18. Bougea, A.; Efthymiopoulou, E.; Spanou, I.; Zikos, P. A Novel Machine Learning Algorithm Predicts Dementia with Lewy Bodies Versus Parkinson's Disease Dementia Based on Clinical and Neuropsychological Scores. *J. Geriatr. Psychiatry Neurol.* **2021**, 891988721993556. [CrossRef]
19. Gurevich, P.; Stuke, H.; Kastrup, A.; Stuke, H.; Hildebrandt, H. Neuropsychological Testing and Machine Learning Distinguish Alzheimer's Disease from Other Causes for Cognitive Impairment. *Front. Aging Neurosci.* **2017**, *9*, 114. [CrossRef]
20. Zhang, Z.; Hong, X.; Li, H.; Zhao, J.H.; Huang, J.B.; Wei, J.; Wang, J.M.; Li, S.W.; Yang, E.L.; Wu, J.X. The mini-mental state examination in the Chinese residents population aged 55 years and over in the urban and rural areas of Beijing. *Chin. J. Neurol.* **1999**, *32*, 149–153.
21. Katzman, R.; Zhang, M.Y.; Ouang, Y.Q.; Wang, Z.; Liu, W.T.; Yu, E.; Wong, S.-C.; Salmon, D.P.; Grant, I. A Chinese version of the mini-mental state examination; Impact of illiteracy in a Shanghai dementia survey. *J. Clin. Epidemiol.* **1988**, *41*, 971–978. [CrossRef]
22. Xu, G.; Meyer, J.S.; Huang, Y.; Du, F.; Chowdhury, M.; Quach, M. Adapting Mini-Mental State Examination for dementia screening among illiterate or minimally educated elderly Chinese. *Int. J. Geriatr. Psychiatry* **2003**, *18*, 609–616. [CrossRef] [PubMed]
23. Zhang, M.; Yu, E.; He, Y. Tools for dementia epidemiological investigations and their applications. *Shanghai Arch. Psychiatry* **1995**, *7*, 1–62.
24. Lawton, M.P.; Brody, E.M. Assessment of older people: Self-maintaining and instrumental activities of daily living. *Gerontologist* **1969**, *9*, 179–186. [CrossRef]
25. Zigmond, A.S.; Snaith, R.P. The Hospital Anxiety and Depression Scale. *Acta Psychiatr. Scand.* **1983**, *67*, 361–370. [CrossRef] [PubMed]
26. Chan, A.S.; Poon, M.W. Performance of 7- to 95-year-old individuals in a Chinese version of the category fluency test. *J. Int. Neuropsychol. Soc.* **1999**, *5*, 525–533. [CrossRef] [PubMed]
27. Gong, Y. *Manual of Modified Wechsler Adult Intelligence Scale (WAIS-RC)*; Hunan Med College: Changsha, China, 1982; pp. 45–48.
28. Gong, Y. The Chinese revision of Halstead-Reitan Neuropsychological Test Battery for Adults. *Acta Psychol. Sin.* **1986**, *18*, 433–442.
29. Xu, S.; Wu, Z. The construction of "The Clinical Memory Test". *Acta Psychol. Sin.* **1986**, *18*, 100–108.
30. Gao, S.; Zhu, Y.; Shi, S.; Peng, Y. Standard Aphasia Battery of Chinese. *Chin. Ment. Health J.* **1992**, *6*, 125–128.
31. Luria, A.R. *Higher Cortical Functions in Man*; Springer Science & Business Media: Berlin/Heidelberg, Germany, 2012.
32. Fogel, B.S.; Schiffer, R.B.; Rao, S.M. *Synopsis of Neuropsychiatry*; Lippincott Williams & Wilkins: Philadelphia, PA, USA, 2000.
33. Gong, Y.; Jiang, D.; Deng, J. *Manual of Modified Wechsler Memory Scale (WMS)*; Hunan Med College: Changsha, China, 1989; Volume 19.
34. Guo, Q.H.; Sun, Y.T.; Yu, P.M.; Hong, Z.; Lv, C.Z. Norm of auditory verbal learning test in the normal aged in Chinese community. *Chin. J. Clin. Psychol.* **2007**, *15*, 132–135.
35. Albert, M.S.; DeKosky, S.T.; Dickson, D.; Dubois, B.; Feldman, H.H.; Fox, N.C.; Gamst, A.; Holtzman, D.M.; Jagust, W.J.; Petersen, R.C.; et al. The diagnosis of mild cognitive impairment due to Alzheimer's disease: Recommendations from the National Institute on Aging-Alzheimer's Association workgroups on diagnostic guidelines for Alzheimer's disease. *Alzheimer's Dement.* **2011**, *7*, 270–279. [CrossRef]
36. McKhann, G.M.; Knopman, D.S.; Chertkow, H.; Hyman, B.T.; Jack, C.R., Jr.; Kawas, C.H.; Klunk, W.E.; Koroshetz, W.J.; Manly, J.J.; Mayeux, R.; et al. The diagnosis of dementia due to Alzheimer's disease: Recommendations from the National Institute on Aging-Alzheimer's association workgroups on diagnostic guidelines for Alzheimer's disease. *Alzheimer's Dement.* **2011**, *7*, 263–269. [CrossRef]
37. Jack, C.R., Jr.; Bennett, D.A.; Blennow, K.; Carrillo, M.C.; Dunn, B.; Haeberlein, S.B.; Holtzman, D.M.; Jagust, W.; Jessen, F.; Karlawish, J.; et al. NIA-AA Research Framework: Toward a biological definition of Alzheimer's disease. *Alzheimer's Dement.* **2018**, *14*, 535–562. [CrossRef]
38. Friedman, T.W.; Yelland, G.W.; Robinson, S.R. Subtle cognitive impairment in elders with Mini-Mental State Examination scores within the 'normal' range. *Int. J. Geriatr. Psychiatry* **2011**, *27*, 463–471. [CrossRef]
39. Votruba, K.L.; Persad, C.; Giordani, B. Cognitive Deficits in Healthy Elderly Population with "Normal" Scores on the Mini-Mental State Examination. *J. Geriatr. Psychiatry Neurol.* **2016**, *29*, 126–132. [CrossRef]

40. Graham, S.A.; Lee, E.E.; Jeste, D.V.; Van Patten, R.; Twamley, E.W.; Nebeker, C.; Yamada, Y.; Kim, H.-C.; Depp, C.A. Artificial intelligence approaches to predicting and detecting cognitive decline in older adults: A conceptual review. *Psychiatry Res.* **2019**, *284*, 112732. [CrossRef]
41. Battista, P.; Salvatore, C.; Castiglioni, I. Optimizing Neuropsychological Assessments for Cognitive, Behavioral, and Functional Impairment Classification: A Machine Learning Study. *Behav. Neurol.* **2017**, *2017*, 1850909. [CrossRef]
42. Sarica, A.; Cerasa, A.; Quattrone, A. Random Forest Algorithm for the Classification of Neuroimaging Data in Alzheimer's Disease: A Systematic Review. *Front. Aging Neurosci.* **2017**, *9*, 329. [CrossRef]
43. Breiman, L. Random forests. *Mach. Learn.* **2001**, *45*, 5–32. [CrossRef]
44. Kleiman, M.J.; Barenholtz, E.; Galvin, J.E. Screening for Early-Stage Alzheimer's Disease Using Optimized Feature Sets and Machine Learning. *J. Alzheimer's Dis.* **2021**, *81*, 355–366. [CrossRef]
45. Battista, P.; Salvatore, C.; Berlingeri, M.; Cerasa, A.; Castiglioni, I. Artificial intelligence and neuropsychological measures: The case of Alzheimer's disease. *Neurosci. Biobehav. Rev.* **2020**, *114*, 211–228. [CrossRef]
46. Lins, A.; Muniz, M.T.C.; Garcia, A.N.M.; Gomes, A.V.; Cabral, R.M.; Bastos-Filho, C.J.A. Using artificial neural networks to select the parameters for the prognostic of mild cognitive impairment and dementia in elderly individuals. *Comput. Methods Programs Biomed.* **2017**, *152*, 93–104. [CrossRef]
47. Quintana, M.; Guàrdia, J.; Sánchez-Benavides, G.; Aguilar, M.; Molinuevo, J.L.; Robles, A.; Barquero, M.S.; Antúnez, C.; Martínez-Parra, C.; García, A.F.; et al. Using artificial neural networks in clinical neuropsychology: High performance in mild cognitive impairment and Alzheimer's disease. *J. Clin. Exp. Neuropsychol.* **2012**, *34*, 195–208. [CrossRef]
48. Weakley, A.; Williams, J.A.; Schmitter-Edgecombe, M.; Cook, D.J. Neuropsychological test selection for cognitive impairment classification: A machine learning approach. *J. Clin. Exp. Neuropsychol.* **2015**, *37*, 899–916. [CrossRef]
49. Tunvirachaisakul, C.; Supasitthumrong, T.; Tangwongchai, S.; Hemrunroj, S.; Chuchuen, P.; Tawankanjanachot, I.; Likitchareon, Y.; Phanthumchinda, K.; Sriswasdi, S.; Maes, M. Characteristics of Mild Cognitive Impairment Using the Thai Version of the Consortium to Establish a Registry for Alzheimer's Disease Tests: A Multivariate and Machine Learning Study. *Dement. Geriatr. Cogn. Disord.* **2018**, *45*, 38–48. [CrossRef]
50. Lv, S.; Wang, X.; Cui, Y.; Jin, J.; Sun, Y.; Tang, Y.; Bai, Y.; Wang, Y.; Zhou, L. Application of attention network test and demographic information to detect mild cognitive impairment via combining feature selection with support vector machine. *Comput. Methods Programs Biomed.* **2009**, *97*, 11–18. [CrossRef]
51. Reverberi, C.; Cherubini, P.; Baldinelli, S.; Luzzi, S. Semantic fluency: Cognitive basis and diagnostic performance in focal dementias and Alzheimer's disease. *Cortex* **2014**, *54*, 150–164. [CrossRef]
52. Clark, D.G.; Kapur, P.; Geldmacher, D.S.; Brockington, J.; Harrell, L.; DeRamus, T.; Blanton, P.; Lokken, K.; Nicholas, A.; Marson, D. Latent information in fluency lists predicts functional decline in persons at risk for Alzheimer disease. *Cortex* **2014**, *55*, 202–218. [CrossRef]
53. Zhao, Q.; Lv, Y.; Zhou, Y.; Hong, Z.; Guo, Q. Short-Term Delayed Recall of Auditory Verbal Learning Test Is Equivalent to Long-Term Delayed Recall for Identifying Amnestic Mild Cognitive Impairment. *PLoS ONE* **2012**, *7*, e51157. [CrossRef]
54. Yu, H.; Guo, Q.; Hong, Z.; Lv, C. Logic Memory Test in early detection of Alzheimer's disease. *Nerve Dis. Ment. Hygeine* **2005**, *5*, 89–91.
55. Curiel, R.E.; Crocco, E.; Rosado, M.; Duara, R.; Greig, M.T.; Raffo, A.; Loewenstein, D.A. A Brief Computerized Paired Associate Test for the Detection of Mild Cognitive Impairment in Community-Dwelling Older Adults. *J. Alzheimer's Dis.* **2016**, *54*, 793–799. [CrossRef]
56. Duchek, J.M.; Cheney, M.; Ferraro, F.R.; Storandt, M. Paired Associate Learning in Senile Dementia of the Alzheimer Type. *Arch. Neurol.* **1991**, *48*, 1038–1040. [CrossRef]
57. Wang, L.; Nie, K.; Zhao, X.; Feng, S.; Xie, S.; He, X.; Ma, G.; Wang, L.; Huang, Z.; Huang, B.; et al. Characteristics of gray matter morphological change in Parkinson's disease patients with semantic abstract reasoning deficits. *Neurosci. Lett.* **2018**, *673*, 85–91. [CrossRef]

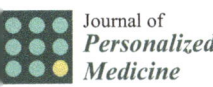

Article

Facial Recognition Intensity in Disease Diagnosis Using Automatic Facial Recognition

Danning Wu [1,2], Shi Chen [2], Yuelun Zhang [3], Huabing Zhang [2], Qing Wang [4], Jianqiang Li [5], Yibo Fu [1], Shirui Wang [2], Hongbo Yang [2], Hanze Du [2], Huijuan Zhu [2], Hui Pan [6,*] and Zhen Shen [7,8,*]

1. Eight-Year Program of Clinical Medicine, Peking Union Medical College Hospital, Peking Union Medical College, Chinese Academy of Medical Sciences, Beijing 100730, China; danie_wu@student.pumc.edu.cn (D.W.); pumcfyb@163.com (Y.F.)
2. Department of Endocrinology, Key Laboratory of Endocrinology of National Health Commission, Translation Medicine Centre, Peking Union Medical College Hospital, Peking Union Medical College, Chinese Academy of Medical Sciences, Beijing 100730, China; cs0083@126.com (S.C.); huabingzhangchn@163.com (H.Z.); wangsr13@126.com (S.W.); yanghb@pumch.cn (H.Y.); vespasian_du@126.com (H.D.); shengxin2004@163.com (H.Z.)
3. Medical Research Center, Peking Union Medical College Hospital, Peking Union Medical College, Chinese Academy of Medical Sciences, Beijing 100730, China; yuelunzhang@outlook.com
4. Department of Automation, Tsinghua University, Beijing 100084, China; qing.wang@tsinghua.edu.cn
5. School of Software Engineering, Beijing University of Technology, Beijing 100124, China; lijianqiang@bjut.edu.cn
6. Key Laboratory of Endocrinology of National Health Commission, Department of Endocrinology, State Key Laboratory of Complex Severe and Rare Diseases Peking Union Medical College Hospital, Chinese Academy of Medical Sciences and Peking Union Medical College, Beijing 100730, China
7. State Key Laboratory for Management and Control of Complex Systems, Beijing Engineering Research Center of Intelligent Systems and Technology, Institute of Automation, Chinese Academy of Sciences, Beijing 100190, China
8. Qingdao Academy of Intelligent Industries, Qingdao 266109, China
* Correspondence: panhui20111111@163.com (H.P.); zhen.shen@ia.ac.cn (Z.S.)

Abstract: Artificial intelligence (AI) technology is widely applied in different medical fields, including the diagnosis of various diseases on the basis of facial phenotypes, but there is no evaluation or quantitative synthesis regarding the performance of artificial intelligence. Here, for the first time, we summarized and quantitatively analyzed studies on the diagnosis of heterogeneous diseases on the basis on facial features. In pooled data from 20 systematically identified studies involving 7 single diseases and 12,557 subjects, quantitative random-effects models revealed a pooled sensitivity of 89% (95% CI 82% to 93%) and a pooled specificity of 92% (95% CI 87% to 95%). A new index, the facial recognition intensity (FRI), was established to describe the complexity of the association of diseases with facial phenotypes. Meta-regression revealed the important contribution of FRI to heterogeneous diagnostic accuracy ($p = 0.021$), and a similar result was found in subgroup analyses ($p = 0.003$). An appropriate increase in the training size and the use of deep learning models helped to improve the diagnostic accuracy for diseases with low FRI, although no statistically significant association was found between accuracy and photographic resolution, training size, AI architecture, and number of diseases. In addition, a novel hypothesis is proposed for universal rules in AI performance, providing a new idea that could be explored in other AI applications.

Keywords: artificial intelligence; computer-aided diagnosis; facial phenotypes; machine learning; complexity theory

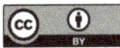

1. Introduction

Many diseases display distinctive facial manifestations, especially endocrine diseases and genetic diseases, including monogenic disorders, chromosomal diseases, and thousands of rare diseases [1]. Recognition by the human eye often causes misjudgment and delays diagnosis due to inconspicuous early facial symptoms associated with these diseases, large individual facial differences, and lack of physicians' knowledge of rare diseases. With the development of artificial intelligence (AI) technology, AI methods have been widely applied in different fields [2–6]. Automatic image recognition based on AI could identify image features for the diagnosis and screening of various diseases, with satisfactory performance for the diagnosis of pulmonary nodules, tumors, fundus diseases, even COVID-19 [7–10]. Among these AI techniques, facial recognition based on artificial intelligence enables computers to detect underlying facial patterns and has played an important role in the diagnosis and screening of diseases with facial phenotypes or changes in recent years [11,12]. It is assumed that artificial intelligence could help to improve diagnostic accuracy and to avoid delayed diagnosis, leading to earlier intervention, conservation of social healthcare resources, and implementation of health policies in the future [12–14]. Different models and systems have been developed to provide possible improvement for diagnostic accuracy [15].

However, there remains a lack of exploration of the factors influencing AI performance or of universal rules to reduce heterogeneity [14]. As has been shown before, diagnostic accuracy of facial recognition for Turner syndrome tended to be lower than that of Down syndrome, although a larger sample size helped to improve it [16,17]. However, the heterogeneity of diseases and AI methods studied and the limited number of works on rare diseases makes it difficult to review and summarize individual studies in a unified manner. Since the complexity theory could be applied to quantitatively describe facial features, this theory needs to be developed to explore the universal rules determining the diagnostic performance of AI based on facial features for heterogeneous diseases.

This is the first study that conducted a systematic review and meta-analysis to summarize the data regarding the diagnosis of heterogeneous diseases on the basis of facial features and explored the universal rules governing the application of facial recognition based on AI in the field of medical diagnosis. We aimed to quantitatively analyze the diagnostic accuracy of facial recognition based on AI, as well as the factors influencing the diagnostic performance and to provide a potential reference for clinical practice. In addition, our study proposes a potential hypothesis for evaluating the performance of AI in other fields, such as image recognition based on AI, and provides a new idea for dealing with heterogeneity when reviewing and analyzing the performance of AI applications.

2. Materials and Methods

2.1. Study Identification and Selection

We searched Medline, PubMed, IEEE, Cochrane Library, EMBASE to identify potential eligible studies published from 1 January 2010 to 15 August 2021. The references of relevant publications were also checked manually. The detailed search strategy containing the index test (facial recognition) and the target condition (diagnosis) is shown in Supplementary Table S1.

Studies were included if they evaluated facial recognition by algorithms of artificial intelligence for the diagnosis of diseases based on facial phenotypes or deformities using photographs and provided sufficient information for quantitative data synthesis. Studies were excluded of they were reviews, lacked a control group, or identified more than one possible disease as a diagnostic result by facial recognition. The titles and the abstracts were screened by two reviewers independently (DW and SC), and the full texts of potentially eligible studies were further screened.

2.2. Data Extraction and Quality Assessment

The data obtained from each study included publication characteristics (authors and year of publication); characteristics of the targeted disease (number of diseases and specific facial features); characteristics of the sample set (data sources, age, sex, and resolution of photographs); characteristics of the index test (algorithms, and number of images used in model training); characteristics of the reference standard (diagnostic criteria); accuracy data (number of true positives, true negatives, false positives, and false negatives). Supplements in each study were also reviewed if available.

Quality Assessment of Diagnostic Accuracy Studies-2 (QUADAS-2) was used to assess the risk of bias in patient selection, index test, reference standard, and flow and timing of the included studies. Publication bias was not assessed in our study because there is not a universally accepted method for the review of diagnostic studies to detect publication bias according to the Cochrane Handbook for Diagnostic Tests Review.

2.3. Definition and Calculation of FRI

We defined facial recognition intensity (FRI) as an index to describe the difference of facial features between a studied disease and healthy controls. FRI is calculated as shown in Equation (1) by multiplying the number of independent facial phenotypes of a disease and the maximum penetrance among these facial features.

$$FRI = N_f \times P_{max} \qquad (1)$$

In Equation (1), N_f represents the number of facial phenotypes relevant to a disease, and P_{max} is the maximum penetrance among these facial features, representing the percentage of individuals in a group of patients who exhibited a specific facial phenotype. The facial features and the penetrance of facial phenotypes were collected from the original articles and relevant reviews. If a facial phenotype was associated with a specific group of patients, penetrance was defined to be 100%. Since some of the facial phenotypes were correlated, such as small jaws and crowded teeth, associated phenotypes were counted only once to calculate FRI. For example, Down syndrome displayed nine independent facial phenotypes, and the maximum penetrance of these facial phenotypes was 100% [18]; hence, FRI of Down syndrome was calculated by multiplying 9 by 100%, resulting in 9. FRI was defined to summarize the common characteristics of objects, e.g., facial phenotypes in the presence of different diseases, and to minimize heterogeneity among objects analyzed by AI methods so to make them comparable in the subsequent analysis of performance of facial recognition based on AI for disease diagnosis.

2.4. Statistical Methods

Extracted two-by-two data are graphically shown in a forest plot with the point estimate of sensitivity and specificity and their 95% CIs. Considering the unclear and heterogeneous thresholds for diagnosing different disease with facial phenotypes by facial recognition methods, we used a quantitative random-effects model with bivariate mixed-effects binary regression to combine the sensitivity and specificity and to estimate the summary receiver operating characteristic (SROC) curve. The combined SROC curve and the optimum diagnostic threshold with 95% confidence region and 95% prediction region were plotted. Subgroup analyses and meta-regression were used to explore the heterogeneity between studies. Facial recognition intensity (FRI) and sample size of the training set were analyzed as covariates in meta-regression to explore quantitative relationships with diagnostic accuracy of facial recognition. The result of the meta-regression is shown in a bubble chart and demonstrates a fitting straight line. In addition to FRI and sample size of the training set, we also estimated the following covariates in subgroup analysis: resource of the control group, photo resolution, number of included diseases, and model of facial recognition. Covariates with statistically significant coefficients were regarded as a source of heterogeneity. The robustness of the main results was evaluated by sensitivity analyses. We explored the effect of excluding studies not reporting the model of facial recognition or gold standard of targeted conditions and those using internal validation to evaluate the models.

Data analysis for this paper was performed using Stata Statistical Software 16 (StataCorp., College Station, TX, USA) with two-tailed probability of Type I error of 0.05 ($\alpha = 0.05$).

3. Results

3.1. Systematic Review

Figure 1 shows the flow diagram for filtering articles. We identified 2534 records by electronic search and 29 by hand search. In total, 141 full-text articles were assessed for eligibility, and 20 studies in 14 publications met our criteria for inclusion. Ozdemir et al. [19] included three studies, and Basel-Vanagaite et al. [20], Gurovich et al. [2], Zhao et al. [17], and Saraydemir et al. [16] included two studies using different sample sets in one publication.

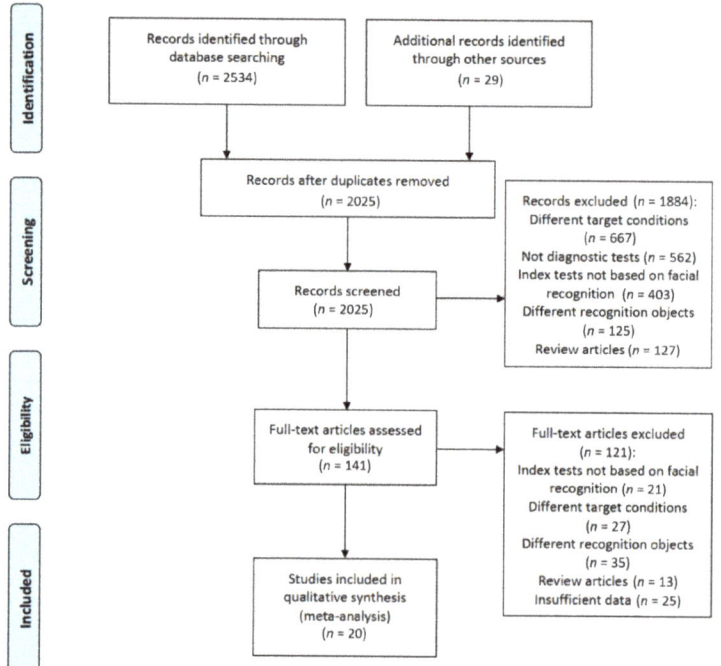

Figure 1. Flow chart for study inclusion and exclusion. The titles and the abstracts were screened by two reviewers independently, and the full texts of potentially eligible studies were further screened.

The detailed characteristics of the eligible studies are shown in Supplementary Table S2. The total number of subjects tested in the included studies was 12,557. A single disease was targeted in 16 studies, including 3 studies on Cornelia de Lange syndrome [2,20], 2 on Turner syndrome [21,22], 3 on Down syndrome [16,17], 1 on Angelman syndrome [2], 4 on acromegaly [23–26], 2 on Cushing's syndrome [27,28], and 1 study on fetal alcohol spectrum disorders (FASD) [29], as multiple diseases were detected in 4 studies [17,19]. Nine studies used photographs from public databases and web pages [2,25,27], and 11 studies obtained their photographs in local hospitals [20–24]. Ten studies described the demographic characteristics of their study population, reporting a percentage of males ranging from 0 to 66.2% [16,17,21,22,24–26]. The diagnostic criteria of the targeted diseases were reported in 12 studies and included analysis of gene mutation [2,20] and karyotype [16,17,21,22], success of previous treatment [23], experts' opinions [26], diagnostic tests [24,27,29]. An internal validation set was used for evaluation of the model in 12 studies [16,17,19,21,26–29], and an external validation set was reported in 8 studies [2,20,22–25]. Nine studies included a healthy control group [2,17,19,20,22], and patients with other diseases were included in 11 studies as a control group [16,17,21,23–29]. Apart from 5 studies not reporting the used AI architecture [17,19,20,26,27], several types of machine learning models were applied in 15 studies, including 7 studies using algorithms of deep learning and neural network [2,20,22,28,29] or a combination of neural network and other models [24]. The following models were also reported: SVM [16,21,23], Haar cascade classifier [25], hierarchical decision tree [19], k-NN [16,19] and combination of conventional models [11]. Fourteen studies reported a resolution of photographs ranging from 100 × 100 to 1500 × 1000 pixels [2,16,17,19,21,22,24–26,28]. The number of photographs used to train the model was reported in 20 studies and ranged from 30 to 3465, whereas the number of photographs in the testing set ranged from 17 to 242 [2,16,17,19–29].

3.2. Risk of Bias Assessment of the Eligible Studies

Supplementary Tables S2 and S3 show the results of the risk of bias assessment of the included studies. Regarding patient selection, risk of bias was unclear in 4 studies due to the insufficient information describing the sampling method [2,20] and high in 16 studies with a case–control design [16,17,19,21–29]. With respect to the index test, facial recognition was based on artificial intelligence algorithms without knowledge of the clinical diagnosis in all studies. As for the reference standard, risk of bias was low in 15 studies [2,16,17,20–22,24,26–29] and unclear in 5 studies that did not report the reference standard or an interpretation [19,23,25]. In the domain of flow and timing, risk of bias was low in 16 studies [2,16,17,20–23,25–29], unclear in 3 studies that did not report the reception of the reference standard [19], and high in 1 study because not all patients were subjected to the two tests assessed in the study [24].

3.3. Meta-Analysis

Figure 2 shows the paired forest plot for sensitivity and specificity with the corresponding 95% CIs for each study. Eligible studies were further combined, and the summary receiver operating characteristic (SROC) curve is shown in Figure 3 with the 95% confidence region and 95% prediction region. We calculated the following summarized estimates using random-effects models with 95% confidence interval (CI): sensitivity 89% (95% CI 82% to 93%), specificity 92% (95% CI 87% to 95%), positive likelihood ratio 11.1 (95% CI 6.5 to 18.8), negative likelihood ratio 0.12 (95% CI 0.08 to 0.20), and diagnostic odds ratio (OR) 90 (95% CI 35 to 230).

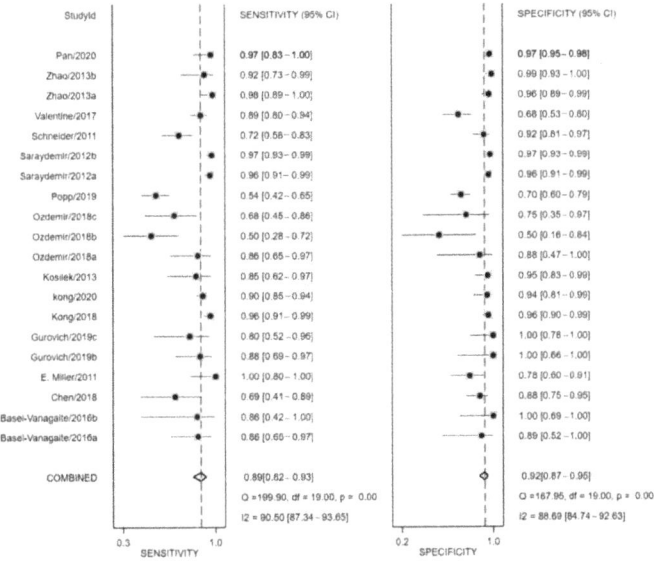

Figure 2. Forest plots of sensitivity and specificity in automatic diagnosis by facial recognition.

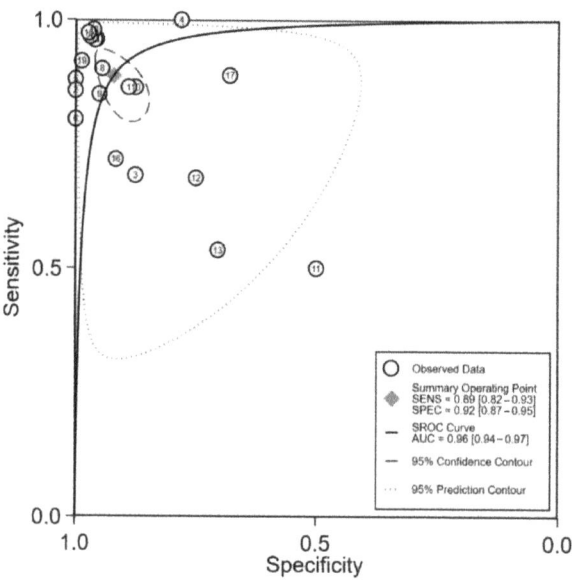

Figure 3. Summary receiver operating characteristics (SROC) curves of eligible studies. The dashed line indicates the 95% confidence region, and the dotted line indicates the 95% prediction region.

3.4. Sensitivity Analysis

After excluding eight studies that evaluated the models with an external validation set [2,20,22–25], pooled sensitivity was 86% (95% CI 75% to 93%), and specificity was 90% (95% CI 82% to 95%). After excluding studies with unclear models [17,19,20,26,27], pooled sensitivity was 90% (95% CI 83% to 94%), and specificity was 91% (95% CI 84% to 96%). After excluding studies with an unclear reference standard [17,20,25,28], pooled sensitivity was 89.0% (95% CI 82.0% to 94.0%), and specificity was 93.0% (95% CI 88.0% to 96.0%). Since these estimates were similar to the main results for the whole dataset, we did not find evidence that the overall combined estimates were influenced by external validation sets, unclear models, or unclear reference standards.

3.5. Evaluation of Facial Recognition Intensity (FRI)

Table 1 shows the prevalence, facial phenotypes of disease, and maximum penetrance of the phenotypes in the eligible studies. Among 16 studies targeting a single disease, Down syndrome showed 9 specific facial phenotypes, and the maximum penetrance of the facial phenotypes was 100% [18]; hence, the calculated FRI of Down syndrome was 9. As for Cornelia de Lange syndrome [2,20], it showed nine facial phenotypes, and the maximum penetrance was 82.7% according to the international consensus statement [30]. After calculation, FRI of Cornelia de Lange syndrome was 7.443. Angelman syndrome showed six facial features, with maximum penetrance of facial phenotypes of 100% and FRI of 8. Turner syndrome showed six facial phenotypes and the maximum penetrance of facial phenotypes was 56% [31]; therefore, FRI of Turner syndrome was 3.36. Fetal alcohol spectrum disorders (FASD) were associated with four facial phenotypes with maximum penetrance of 100% [29], resulting in FRI of 4.

Table 1. Assessment of facial recognition intensity (FRI) of diseases in the eligible studies.

Disease	Prevalence	Maximum Penetrance (Pmax)	Facial Phenotypes		Facial Recognition Intensity (FRI)
			Independent Facial Phenotypes	Number of Facial Phenotypes (Nf)	
Down syndrome [16,17]	1/300~1000	100%	Short face Upward slanting eyes Epicanthus Brushfield spots (white spots on the colored part of the eyes) Low-set ears Small ears Flattened nose Small mouth Protruding tongue	9	9
Acromegaly [23–26]	7/1000	100%	Forehead bulge Prominent jaw Prominent zygomatic arch Deep nasolabial folds Enlarged nose Enlarged brow Enlarged ear Enlarged lip	8	8
Cornelia de Lange Syndrome [2,20]	1/10,000~1/30,000	82.7%	Short face Small jaw Arched eyebrows Joined eyebrows Short nose Forward nostril Long philtrum Thin upper lip Upturned corners of the mouth	9	7.443
Angelman syndrome [2]	1/20,000~1/12,000	100%	Narrow bifrontal diameter Huge jaw Almond-shaped palpebral fissures Narrow nasal bridge Thin upper lip Protruding tongue	6	6
Cushing's syndrome [27,28]	4/100,000	100%	Red face Full moon face Acne Excessive hair Chemosis conjunctiva	5	5
Fetal alcohol spectrum disorders (FASDs) [29]	7.7/1000	100%	Small head Short palpebral fissures Smooth philtrum Thin vermilion border of the upper lip	4	4
Turner syndrome [21,22]	1/2500	56%	Small jaw Epicanthus Ptosis Ocular hypertelorism Low-set ears Multiple facial nevi	6	3.36

Among endocrine diseases, acromegaly showed eight facial phenotypes [28]. Since the maximum penetrance was 100%, FRI of acromegaly was 8. Cushing's syndrome showed five facial phenotypes and maximum penetrance of facial phenotypes of 100% [27,28], resulting in FRI of 5.

3.6. Effect of FRI on the Accuracy of Facial Recognition

Table 2 shows the results of random-effects model meta-regression analysis exploring the relationship between facial recognition intensity (FRI), sample size of the training set, and diagnostic accuracy of facial recognition. The coefficient of FRI in the model was 0.4868 (95% CI 0.0935 to 0.8800, $p = 0.015$), revealing a significant association with natural logarithms of OR of automatic diagnosis by facial recognition. Meanwhile, the sample size of the training set was not associated with diagnostic accuracy of facial recognition, indicating no significant contribution to the heterogeneity between studies.

Table 2. Meta-regression between FRI, sample size of the training set, and ln(OR) of automatic diagnosis by facial recognition. FRI = facial recognition intensity, OR = diagnostic odds ratio. FRI and sample size of the training set were analyzed as covariates in a meta-regression model to explore the heterogeneity between studies. Their coefficient and 95% confidence interval in the model are shown with two-tailed probability of type I error of 0.05 ($\alpha = 0.05$).

Covariate	Coefficient [95 CI]	p Value
Facial recognition intensity (FRI)	0.4939 [0.0710, 0.9169]	0.022
Sample size of the training set	0.0004 [−0.0006, 0.0014]	0.467

Therefore, after excluding the sample size of the training set from the model, the relationship between facial recognition intensity and diagnostic accuracy of facial recognition was determined as shown in Figure 4. The model with FRI as a variable showed significant association with natural logarithms of OR of automatic diagnosis, with the coefficient of FRI corresponding to 0.4960 (95% CI 0.0748 to 0.9171, $p = 0.021$), indicating that a larger FRI value of a disease was significantly associated with a higher diagnostic accuracy by facial recognition. The relationship between FRI value for a disease and diagnostic accuracy is shown in Equation (2):

$$\ln(OR) = \ln[Se\, Sp/((1 - Se) \times (1 - Sp))] = 0.4960 \times FRI + 1.459 \qquad (2)$$

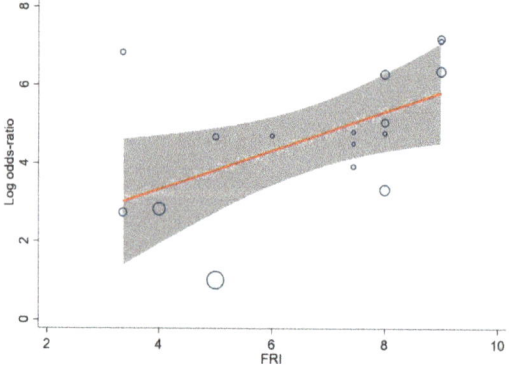

Figure 4. Bubble plots of meta-regression between FRI and ln(OR) of automatic diagnosis by facial recognition. FRI = facial recognition intensity, OR = diagnostic odds ratio. The straight line indicates linear prediction in the meta-regression model between FRI and diagnostic accuracy. The gray zone indicates the 95% confidence region, and the round bubbles represent the eligible studies. The size of the bubbles indicates the impact on the model.

According to Equation (2), Table 3 shows the quantitative association between FRI and accuracy of automatic diagnosis by facial recognition. When both sensitivity and specificity reached 85%, it was required that the FRI value of a disease reached 4.05. When sensitivity and specificity rose to 90%, FRI should correspondingly increase to 5.92. FRI needed to reach 8.93 to ensure that the sensitivity and specificity reached 95%.

Table 3. Association between FRI and accuracy of automatic diagnosis by facial recognition. FRI = facial recognition intensity, OR = diagnostic odds ratio. Quantitative relationship between FRI and diagnostic accuracy (including Figure 2. in meta-analysis. $\ln(OR) = \ln[Se\,Sp/(1-Se)(1-Sp)] = 0.4951 \times FRI + 1.46$.

Sensitivity	Specificity	OR	ln(OR)	FRI
85%	85%	32.11	3.47	4.05
90%	85%	51.00	3.93	4.98
90%	90%	81.00	4.39	5.92
95%	90%	171.00	5.14	7.42
95%	95%	361.00	5.89	8.93

3.7. Effect of Sample Size of the Training Set and AI Model on the Accuracy of Facial Recognition

Table 4 lists the range of FRI, sample sizes of the training set, AI models, as well as relative median and range of diagnostic accuracy by facial recognition. As for the sample size of the training set, which ranged from 30 to 3465 in the eligible studies, it was shown that the diagnostic accuracy of diseases with FRI higher than 8 was greater than 0.95, even if the sample size of the training set was lower than 100, with the minimum sample size being 30. Diseases with FRI ranging from 6 to 8 showed relatively low diagnostic accuracy when the sample size of the training set was lower than 100, with the minimum sample size being 49, and the accuracy increased with the sample size. The minimum training size for diseases with FRI lower than 6 was 60, and a sample size greater than 1000 significantly improved the diagnostic accuracy of facial recognition, indicating that a modest increase in the sample size of the training set played an important role in improving the diagnostic accuracy of diseases with low FRI.

Table 4. Association between FRI, sample size of the training set, AI models, and accuracy of automatic diagnosis by facial recognition. FRI = facial recognition intensity, DL = deep learning. The diagnostic accuracy is shown as median (minimum, maximum).

FRI	Minimum Sample Size of Training Set	Range of Sample Size of Training Set	Range of Accuracies Sensitivities	Range of Accuracies Specificities	AI Models	Range of Accuracies Sensitivities	Range of Accuracies Specificities
>8	30	<100 100~200	0.967 (0.960~0.973) 0.977	0.967 (0.960~0.973) 0.962	Non-DL	0.973 (0.960~0.977)	0.962 (0.960~0.973)
6~8	49	<100 100~1000 >1000	0.710 0.790 (0.719~0.860) 0.901 (0.800~0.960)	1.000 0.903 (0.890~0.915) 1.000 (0.944~1.000)	Non-DL DL	0.810 (0.719~0.901) 0.860 (0.800~0.960)	0.972 (0.944~1.000) 1.000 (0.890~1.000)
<6	60	<100 100~1000 >1000	0.769 (0.688~0.850) 0.714 (0.537~0.890) 0.967	0.913 (0.875~0.950) 0.697 (0.690~0.704) 0.970	Non-DL DL	0.688 0.929 (0.890~0.967)	0.875 0.830 (0.690~0.970)

AI methods also showed a similar trend. Diagnostic accuracy of AI reached more than 0.95 with non-deep learning models for diseases with FRI higher than 8, and the application of deep learning models contributed to a higher sensitivity for diseases with lower FRI. Especially for diseases with FRI lower than 6, the median sensitivity improved from 0.688 to 0.929 by using deep learning models. However, the specificity was not influenced by the use of deep learning models.

3.8. Sources of Heterogeneity

Table 5 shows the detailed results of subgroup analyses exploring the potential source of between-study heterogeneity. Facial feature strength was significantly associated with diagnostic accuracy by facial recognition ($p = 0.003$). However, we found no association between facial recognition's accuracy and photographic resolution, sample size of training sets, model of machine learning, number of targeted diseases, and selection of the control group.

Table 5. Subgroup analyses for the accuracy of automatic diagnosis by facial recognition. Image resolution was calculated by multiplying column pixels by row pixels. If images of different resolution were used, the average resolution was calculated. The two-tailed probability of type I error was 0.05 ($\alpha = 0.05$).

Subgroup Variables	Numbers of Eligible Studies	Sensitivity, % [95 CI]	Specificity, % [95 CI]	p for Interaction
Image resolution				0.415
<30,000 pixels	7	0.85 [0.73–0.97]	0.90 [0.82–0.98]	
≥30,000 pixels	7	0.90 [0.82–0.98]	0.94 [0.89–0.98]	
Sample size of training set				0.145
<1000	14	0.87 [0.80–0.93]	0.89 [0.84–0.95]	
≥1000	6	0.92 [0.86–0.99]	0.97 [0.93–1.00]	
Model/system of AI				0.802
Neural network	7	0.91 [0.83–0.99]	0.93 [0.85–1.00]	
Non-neural network	8	0.92 [0.86–0.97]	0.92 [0.86–0.98]	
Number of diseases				0.930
1	16	0.90 [0.86–0.95]	0.78 [0.60–0.97]	
>1	4	0.93 [0.89–0.97]	0.88 [0.74–1.00]	
Selection of control group				0.573
Healthy	9	0.85 [0.75–0.95]	0.94 [0.89–0.99]	
Other diseases	11	0.90 [0.84–0.96]	0.91 [0.86–0.97]	
Facial recognition intensity (FRI)				0.003
≤6	7	0.81 [0.71–0.90]	0.90 [0.83–0.96]	
>6	9	0.95 [0.92–0.98]	0.95 [0.91–0.98]	

4. Discussion

At present, artificial intelligence methods have been widely applied in different fields. However, studies exploring factors influencing the diagnostic accuracy of these methods, as well as systematic reviews and meta-analyses summarizing AI application in the diagnosis of heterogeneous diseases are still lacking. To our knowledge, this is the first study that fills this gap by summarizing heterogeneous studies on the automatic diagnosis of diseases on the basis of facial features and quantitatively analyzes the diagnostic capability of facial recognition based on AI. The review and meta-analysis were conducted strictly following the guidelines for diagnostic reviews [32]. Comprehensive and large-scale studies published so far were included, searched in both medical databases and engineering and technology databases. Representative and high-quality studies focused on different diseases using various known AI methods and were conducted in different countries. Our study summarized and quantitatively analyzed heterogeneous studies on the automatic diagnosis of different diseases based on facial features, showing a pooled sensitivity of 89% (95% CI 82% to 93%) and a specificity of 92% (95% CI 87% to 95%), similar to the results of previous meta-analyses on automatic image recognition for diabetic retinopathy screening [8,33,34], colorectal neoplasia, and breast cancer [35–38], indicating a promising diagnostic performance of facial recognition based on AI for heterogeneous diseases. A sensitivity analysis was conducted to evaluate the robustness of the results. The results were interpreted logically and adapted to clinical applications.

We propose a new index, facial feature intensity (FRI), to reflect the complexity of facial features associated with a targeted object. FRI was defined to minimize the heterogeneity across objects in AI applications and is calculated by multiplying the number of independent facial phenotypes by the maximum penetrance of these facial phenotypes. The number of details in facial features determines the complexity that distinguishes facial features of the targeted object from those of other objects, and the penetrance is the proportion of patients showing a certain complexity of facial features. Since FRI was revealed as the most important influencing factor for the diagnostic accuracy of facial recognition based on AI, the complexity of a targeted object plays the most important role in AI performance, rather than AI technology itself. According to Equation (2) in the meta-regression analysis, the expected accuracy of facial recognition for detecting a disease with the known FRI value could be predicted by calculation, which is of great clinical value.

The interactions between AI parameters and FRI were also taken into consideration, including sample size of the training set and AI architecture. The results revealed that, although larger training size and selection of deep-learning models did not contribute significantly to the heterogeneity between studies in either meta-regression or subgroup analysis, they showed a trend indicating improved diagnostic accuracy for diseases with lower FRI. An appropriate increase in the size of the training samples and the use of deep-learning models improved the accuracy of facial recognition, revealing that the improvement of AI parameters contributed to a better performance of AI for objects with low complexity. This finding is also supported by results on the detection of breast cancer, showing that increasing the training set size would not increase the diagnostic accuracy continuously [38]. Since the number of patients with rare diseases is limited, this finding is clinically significant as it indicates that the sample size of the training set can be within reasonable limits in AI applications. Moreover, the existing AI models have still to be improved to increase the diagnostic accuracy by facial recognition. Therefore, technology innovation is needed, and new AI methods might show better diagnostic accuracy by facial recognition.

Moreover, according to our findings, we propose a new hypothesis regarding AI application, that we named object's complexity theory (OCT) and that could be expanded to the application of AI technology in other fields. According to OCT, within the limits of a reasonable research design, the complexity of the targeted objects determines the complexity of AI processing and plays the most important role in AI performance, while improvement of AI parameters contributes to a better performance of AI for objects with low complexity. The hypothesis is consistent with existing evidence and is supported by previous theorems. According to the complexity theory proposed by J. Hartmanis and R. E. Stearns in 1965, the deep commonalities typical of complex systems determine the process of solving problems, which is relevant in diverse fields [39]. OCT represents the development and extension of the complexity theory regarding the performance of AI applications. According to the No Free Lunch Theorem (NFLT) for artificial intelligence proposed by David Wolpert and William Macready in 1996 [40] and optimized in 1997 [41], an algorithm performing well on a certain object paid with degraded performance on all remaining objects. If we use i to index the examined objects arbitrarily and O_i to represent an object, the NFLT is represented by Equation (3)

$$\sum_k f(O_k, a_i) = \sum_k f(O_k, a_j), \quad \forall i, j \tag{3}$$

where a_i and a_j are algorithms, and $f(O_k, a_i)$ is the performance of a_i on the object O_k. The equation shows that the overall performances of all the algorithms were the same. The only way a strategy could outperform another is to specialize the structure of the specific object under consideration [42]. As for our hypothesis, OCT, based on the application in facial recognition, we can establish Equation (4), on the basis of NFLT:

$$f(O_k, a_i) = g(O_k, \text{FRI}_k), \quad \forall i, \text{ if FRI}_k \geq 6 \tag{4}$$

where $g(O_k, FRI_k)$ is the performance of the algorithm a_i on the k-th object. The equation revealed that the structure of the object is reflected in the FRI. For objects with a large enough FRI, independently of the parameters of AI technology, the performances are more or less the same. The theory provides a new idea, suggesting that more indices for the evaluation of the complexity of targeted objects should be explored and developed in further studies to better determine AI performance in other fields.

Moreover, OCT and its application in facial recognition provide a new idea to deal with heterogeneity in studies and to evaluate the complexity of targeted objects. OCT should be applied and developed in further studies to determine AI performance in other fields. For image recognition based on AI, facial feature intensity (FRI) could also be converted into image feature intensity (IRI) to describe the characteristics of images related to more diseases. IRI might be the most important factor for AI performance within the limits of a reasonable sample size and of the study design. Previous studies have demonstrated that the image characteristics of diseases play an important role in the performance of image recognition by AI methods [43], including the automatic screening of pulmonary nodules [7,44,45], referable glaucomatous optic neuropathy (GON) [46], colorectal adenoma and polyps [47,48], which also indicates that IRI describes image characteristics of diseases and is critical for AI performance in automatic image recognition. As has been shown before for diabetic retinopathy screening, no statistically significant contribution to heterogeneous diagnostic accuracy has been demonstrated for sample size of the training sets and architecture of convolutional neural networks [34]. Therefore, the complexity theory explains the relationship between complexity of a disease and AI performance and should be extended to other AI applications.

There are some limitations in our study. First, the photographs overlapped in several studies using the same data sources, and it was difficult to eliminate this and evaluate its influence. Second, the risk of bias for the domain of patient selection was high or unclear in several studies. More than half of the studies had a case–control design, due to the limited number of patients with rare diseases. In addition, no traditional thresholds were mentioned in these studies, and we could only compare the sensitivity and specificity by finding the best cut-off point.

5. Conclusions

We quantitatively analyzed studies on the association of heterogeneous diseases with facial features and revealed the promising diagnostic performance of facial recognition based on AI in detecting diseases on the basis of facial features. A new index, facial feature intensity (FRI), was proposed to describe the complexity with facial features associated with different diseases, which was proved to be the most important factor influencing diagnostic accuracy by facial recognition. In addition, we explored the universal rules governing facial recognition based on AI in the field of medical diagnosis and provide a potential reference to solve practical problems in AI applications. An appropriate increase in training sample size and the use of deep learning models might play a role in improving the diagnostic accuracy for diseases with lower FRI. Our study firstly proposes a new hypothesis, the object's complexity theory (OCT), on the performance of AI and provides a new idea for dealing with heterogeneity when evaluating AI performance in other applications.

Supplementary Materials: The following are available online at https://www.mdpi.com/article/10.3390/jpm11111172/s1, Table S1: Search strategy (Medline), Table S2: Characteristics of included studies, Table S3: Methodological quality assessment of included studies using QUADAS-2.

Author Contributions: S.C. and D.W. contributed equally to this work. S.C., D.W., H.P. and Z.S. designed the study. D.W. and S.C. performed the literature search and appraised the articles. D.W. and Y.Z. performed the analysis with support from Y.F., S.W., H.Y. and H.D., S.C. and D.W. wrote the first draft. H.Z. (Huabing Zhang), Q.W., J.L., H.Z. (Huijuan Zhu), H.P. and Z.S. revised, edited, and finalized the manuscript. All authors have read and agreed to the published version of the manuscript.

Funding: This work was supported by the Beijing Municipal Natural Science Foundation (Grant No. 7192153) and the National Natural Science Foundation of China (Grants 61773382, 61872365, U1909218).

Institutional Review Board Statement: Not applicable.

Informed Consent Statement: Not applicable.

Data Availability Statement: Data from this study will be made available upon request from the authors.

Conflicts of Interest: The authors declare that they have no competing interest or personal relationships that could be perceived as prejudicing the impartiality of this study.

References

1. Hurst, A.C.E. Facial recognition software in clinical dysmorphology. *Curr. Opin. Pediatrics* **2018**, *30*, 701–706. [CrossRef]
2. Gurovich, Y.; Hanani, Y.; Bar, O.; Nadav, G.; Fleischer, N.; Gelbman, D.; Basel-Salmon, L.; Krawitz, P.M.; Kamphausen, S.B.; Zenker, M.; et al. Identifying facial phenotypes of genetic disorders using deep learning. *Nat. Med.* **2019**, *25*, 60–64. [CrossRef]
3. Miller, D.D.; Brown, E.W. Artificial Intelligence in Medical Practice: The Question to the Answer? *Am. J. Med.* **2018**, *131*, 129–133. [CrossRef]
4. Huang, S.; Yang, J.; Fong, S.; Zhao, Q. Artificial intelligence in cancer diagnosis and prognosis: Opportunities and challenges. *Cancer Lett.* **2020**, *471*, 61–71. [CrossRef]
5. Loftus, T.J.; Tighe, P.J.; Filiberto, A.C.; Efron, P.A.; Brakenridge, S.C.; Mohr, A.M.; Rashidi, P.; Upchurch, G.R., Jr.; Bihorac, A. Artificial Intelligence and Surgical Decision-making. *JAMA Surg.* **2020**, *155*, 148–158. [CrossRef]
6. Liu, G.; Wei, Y.; Xie, Y.; Li, J.; Qiao, L.; Yang, J.-J. A computer-aided system for ocular myasthenia gravis diagnosis. *Tsinghua Sci. Technol.* **2021**, *26*, 749–758. [CrossRef]
7. Zheng, G.; Han, G.; Soomro, N.Q. An inception module CNN classifiers fusion method on pulmonary nodule diagnosis by signs. *Tsinghua Sci. Technol.* **2020**, *25*, 368–383. [CrossRef]
8. Kaushik, H.; Singh, D.; Kaur, M.; Alshazly, H.; Zaguia, A.; Hamam, H. Diabetic Retinopathy Diagnosis from Fundus Images Using Stacked Generalization of Deep Models. *IEEE Access* **2021**, *9*, 108276–108292. [CrossRef]
9. Alshazly, H.; Linse, C.; Abdalla, M.; Barth, E.; Martinetz, T. COVID-Nets: Deep CNN architectures for detecting COVID-19 using chest CT scans. *PeerJ Comput. Sci.* **2021**, *7*, e655. [CrossRef]
10. Alshazly, H.; Linse, C.; Barth, E.; Martinetz, T. Explainable COVID-19 Detection Using Chest CT Scans and Deep Learning. *Sensors* **2021**, *21*, 455. [CrossRef]
11. Hong, N.; Park, H.; Rhee, Y. Machine Learning Applications in Endocrinology and Metabolism Research: An Overview. *Endocrinol. Metab.* **2020**, *35*, 71–84. [CrossRef] [PubMed]
12. Marwaha, A.; Chitayat, D.; Meyn, M.S.; Mendoza-Londono, R.; Chad, L. The point-of-care use of a facial phenotyping tool in the genetics clinic: Enhancing diagnosis and education with machine learning. *Am. J. Med. Genet. Part A* **2021**, *185*, 1151–1158. [CrossRef] [PubMed]
13. Elmas, M.; Gogus, B. Success of Face Analysis Technology in Rare Genetic Diseases Diagnosed by Whole-Exome Sequencing: A Single-Center Experience. *Mol. Syndromol.* **2020**, *11*, 4–14. [CrossRef]
14. Dias, R.; Torkamani, A. Artificial intelligence in clinical and genomic diagnostics. *Genome Med.* **2019**, *11*, 70. [CrossRef] [PubMed]
15. Saraydemir, S.; Taşpınar, N.; Eroğul, O.; Kayserili, H.; Dinçkan, N. Down syndrome diagnosis based on Gabor Wavelet Transform. *J. Med. Syst.* **2012**, *36*, 3205–3213. [CrossRef] [PubMed]
16. Zhao, X.; Wang, Z.; Gao, L.; Li, Y.; Wang, S. Incremental face clustering with optimal summary learning via graph convolutional network. *Tsinghua Sci. Technol.* **2021**, *26*, 536–547. [CrossRef]
17. Zhao, Q.; Rosenbaum, K.; Okada, K.; Zand, D.J.; Sze, R.; Summar, M.; Linguraru, M.G. Automated Down syndrome detection using facial photographs. In Proceedings of the 2013 35th Annual International Conference of the IEEE Engineering in Medicine and Biology Society (EMBC), Osaka, Japan, 3–7 July 2013; pp. 3670–3673. [CrossRef]
18. Devlin, L.; Morrison, P.J. Accuracy of the clinical diagnosis of Down syndrome. *Ulst. Med. J.* **2004**, *73*, 4–12.
19. Özdemir, M.E.; Telatar, Z.; Eroğul, O.; Tunca, Y. Classifying dysmorphic syndromes by using artificial neural network based hierarchical decision tree. *Australas. Phys. Eng. Sci. Med.* **2018**, *41*, 451–461. [CrossRef]
20. Basel-Vanagaite, L.; Wolf, L.; Orin, M.; Larizza, L.; Gervasini, C.; Krantz, I.D.; Deardoff, M.A. Recognition of the Cornelia de Lange syndrome phenotype with facial dysmorphology novel analysis. *Clin. Genet.* **2016**, *89*, 557–563. [CrossRef]
21. Chen, S.; Pan, Z.X.; Zhu, H.J.; Wang, Q.; Yang, J.J.; Lei, Y.; Li, J.Q.; Pan, H. Development of a computer-aided tool for the pattern recognition of facial features in diagnosing Turner syndrome: Comparison of diagnostic accuracy with clinical workers. *Sci. Rep.* **2018**, *8*, 9317. [CrossRef] [PubMed]
22. Pan, Z.; Shen, Z.; Zhu, H.; Bao, Y.; Liang, S.; Wang, S.; Li, X.; Niu, L.; Dong, X.; Shang, X.; et al. Clinical application of an automatic facial recognition system based on deep learning for diagnosis of Turner syndrome. *Endocrine* **2020**, *72*, 865–873. [CrossRef] [PubMed]

23. Miller, R.E.; Learned-Miller, E.G.; Trainer, P.; Paisley, A.; Blanz, V. Early diagnosis of acromegaly: Computers vs clinicians. *Clin. Endocrinol.* **2011**, *75*, 226–231. [CrossRef]
24. Kong, X.; Gong, S.; Su, L.; Howard, N.; Kong, Y. Automatic Detection of Acromegaly from Facial Photographs Using Machine Learning Methods. *EBioMedicine* **2018**, *27*, 94–102. [CrossRef]
25. Kong, Y.; Kong, X.; He, C.; Liu, C.; Wang, L.; Su, L.; Gao, J.; Guo, Q.; Cheng, R. Constructing an automatic diagnosis and severity-classification model for acromegaly using facial photographs by deep learning. *J. Hematol. Oncol.* **2020**, *13*, 88. [CrossRef] [PubMed]
26. Schneider, H.J.; Kosilek, R.P.; Günther, M.; Roemmler, J.; Stalla, G.K.; Sievers, C.; Reincke, M.; Schopohl, J.; Würtz, R.P. A novel approach to the detection of acromegaly: Accuracy of diagnosis by automatic face classification. *J. Clin. Endocrinol. Metab.* **2011**, *96*, 2074–2080. [CrossRef]
27. Kosilek, R.P.; Schopohl, J.; Grunke, M.; Reincke, M.; Dimopoulou, C.; Stalla, G.K.; Würtz, R.P.; Lammert, A.; Günther, M.; Schneider, H.J. Automatic face classification of Cushing's syndrome in women—A novel screening approach. *Exp. Clin. Endocrinol. Diabetes* **2013**, *121*, 561–564. [CrossRef]
28. Popp, K.H.; Kosilek, R.P.; Frohner, R.; Stalla, G.K.; Athanasoulia-Kaspar, A.; Berr, C.; Zopp, S.; Reincke, M.; Witt, M.; Würtz, R.P.; et al. Computer Vision Technology in the Differential Diagnosis of Cushing's Syndrome. *Exp. Clin. Endocrinol. Diabetes* **2019**, *127*, 685–690. [CrossRef]
29. Valentine, M.; Bihm, D.C.J.; Wolf, L.; Hoyme, H.E.; May, P.A.; Buckley, D.; Kalberg, W.; Abdul-Rahman, O.A. Computer-Aided Recognition of Facial Attributes for Fetal Alcohol Spectrum Disorders. *Pediatrics* **2017**, *140*, e20162028. [CrossRef]
30. Kline, A.D.; Moss, J.F.; Selicorni, A.; Bisgaard, A.M.; Deardorff, M.A.; Gillett, P.M.; Ishman, S.L.; Kerr, L.M.; Levin, A.V.; Mulder, P.A.; et al. Diagnosis and management of Cornelia de Lange syndrome: First international consensus statement. *Nat. Rev. Genet.* **2018**, *19*, 649–666. [CrossRef]
31. Kruszka, P.; Addissie, Y.A.; Tekendo-Ngongang, C.; Jones, K.L.; Savage, S.K.; Gupta, N.; Sirisena, N.D.; Dissanayake, V.H.W.; Paththinige, C.S.; Aravena, T.; et al. Turner syndrome in diverse populations. *Am. J. Med. Genet. Part A* **2020**, *182*, 303–313. [CrossRef] [PubMed]
32. Higgins, J.P.T.; Thomas, J.; Chandler, J.; Cumpston, M.; Li, T.; Page, M.J.; Welch, V.A. *Cochrane Handbook for Systematic Reviews of Interventions*, 2nd ed.; John Wiley & Sons: Chichester, UK, 2019.
33. Wu, H.Q.; Shan, Y.X.; Wu, H.; Zhu, D.R.; Tao, H.M.; Wei, H.G.; Shen, X.Y.; Sang, A.M.; Dong, J.C. Computer aided diabetic retinopathy detection based on ophthalmic photography: A systematic review and Meta-analysis. *Int. J. Ophthal.* **2019**, *12*, 1908–1916. [CrossRef] [PubMed]
34. Wang, S.; Zhang, Y.; Lei, S.; Zhu, H.; Li, J.; Wang, Q.; Yang, J.; Chen, S.; Pan, H. Performance of deep neural network-based artificial intelligence method in diabetic retinopathy screening: A systematic review and meta-analysis of diagnostic test accuracy. *Eur. J. Endocrinol.* **2020**, *183*, 41–49. [CrossRef] [PubMed]
35. Posso, M.; Puig, T.; Carles, M.; Rué, M.; Canelo-Aybar, C.; Bonfill, X. Effectiveness and cost-effectiveness of double reading in digital mammography screening: A systematic review and meta-analysis. *Eur. J. Radiol.* **2017**, *96*, 40–49. [CrossRef]
36. Dorrius, M.D.; Jansen-van der Weide, M.C.; van Ooijen, P.M.; Pijnappel, R.M.; Oudkerk, M. Computer-aided detection in breast MRI: A systematic review and meta-analysis. *Eur. Radiol.* **2011**, *21*, 1600–1608. [CrossRef]
37. Hassan, C.; Spadaccini, M.; Iannone, A.; Maselli, R.; Jovani, M.; Chandrasekar, V.T.; Antonelli, G.; Yu, H.; Areia, M.; Dinis-Ribeiro, M.; et al. Performance of artificial intelligence in colonoscopy for adenoma and polyp detection: A systematic review and meta-analysis. *Gastrointest. Endosc.* **2021**, *93*, 77–85.e76. [CrossRef]
38. Hughes, K.S.; Zhou, J.; Bao, Y.; Singh, P.; Wang, J.; Yin, K. Natural language processing to facilitate breast cancer research and management. *Breast J.* **2020**, *26*, 92–99. [CrossRef]
39. Hartmanis, J.; Stearns, R.E. On the computational complexity of algorithms. *Trans. Am. Math. Soc.* **1965**, *117*, 285–306. [CrossRef]
40. Wolpert, D.H. The Lack of a Priori Distinctions between Learning Algorithms. *Neural Comput.* **1996**, *8*, 1341–1390. [CrossRef]
41. Wolpert, D.H.; Macready, W.G. No free lunch theorems for optimization. *IEEE Trans. Evol. Comput.* **1997**, *1*, 67–82. [CrossRef]
42. Ho, Y.C.; Pepyne, D.L. Simple explanation of the no-free-lunch theorem and its implications. *J. Optim. Theory Appl.* **2002**, *115*, 549–570. [CrossRef]
43. Tagliafico, A.S.; Piana, M.; Schenone, D.; Lai, R.; Massone, A.M.; Houssami, N. Overview of radiomics in breast cancer diagnosis and prognostication. *Breast* **2020**, *49*, 74–80. [CrossRef] [PubMed]
44. Gong, J.; Liu, J.; Hao, W.; Nie, S.; Wang, S.; Peng, W. Computer-aided diagnosis of ground-glass opacity pulmonary nodules using radiomic features analysis. *Phys. Med. Biol.* **2019**, *64*, 135015. [CrossRef]
45. Beig, N.; Khorrami, M.; Alilou, M.; Prasanna, P.; Braman, N.; Orooji, M.; Rakshit, S.; Bera, K.; Rajiah, P.; Ginsberg, J.; et al. Perinodular and Intranodular Radiomic Features on Lung CT Images Distinguish Adenocarcinomas from Granulomas. *Radiology* **2019**, *290*, 783–792. [CrossRef]
46. Phene, S.; Dunn, R.C.; Hammel, N.; Liu, Y.; Krause, J.; Kitade, N.; Schaekermann, M.; Sayres, R.; Wu, D.J.; Bora, A.; et al. Deep Learning and Glaucoma Specialists: The Relative Importance of Optic Disc Features to Predict Glaucoma Referral in Fundus Photographs. *Ophthalmology* **2019**, *126*, 1627–1639. [CrossRef]

47. Aziz, M.; Fatima, R.; Dong, C.; Lee-Smith, W.; Nawras, A. The impact of deep convolutional neural network-based artificial intelligence on colonoscopy outcomes: A systematic review with meta-analysis. *J. Gastroenterol. Hepatol.* **2020**, *35*, 1676–1683. [CrossRef]
48. Wang, P.; Berzin, T.M.; Glissen Brown, J.R.; Bharadwaj, S.; Becq, A.; Xiao, X.; Liu, P.; Li, L.; Song, Y.; Zhang, D.; et al. Real-time automatic detection system increases colonoscopic polyp and adenoma detection rates: A prospective randomised controlled study. *Gut* **2019**, *68*, 1813–1819. [CrossRef]

MDPI
St. Alban-Anlage 66
4052 Basel
Switzerland
Tel. +41 61 683 77 34
Fax +41 61 302 89 18
www.mdpi.com

Journal of Personalized Medicine Editorial Office
E-mail: jpm@mdpi.com
www.mdpi.com/journal/jpm

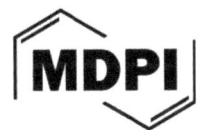

www.ingramcontent.com/pod-product-compliance
Lightning Source LLC
LaVergne TN
LVHW070746100526
838202LV00013B/1314